ICD-10-CM
Coder Training Manual
2014

Prepared by the
HIM Practice Excellence Team
American Health Information
Management Association

Contributing Authors
Kathryn DeVault, RHIA, CCS, CCS-P
Ann Barta, MSA, RHIA, CDIP
Melanie Endicott, MBA/HCM, RHIA, CDIP, CCS,
CCS-P, FAHIMA

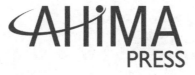

AHIMA
PRESS

AHIMA Product No.: AC206814
ISBN: 978-1-58426-428-6

AHIMA Staff:
Angie Comfort, RHIT, CDIP, CCS, Technical Review
Katherine M. Greenock, MS, Production Development Editor
Jessica Block, MA, Assistant Editor
Jason O. Malley, Director, Creative Content Development
Pamela Woolf, Managing Editor

American Health Information Management Association
233 North Michigan Avenue, 21st Floor
Chicago, Illinois 60601-5809
www.ahima.org

Contents

iii

About the Authors

Kathryn DeVault, RHIA, CCS, CCS-P, is senior director of HIM Practice Excellence for AHIMA. In her role, she provides professional expertise to AHIMA members, the media, and outside organizations on professional practice issues. In addition, she authors materials for and supports AHIMA online coding education, including the AHIMA Coding Basics program. Ms. DeVault also serves as a technical advisor for the association on ICD-9-CM, ICD-10, and CPT coding publications. Ms. DeVault also serves as author and faculty for the AHIMA ICD-10-CM/PCS Academies.

Prior to joining AHIMA in 2008, Ms. DeVault served as data quality analyst for coding in a regional healthcare system. For the past eight years, she has been a coding educator at a local community college. Ms. DeVault has authored many articles and has presented numerous seminars and educational sessions on coding and HIM-related topics.

As an AHIMA member, Ms. DeVault has participated in numerous leadership roles at both the state and regional level through the Colorado Health Information Management Association. She received her bachelor's degree in liberal arts from the University of Colorado.

Ann Barta, MSA, RHIA, CDIP is a director of HIM Practice Excellence for AHIMA. In her role, she provides professional expertise to AHIMA members, the media, and outside organizations on professional practice issues. In addition, she authors materials for and supports AHIMA online coding education, including the AHIMA Coding Basics program. Ms. Barta also serves as faculty for the AHIMA ICD-10-CM/PCS Academies.

Prior to joining AHIMA, Ms. Barta participated in a one-year contract between the AHIMA Foundation of Research and Education and Centers for Medicare and Medicaid Services (CMS) to determine potential impacts to CMS when converting from ICD-9-CM to ICD-10-CM/PCS coding systems. Prior to that, Ms. Barta served as a corporate coding manager for a large healthcare system. She has more than 30 years experience as an HIM director and coding consultant. She has been an educator of coding and HIM for more than 15 years, served as an associate dean for health sciences, and was system coordinator for an RHIT program.

As an AHIMA member, Ms. Barta participated in various leadership positions. She has served on various RHIT Program Advisory Boards. Additionally, she was actively involved with the Illinois Health Information Management Association, serving on the Education Committee and as a state coding instructor with the implementation of ICD-9-CM. Ms. Barta received her master of science in health services administration from Central Michigan University in Mt. Pleasant.

Melanie Endicott, MBA/HCM, RHIA, CDIP, CCS, CCS-P, FAHIMA is a director of HIM Practice Excellence for AHIMA providing professional expertise to AHIMA members on professional practice issue. She also authors and supports AHIMA online coding education, including the Coding Basics program. Ms. Endicott is also an AHIMA ICD-10-CM/PCS Academy faculty member.

Prior to joining AHIMA in 2004, Ms. Endicott served as health information analyst for coding in a large acute-care facility. She has been an educator of health information technology and health information administration for several years at several colleges and universities. She has presented numerous seminars and educational sessions on coding and HIM-related topics at the local, state, and regional levels.

As an AHIMA member, Ms. Endicott also participated in numerous leadership roles at both the state and regional level through the Washington State Health Information Management Association. She received her bachelor's degree in health information management from Carroll College and her master's degree in business administration and healthcare management from the University of Phoenix.

Acknowledgments

The exercises in this book were created using several AHIMA resources as a base. All of the adapted materials underwent a vigorous review to bring them into alignment with the latest versions of the ICD-10-CM code sets and guidelines which were available at the time of publication.

The author team adapted many of the application exercises in this book from case scenarios originally created by Anita Hazelwood, MLS, RHIA, FAHIMA and Carol Venable, MPH, RHIA, FAHIMA. The authors also would like to thank Sue Bowman, RHIA, CCS, FAHIMA for her contribution to the content and review of this publication. In addition, the authors would like to thank June Bronnert, RHIA, CCS, CCS-P; Ann Zeisset, RHIT, CCS, CCS-P; Anita Majerowicz, MS, RHIA; and Lynn Kuehn, MS, RHIA, CCS-P, FAHIMA for their contributions.

Preface to the Training Manual

On January 16, 2009, the US Department of Health and Human Services (HHS) published a Final Rule for the adoption of ICD-10-CM and ICD-10-PCS code sets to replace the 30-year-old ICD-9-CM code sets under rules 45 CFR Parts 160 and 162 of the Health Insurance Portability and Accountability Act of 1996 (HIPAA). The initial compliance date for the two classification sets was established as October 1, 2013 and this has subsequently been revised with an updated compliance date of October 1, 2014. A second rule related to the HIPAA transaction standards—X12 version 5010 and NCPDP version D.0—establishes earlier effective dates. The HIPAA transactions software must be updated to accommodate the use of the ICD-10-CM and ICD-10-PCS code sets by January 1, 2012 with the exception of Medicaid Pharmacy Subrogation Transactions, which have an effective date of January 1, 2013.

To read the final rules published in the *Federal Register*, please go to the following websites:

- Modifications to the Health Insurance Portability and Accountability Act (HIPAA) Electronic Transaction Standards:
  http://edocket.access.gpo.gov/2009/pdf/E9-740.pdf
- HIPAA Administrative Simplification: Modifications to Medical Data Code Set Standards To Adopt ICD–10–CM and ICD–10–PCS:
  http://edocket.access.gpo.gov/2009/pdf/E9-743.pdf
- ICD–10–CM/PCS final compliance date:
  http://www.gpo.gov/fdsys/pkg/FR-2012-09-05/pdf/2012-21238.pdf

The adoption of ICD-10-CM (diagnoses) will affect all components of the healthcare industry. However, the adoption of ICD-10-PCS will affect only those components of the healthcare industry that currently utilize ICD-9-CM Volume 3—inpatient procedures. Therefore, CPT® and HCPCS Level II will continue to be used for reporting physician and other professional services in addition to procedures performed in hospital outpatient departments and other outpatient facilities.

The three key issues HHS believes necessitate the need to update from ICD-9-CM to ICD-10-CM and ICD-10-PCS are

- ICD-9-CM is out of date and running out of space for new codes.
- ICD-10 is the international standard to report and monitor diseases and mortality, making it important for the United States to adopt ICD-10-based classifications for reporting and surveillance.
- ICD codes are core elements of many health information technology (HIT) systems, making the conversion to ICD-10-CM/PCS necessary to fully realize benefits of HIT adoption.

The use of ICD-10-CM will offer greater detail and granularity and will greatly enhance HHS's capability to measure quality outcomes, such as the quality performance outcome measures used in the hospital pay-for-reporting program. The greater detail and granularity of ICD-10-CM/PCS will also provide more precision for claims-based, value-based purchase initiatives such as the hospital-acquired condition (HAC) payment policy.

In addition, the transition to ICD-10-CM/PCS will ultimately facilitate realizing the benefits of using interoperability standards specified by the Healthcare Information Technology Standards Panel (HITSP), including SNOMED CT®. The benefits of using SNOMED CT increase if such use is linked to classification systems such as ICD-10-CM and ICD-10-PCS. Mapping would be used to link SNOMED CT to these new code sets, and plans are underway to develop these maps.

How to Use This Manual

The AHIMA Academy for ICD-10-CM Trainers is primarily designed to prepare individuals to train others in ICD-10-CM through course content that focuses on instruction in the code set. The *ICD-10-CM Coder Training Manual 2014* is designed to be used by students who are trained by AHIMA Academy ICD-10-CM trainers to build upon their basic knowledge of ICD-10-CM fundamentals. Although the implementation date for ICD-10-CM/PCS is several years away, it is necessary that individuals responsible for training are fully knowledgeable of the code sets in order to prepare students and the workforce for the transition. Transitioning curriculum from ICD-9-CM to ICD-10-CM/PCS will present unique challenges for academicians. Educating the workforce will also require that the healthcare industry begin planning and preparing for the new code sets.

The content of the *ICD-10-CM Coder Training Manual 2014* is based on the July, 2013 release of the *International Classification of Diseases, Tenth Revision, Clinical Modification* (ICD-10-CM), which can be downloaded from the following website: http://www.cdc.gov/nchs/icd/icd10cm.htm.

The ICD-10-CM Coder *Training Manual 2014* contains many references to and explanations of ICD-10-CM coding guidelines and conventions. It includes ICD-10-CM coding exercises at the basic, intermediate, and advanced level as well as beginner, intermediate, and advanced coding exercises. These coding exercises emphasize all aspects of the coding classification system so students can apply their knowledge of coding principles and definitions. Answers to the coding exercises are provided.

Students should recognize that additional, self-directed study will be required to master the guidelines and principles of ICD-10-CM coding beyond the materials provided in this manual. In addition, many students will require additional coursework to increase their level of knowledge in anatomy, physiology, pathophysiology, pharmacology, and medical terminology. Because ICD-10-CMS requires a stronger background in the biomedical sciences, instructors should develop plans for assessing their students' strengths/weaknesses in these areas. Identifying students' learning needs and levels of knowledge is crucial to preparing a solid educational transition plan.

In addition to this text, students of the AHIMA Academy will use the 2014 *ICD-10-CM* code book to complete the practice exercises.

Introduction: ICD-10-CM Overview

Section 1 – Introduction to the ICD-10-CM Classification System

History

The *International Classification of Diseases, Tenth Revision, Clinical Modification (ICD-10-CM)* is the United States' clinical modification to the World Health Organization's (WHO) *International Classification of Diseases, Tenth Revision (ICD-10)*. ICD-10 was adopted by the World Health Assembly in 1990. Following the publication of ICD-10, a number of countries performed an analysis to determine if the WHO classification would meet their needs given the changes to the roles of ICD since the *Ninth Revision*.

The first modification to ICD-10 was published in 1998. The Australian National Centre for Classification in Health (NCCH) published the *International Statistical Classification of Diseases and Related Health Problems, Tenth Revision, Australian Modification* (ICD-10-AM). Subsequent editions have been made available every two years.

In 2001, the Canadian Institute for Health Information (CIHI), through the work of an Expert Panel, published the *International Statistical Classification of Diseases and Related Health Problems, Tenth Revision, Canada* (ICD-10-CA).

The United States remains the only industrialized nation that has not yet implemented ICD-10 (or a clinical modification) for morbidity, meaning diseases or causes of illness typically coded in a healthcare facility. Since 1999, however, the United States has used ICD-10 for mortality reporting—the coding of death certificates (typically done by a vital statistics office, not the healthcare facility). Implementing ICD-10-CM will maintain data comparability internationally and between mortality and morbidity data in the United States.

> **Activity – History of ICD-10**
> To learn more about the processes involved with ICD-10, visit the World Health Organization website (http://www.who.int/classifications/icd/en/).
>
> Review the information on ICD-10 with special attention to the implementation of ICD-10.

> **NOTE:** There is an ICD-10 training tool on the WHO website that you are welcome to peruse; however, remember that this information pertains to ICD-10 and not to the US modification of ICD-10-CM.

Development of ICD-10-CM

In 1994, under the leadership of the National Center for Health Statistics (NCHS), the United States began their process of determining whether an ICD-10 modification should be developed. NCHS awarded a contract to the Center for Health Policy Studies to decide if a clinical modification was necessary. A Technical Advisory Panel (TAP) was formed and their recommendation was to create a clinical modification. In 1997, the entire draft of the Tabular List of ICD-10-CM and the preliminary crosswalk between ICD-9-CM and ICD-10-CM were made available on the NCHS website for public comments. The public comment period ran from December 1997 through February 1998. Since that time revisions were based on further study and the comments submitted. Draft versions of ICD-10-CM were made available in 2002, 2007, 2009, 2010, 2011, 2012, and 2013. One last limited code update will be made to the

ICD-10-CM code set in 2014. Beginning October 1, 2015, ICD-10-CM will have regular annual updates which go into effect on October 1 of each year.

While ICD-10 provides many more categories for diseases and other health-related conditions than previous revisions, the clinical modifications thus far to ICD-10 offer a higher level of specificity by including separate codes for laterality and additional characters for expanded detail. In addition, other changes include combining etiology and manifestations, poisoning and external cause, or diagnosis and symptoms into a single code. ICD-10-CM also provides code titles and language that complement accepted clinical practice. ICD-10-CM codes have the potential to reveal more about quality of care, so that data can be used in a more meaningful way to better understand complications, better design clinically robust algorithms, and better track the outcomes of care. ICD-10-CM incorporates greater specificity and clinical detail to provide information for clinical decision making and outcome research.

The long-awaited official Notice of Proposed Rule Making (NPRM) related to the adoption of the ICD-10-CM and ICD-10-PCS classifications was published in the Federal Register on August 22, 2008. Additional information is available on the CMS website. On January 16, 2009, the Centers for Medicare and Medicaid Services (CMS) published a Health and Human Services (HHS) compliance date of October 1, 2013, for the two code sets. This compliance date has subsequently been delayed until October 1, 2014, and is based on the date of discharge for inpatient claims and the date of service for outpatient claims.

> **Note:** Additional information about the development of ICD-10-CM and the final rule can be found on the CMS website (https://www.cms.gov/icd10/).

This rule will modify two of the medical data code set standards adopted in the Transactions and Code Sets final rule published in the *Federal Register*. It would also implement certain provisions of the Administrative Simplification subtitle of the Health Insurance Portability and Accountability Act (HIPAA) of 1996. Specifically, the rule would modify the standard code sets for coding diagnoses and inpatient hospital procedures by concurrently adopting the *International Classification of Diseases, Tenth Revision, Clinical Modification* (ICD-10-CM) for diagnosis coding, and the *International Classification of Diseases, Tenth Revision, Procedure Coding System* (ICD-10-PCS) for inpatient hospital procedure coding. These new codes will replace the *International Classification of Diseases, Ninth Revision, Clinical Modification* (ICD-9-CM) Volumes 1 and 2 and the *International Classification of Diseases, Ninth Revision, Clinical Modification* (CM) Volume 3 for diagnosis and procedure codes respectively.

> **Note:** CPT® will continue to be used by all providers currently using it.

Organizational and Structural Changes in ICD-10-CM

ICD-10-CM represents a significant improvement over ICD-9-CM. ICD-10-CM continues to have the same hierarchical structure as ICD-9-CM where the first three characters are the category of the code and all codes within the same category have similar traits. Although the hierarchical structure is the same, differences are seen in the organization of ICD-10-CM, including

- ICD-10-CM consists of 21 chapters compared to 17 chapters in ICD-9-CM
- ICD-9-CM's V and E code supplemental classifications are incorporated into the main classification in ICD-10-CM
- Diseases and conditions of the sense organs (eyes and ears) have been separated from the nervous system diseases and conditions and have their own chapters in ICD-10-CM

- To reflect current medical knowledge, certain diseases have been reclassified (or reassigned) to a more appropriate chapter in ICD-10-CM. For example, gout has been reclassified from the endocrine chapter in ICD-9-CM to the musculoskeletal chapter in ICD-10-CM
- In contrast to ICD-9-CM, which classifies injuries by type, ICD-10-CM groups injuries first by specific site (e.g., head, arm, leg), and then by type of injury (e.g., fracture, open wound)
- Postoperative complications have been moved to procedure-specific body system chapters
- ICD-10-CM codes are alphanumeric and can be up to seven characters in length; ICD-9-CM codes are only three to five characters in length
- ICD-10-CM includes full code titles for all codes (no reference back to common fourth and fifth digits)
- Addition of a sixth character in some chapters
- Addition of seventh characters for obstetrics, injuries, and external causes of injuries
- Addition of placeholder X

New Features in ICD-10-CM

The numerous new features in ICD-10-CM allow for a greater level of specificity and clinical detail. These new features include

- Combination codes for conditions and common symptoms or manifestations

---

Examples:
- ➤ E10.21, Type 1 diabetes mellitus with diabetic nephropathy
- ➤ I25.110, Atherosclerotic heart disease of native coronary artery with unstable angina pectoris
- ➤ K50.112, Crohn's disease of large intestine with intestinal obstruction

---

- Combination codes for poisonings and external causes

Examples:
- ➤ T36.0X1D, Poisoning by penicillins, accidental (unintentional), subsequent encounter
- ➤ T42.4X5A, Adverse effect of benzodiazepines, initial encounter

---

- Added laterality

Examples:
- ➤ H60.332, Swimmer's ear, left ear
- ➤ M94.211, Chondromalacia, right shoulder
- ➤ S40.259A, Superficial foreign body of unspecified shoulder, initial encounter

---

- Added seventh-characters for episode of care

Examples:
- ➤ M80.051A, Age-related osteoporosis with current pathological fracture, right femur, initial encounter for fracture
- ➤ S06.0X1A, Concussion with loss of consciousness of 30 minutes or less, initial encounter
- ➤ S52.132B, Displaced fracture of neck of left radius, initial encounter for open fracture Type I or II or initial encounter for open fracture NOS

- Expanded codes (injuries, diabetes, alcohol and substance abuse, postoperative complications)

Examples:
- ➤ E11.341, Type 2 diabetes mellitus with severe nonproliferative diabetic retinopathy with macular edema
- ➤ F14.221, Cocaine dependence with intoxication delirium
- ➤ K91.71, Accidental puncture and laceration of a digestive system organ or structure during a digestive system procedure

---

- Inclusion of trimesters in obstetrics codes (and elimination of fifth digits for episode of care)

Examples:
- ➤ O10.012, Pre-existing essential hypertension complicating pregnancy, second trimester
- ➤ O99.013, Anemia complicating pregnancy, third trimester

- Changes in time frames specified in certain codes

Examples:
- ➤ Acute myocardial infarction—time period changed from 8 weeks to 4 weeks
- ➤ Time frame for abortion versus fetal death changed from 22 weeks to 20 weeks

---

- Added standard definitions for two types of "excludes" notes

---

Examples:
- ➤ *Excludes1* note indicates "not coded here." The code being excluded is never used with the code. The two conditions cannot occur together.
  Example: B06, Rubella (German measles) has an *Excludes1* of congenital rubella (P35.0)
- ➤ *Excludes2* note indicates "not included here." The excluded condition is not part of the condition represented by the code. It is acceptable to use both codes together if the patient has both conditions.
  Example: J04.0, Acute laryngitis has an *Excludes2* of chronic laryngitis (J37.0)

Activity – New Features in ICD-10-CM
Answer each of the following questions.

1. True or false? V and E codes are supplemental classifications in ICD-10-CM.

2. True or false? In ICD-10-CM, injuries are grouped by anatomical site rather than injury category.

3. How are obstetric cases classified in ICD-10-CM?

4. What is the maximum number of characters in ICD-10-CM?

5. How many chapters does ICD-10-CM contain?

General Equivalence Mappings (GEMs)

Mappings between ICD-9-CM and ICD-10-CM classification systems have been developed to facilitate the transition from one code set to another. Public domain diagnosis code reference mapping files referred to as Diagnosis Code Set General Equivalence Mappings (GEMs) have been released by NCHS. There are two GEMs files available allowing for bidirectional mappings, ICD-9-CM to ICD-10-CM and ICD-10-CM to ICD-9-CM. The GEMs, along with documentation and a user's guide, are available on the NCHS website (http://www.cdc.gov/nchs/icd/icd10cm.htm) and the CMS website (http://www.cms.hhs.gov/ICD10).

Appropriate Usage of GEMs:
- Convert multiple databases from ICD-9-CM to ICD-10-CM
- Variety of research applications involving trend data

Inappropriate Usage of GEMs:
- Crosswalks
  There is not a one-to-one match between ICD-9-CM and ICD-10-CM codes, for a multitude of reasons (e.g., new concepts in ICD-10-CM, a single ICD-9-CM code may map to multiple ICD-10-CM codes).

Optional Resources:

Effectiveness of ICD-10-CM in Capturing Public Health Diseases:
http://library.ahima.org/xpedio/groups/public/documents/ahima/bok1_034294.pdf

ICD-10-CM Enhancements:
http://library.ahima.org/xpedio/groups/public/documents/ahima/bok1_042626.hcsp

ICD-10-CM Primer:
http://library.ahima.org/xpedio/groups/public/documents/ahima/bok1_038084.hcsp

Mortality Coding Marks 10 Years of ICD-10:
http://library.ahima.org/xpedio/groups/public/documents/ahima/bok1_043992.hcsp

Putting the ICD-10-CM/PCS GEMs into Practice:
http://library.ahima.org/xpedio/groups/public/documents/ahima/bok1_046756.hcsp

Why ICD-10 is Worth the Trouble:
http://library.ahima.org/xpedio/groups/public/documents/ahima/bok1_036866.hcsp

Code Structure

The first character of an ICD-10-CM code is an alphabetic letter. All the letters of the alphabet are utilized with the exception of the letter U, which has been reserved by the WHO for the provisional assignment of new diseases of uncertain etiology (U00-U49) and for bacterial agents resistant to antibiotics (U80-U89). Some conditions in ICD-10-CM are not limited to the use of a single letter. For instance, neoplasm codes may begin with the letter C or D. Table 1.1 compares characteristics of ICD-10-CM and ICD-9-CM.

Table 1.1. Comparing ICD-9-CM and ICD-10-CM

ICD-10-CM differs from ICD-9-CM in its organization and structure, code composition, and level of detail.	
ICD-9-CM	**ICD-10-CM**
<ul><li>Consists of three to five digits</li><li>First digit is numeric or alpha (E or V)</li><li>Second, third, fourth, and fifth digits are numeric</li><li>Always at least three digits</li><li>Decimal placed after the first three digits</li><li>Alpha characters are not case-sensitive</li></ul>	<ul><li>Consists of three to seven characters</li><li>First character is alpha</li><li>All letters used except U</li><li>Character 2 always numeric</li><li>Characters 3 through 7 can be alpha or numeric</li><li>Decimal placed after the first three characters</li><li>Alpha characters are not case-sensitive</li></ul>
Code Structure of ICD-10-CM versus ICD-9-CM	
ICD-10-CM codes may consist of up to seven characters, with the seventh character representing visit encounter or sequelae for injuries and external causes.	
ICD-9-CM Code Format	**ICD-10-CM Code Format**
X X X . X X	X X X . X X X X
category / etiology, anatomic site, manifestation	category / etiology, anatomic site, severity / extension

Activity – ICD-10-CM Code Structure Changes

To become more familiar with the differences between ICD-9-CM and ICD-10-CM, go to the ICD-10-CM Tabular List, review the following entries, compare the ICD-10-CM codes to the ICD-9-CM codes, and identify their differences.

ICD-10-CM	ICD-9-CM
L03.313	682.2
S42.311K	733.82
T45.2X5A	E933.5

Organization and Structure of ICD-10-CM

Alphabetic Index

The Alphabetic Index is divided into two parts—the Index to Diseases and Injuries and the Index to External Causes. Similar to ICD-9-CM, within the Index of Diseases and Injury there is a Neoplasm Table and a Table of Drugs and Chemicals.

The Alphabetic Index in ICD-10-CM is formatted the same way as the Index in ICD-9-CM. Main terms set in boldface are listed in alphabetical order. Then, indented beneath the main term, any applicable subterm or essential modifier will be shown in their own alphabetic list. The indented subterm is always read in combination with the main term. Nonessential modifiers appear in parentheses and do not affect the code number assigned. The "-" at the end of an Index entry indicates that additional characters are required.

> *Example:*
> **Aberrant (congenital)** – *see also* Malposition, congenital
> - adrenal gland Q89.1
> - artery (peripheral) Q27.8
> - - basilar NEC Q28.1
> - - cerebral Q28.3
> - breast Q83.8

> **Coding Tip:** These codes would be read:
> Q89.1, Congenital malformations of adrenal gland
> Q27.8, Other specified congenital malformations of peripheral vascular system
> Q28.1, Other malformations of precerebral vessels
> Q28.3, Other malformation of cerebral vessels
> Q83.8, Other congenital malformations of breast

Morphology Codes – Morphology codes are no longer listed in the Alphabetic Index alongside the descriptors and standard ICD-10-CM codes. Additionally, the Morphology codes no longer have a separate appendix in ICD-10-CM as in ICD-9-CM.

> **Note:** The following note appears in the Tabular List at the beginning of Chapter 2: Neoplasms.
> **Morphology [Histology]**
> Chapter 2 classifies neoplasms primarily by site (topography), with broad groupings for behavior, malignant, in situ, benign, etc. The Table of Neoplasms should be used to identify the correct topography code. In a few cases, such as for malignant melanoma and certain neuroendocrine tumors, the morphology (histologic type) is included in the category and codes.

Manifestation Codes – ICD-10-CM Alphabetic Index includes the suggestion of some manifestation codes in the same manner as ICD-9-CM, by including the code as a second code, show in brackets, directly after the underlying or etiology code (which should always be reported first).

Example:
Chorioretinitis – *see also* Inflammation, chorioretinal, disseminated
- Egyptian B76.9 [D63.8]
- histoplasmic B39.9 [H32]

Activity – Alphabetic Index

To become more familiar with the ICD-10-CM Alphabetic Index to Diseases, review the following entries in the ICD-10-CM code book. If you do not have a code book, download the Index file from NCHS's website (http://www.cdc.gov/nchs/icd/icd10cm.htm). Compare the ICD-10-CM Alphabetic Index entries to the ICD-9-CM Alphabetic Index entries for the same terms and identify their similarities.

Main term:	Adenofibroma		
Main term:	Aftercare	Subterm:	involving
Main term:	Anemia	Subterm:	deficiency
		Subterm:	Diamond-Blackfan
Main term:	Failure, failed	Subterm:	heart
Main term:	Pregnancy	Subterm:	complicated by
Main term:	Stone(s)		

Tabular List

The ICD-10-CM Tabular List is divided into 21 chapters. For some chapters, the body or organ system is the axis of the classification. Other chapters, such as Chapter 1: Certain infectious and parasitic diseases, group together conditions by etiology or nature of the disease process. ICD-9-CM has a single chapter for Diseases of the Nervous System and Sense Organs whereas ICD-10-CM places these conditions into three separate chapters. ICD-10-CM also does not separate out the ICD-9-CM codes that explain the External Causes of Injury and Poisonings (E codes) and the Factors Influencing Health Status and Contact with Health Services (V codes) from the core classification.

The order of the ICD-10-CM chapters is a bit different from ICD-9-CM. In ICD-10-CM, disorders of the immune mechanism are included with Diseases of the blood and blood-forming organs. In contrast, the immunity disorders are found in the ICD-9-CM chapter for Endocrine, Nutritional and Metabolic Diseases. In addition, certain chapters are reordered. The ICD-10-CM codes for Diseases of the skin and subcutaneous tissue (Chapter 12) and Diseases of the musculoskeletal system and connective tissue (Chapter 13) follow the chapter for Diseases of the digestive system. Next are chapters for Diseases of the genitourinary system (Chapter 14), Pregnancy, childbirth and the puerperium (Chapter 15), Certain conditions originating in the perinatal period (Chapter 16), and Congenital malformations, deformations and chromosomal abnormalities (Chapter 17).

Note: Within a number of ICD-10-CM chapters, category restructuring and code reorganization have occurred resulting in the classification of certain diseases and disorders different than what is currently seen in ICD-9-CM.

The 21 chapters of the ICD-10-CM classification system are

1. Certain infectious and parasitic diseases (A00-B99)
2. Neoplasms (C00-D49)
3. Diseases of the blood and blood-forming organs and certain disorders involving the immune mechanism (D50-D89)
4. Endocrine, nutritional and metabolic disorders (E00-E89)
5. Mental, behavioral and neurodevelopmental disorders (F01-F99)
6. Diseases of the nervous system (G00-G99)
7. Diseases of the eye and adnexa (H00-H59)
8. Diseases of the ear and mastoid process (H60-H95)
9. Diseases of the circulatory system (I00-I99)
10. Diseases of the respiratory system (J00-J99)
11. Diseases of the digestive system (K00-K95)
12. Diseases of the skin and subcutaneous tissue (L00-L99)
13. Diseases of the musculoskeletal system and connective tissue (M00-M99)
14. Diseases of the genitourinary system (N00-N99)
15. Pregnancy, childbirth and the puerperium (O00-O9A)
16. Certain conditions originating in the perinatal period (P00-P96)
17. Congenital malformations, deformations and chromosomal abnormalities (Q00-Q99)
18. Symptoms, signs and abnormal clinical and laboratory findings, not elsewhere classified (R00-R99)
19. Injury, poisoning and certain other consequences of external causes (S00-T88)
20. External causes of morbidity (V00-Y99)
21. Factors influencing health status and contact with health services (Z00-Z99)

Chapters are further subdivided into subchapters (blocks) that contain three character categories and, similar to ICD-9-CM categories, form the foundation of the code. Each chapter in the Tabular List of ICD-10-CM begins with a summary of the blocks to provide an overview of the categories within the chapter. For example

Chapter 7: Diseases of the eye and adnexa (H00-H59)	
This chapter contains the following blocks:	
H00-H05	Disorders of eyelid, lacrimal system and orbit
H10-H11	Disorders of conjunctiva
H15-H22	Disorders of sclera, cornea, iris and ciliary body
H25-H28	Disorders of lens
H30-H36	Disorders of choroid and retina
H40-H42	Glaucoma
H43-H44	Disorders of vitreous body and globe
H46-H47	Disorders of optic nerve and visual pathways
H49-H52	Disorders of ocular muscles, binocular movement, accommodation and refraction
H53-H54	Visual disturbances and blindness
H55-H57	Other disorders of eye and adnexa
H59	Intraoperative and postprocedural complications and disorders of eye and adnexa, not elsewhere classified

Most, but not all, categories are further subdivided into four- or five-character subcategories. If a category is not further subdivided it is considered to be a valid code, such as P90, Convulsions of newborn.

The fourth character 8, when placed after a decimal point (.8), is used to indicate some "other" specified category, and the fourth character 9 placed after a decimal point (.9) is usually reserved for an unspecified condition. This represents another classification modification with the separation of Not Elsewhere Classified (NEC) and Not Otherwise Specified (NOS) codes. ICD-9-CM sometimes combines these two into a single code. In ICD-10-CM, the Other Specified and Unspecified each have their own code.

Examples:
> ➢ K52.89, Other specified noninfective gastroenteritis and colitis
> ➢ K52.9, Non-infective gastroenteritis and colitis, unspecified

---

Five- and six-character codes provide even greater specificity or additional information about the condition being coded. Similar to ICD-9-CM, ICD-10-CM codes must be used to the highest number of characters available or to the highest level of specificity. When a category has been subdivided into four-, five-, or six-character codes, the code assigned must represent the highest level of specificity represented within ICD-10-CM.

Certain categories have an additional seventh character. The seventh character must always be the seventh and final character of the code. When the code contains fewer than seven characters, placeholder X must be used to fill in the empty character(s).

Example: The code for "Exposure to supersonic waves" is a four-character code (W42.0) that requires a seventh character to describe whether this is the initial or subsequent encounter, or sequela. If this were the initial encounter, this code is written as W42.0XXA.

Tabular List – Activity 1

To become more familiar with the draft ICD-10-CM Tabular List of Diseases and Injuries, review the following entries in the ICD-10-CM code book. If you do not have a code book, download the Tabular file from the NCHS website (http://www.cdc.gov/nchs/icd/icd10cm.htm).

- Find code A54.22, Gonococcal prostatitis. Compare it to code 098.12 in ICD-9-CM.
- Locate codes C41.9, Malignant neoplasm of bone and articular cartilage, unspecified and M90.60, Osteitis deformans in neoplastic disease, unspecified site. Compare codes to 170.9 and 731.1 in ICD-9-CM.

Tabular List – Activity 2

To gain a better understanding of the general classification modifications made to ICD-10-CM, open the ICD-10-CM Tabular List, locate the ICD-10-CM categories, and find the associated ICD-9-CM category. Identify the similarities and the differences.

ICD-10-CM	ICD-9-CM
E10-E13	250
M10	274
D80	279

Another structural similarity is the placement of notes in the ICD-10-CM Tabular List. As in ICD-9-CM, they are located at the beginning of chapters or any of the subdivisions that follow. Their position is important in that the notes that appear at the beginning of a chapter apply to all the categories contained within it. The same rule applies to notes found at the other subdivision levels.

Tabular List – Activity 3

To view examples of notes, go to the Tabular List:

- Locate the note at the beginning of Chapter 18: Symptoms, signs and abnormal clinical and laboratory findings (R00-R99) and compare the note to the note found at the beginning of Chapter 16: Symptoms, Signs and Ill-Defined Conditions (780-799) in ICD-9-CM.
- Find the note for the subchapter on Neoplasms of Uncertain Behavior (D37-D48) and review it against the one found for Neoplasms of Uncertain Behavior (235-238) in ICD-9-CM.

Classification Changes to Chapters 5, 19, and 20

ICD-10 reorganized Chapters 5, 19, and 20, which are integrated into ICD-10-CM.

Chapter 5: Mental and behavioral disorders – This chapter contains more subchapters, categories, and subcategories and codes than ICD-9-CM. Consequently when comparing ICD-10-CM to ICD-9-CM some disorders are classified differently and greater clinical detail is obtainable.

Example:

ICD-9-CM   Chapter 5: Mental Disorders (290-319)

ICD-10-CM   Chapter 5: Mental, behavioral and neurodevelopmental disorders (F01-F99)

Examples:

➢ F10.251, Alcohol dependence with alcohol-induced psychotic disorder with hallucinations

➢ F17.213, Nicotine dependence, cigarettes, with withdrawal

Chapter 19: Injury, poisoning and certain other consequences of external causes – A significant modification was made to the classification of injuries with the publication of ICD-10 and therefore ICD-10-CM. Specific types of injuries found in categories S00-S99 of Chapter 19 of ICD-10-CM are arranged by body region beginning with the head and concluding with the ankle and foot. However, effects of a foreign body, burns, and frostbite are not classified in the body region groups. This chapter also includes codes for poisoning, adverse effects, and other consequences of external causes. In contrast, the type of injury is the axis of classification for the ICD-9-CM Chapter 17: Injury and Poisoning.

Example:

ICD-9-CM   Chapter 17: Injury and Poisoning (800-999)

ICD-10-CM   Chapter 19: Injury, poisoning and certain other consequences of external causes (S00-T88)

Examples:

➢ S32.111A, Minimally displaced Zone I fracture of sacrum, initial encounter for closed fracture

➢ T22.151D, Burn of first degree of right shoulder, subsequent encounter

➢ T45.516A, Underdosing of anticoagulant, initial encounter

Chapter 20: External causes of morbidity – Codes for external causes are no longer located in a supplemental classification in ICD-10-CM. The causes currently located in the ICD-9-CM E code chapter are located either in Chapter 19: Injury, poisoning and certain other consequences of external causes, or Chapter 20: External causes of morbidity. Codes in Chapter 20 capture the cause of the injury or health condition, the intent (unintentional or accidental; or intentional, such as suicide or assault), the place where the event occurred, the activity of the patient at the time of the event, and the person's status (i.e., civilian, military).

Example:	
ICD-9-CM	Supplementary Classification of External Causes of Injury and Poisoning (E800-E999)
ICD-10-CM	Chapter 20: External causes of morbidity (V00-Y99)

Examples:
- ➢ W21.03XA, Struck by baseball, initial encounter
- ➢ Y92.320, Baseball field as the place of occurrence of the external cause
- ➢ Y93.64, Activities involving other sports and athletics played as a team or group: baseball
- ➢ Y99.8, Other external cause status (recreation or sport not for income or while a student)

Section 1 Review Questions

1. Gout is classified to the _____ chapter in ICD-10-CM.
    a.   Certain infectious and parasitic diseases
    b.   Endocrine, nutritional and metabolic diseases
    c.   Musculoskeletal system and connective tissue
    d.   Symptoms, signs and abnormal clinical and laboratory findings, NEC

2. True or false? The United States it the only industrialized nation that has not yet implemented ICD-10-CM.
    a.   True
    b.   False

3. All of the following are structural differences between ICD-9-CM and ICD-10-CM, *except:*
    a.   Addition of a sixth character in some chapters
    b.   Addition of placeholder
    c.   Diseases and conditions of the eyes and ears are classified in the same chapter as diseases of the nervous system
    d.   Postoperative complications have been moved to procedure-specific body system chapters

4. True or false? The WHO version of ICD-10 will be implemented in the United States in 2014.
    a.   True
    b.   False

5. Which of the following is a feature of ICD-10-CM?
    a.   Combination codes have been created for both symptom and diagnosis
    b.   The obstetric codes indicate which trimester the patient is in rather than episode of care
    c.   Codes for postoperative complications have been expanded and a distinction has been made between intraoperative complications and post-procedural disorders
    d.   All of the above

6. Which of the following statements is true?
    a.   All codes in ICD-10-CM include full code titles
    b.   All chapters in ICD-10-CM require the addition of code extensions
    c.   All codes in ICD-10-CM are seven characters in length
    d.   All codes in ICD-10-CM use the placeholder X

7. The ICD-10-CM code to report a disease of the genitourinary system begins with what letter?
    a.   P
    b.   G
    c.   E
    d.   N

8. Which of the following is a true statement regarding ICD-10-CM codes?
    a.   No decimals are used.
    b.   The first character is always an alpha.
    c.   Consist of three to five characters.
    d.   The second and third characters are always numeric.

9. Which of the following is a valid ICD-10-CM code?
    a.   428.9
    b.   L03.313
    c.   T37.0XX1A
    d.   M12X.58

10. True or false? The GEMs are a crosswalk between ICD-9-CM and ICD-10-CM.
    a.   True
    b.   False

Section 2 – ICD-10-CM Conventions and Coding Guidelines

ICD-10-CM Conventions

Correct assignment of ICD-10-CM diagnosis codes is dependent upon the individual understanding certain conventions used in the classification system. Similar to ICD-9-CM, abbreviations, punctuation, symbols, and notes are used as conventions and have special meanings that affect code assignment.

Placeholder Character

ICD-10-CM utilizes a placeholder which is always the letter X and it has two uses:

- As the fifth character for certain six character codes. The X provides for future expansion without disturbing the sixth character structure.

Examples:
- ➤ T37.0X1A, Poisoning by sulfonamides, accidental (unintentional), initial encounter
- ➤ T56.0X2S, Toxic effect of lead and its compounds, intentional self-harm, sequela

---

- When a code has less than six characters and a seventh character is required. The X is assigned for all characters less than six in order to meet the requirement of coding to the highest level of specificity.

Examples:
- ➤ W85.XXXA, Exposure to electric transmission lines, initial encounter
- ➤ S17.0XXA, Crushing injury of larynx and trachea. initial encounter
- ➤ S01.02XA, Laceration with foreign body of scalp, initial encounter

---

Seventh Characters

Some ICD-10-CM categories require a seventh character to provide further specificity about the condition being coded. This seventh character may be a number or letter and must always be the seventh character.

Examples:
- ➤ O64.3XX1, Obstructed labor due to brow presentation, fetus 1
- ➤ S02.110B, Type I occipital condyle fracture, initial encounter for open fracture
- ➤ T17.220D, Food in pharynx causing asphyxiation, subsequent encounter

---

Activity – Placeholders and Seventh Characters

To gain a greater understanding of the purpose of the X placeholder and the seventh character, refer to the Tabular List, locate the following, and determine the use of

- The seventh character for subcategory codes R40.21, R40.22, and R40.23
- The seventh character for category M80
- The X placeholder in subcategory O45.8
- The X placeholder in category X78

Abbreviations

Not Elsewhere Classified (NEC) – ICD-10-CM, like its predecessors, contains codes to classify any and all conditions. A residual category, subdivision, or subclassification provides a location for "other" types of specified conditions that have not been classified anywhere else in the code set. These residual codes may also contain the term "NEC" as part of their descriptor. The Alphabetic Index uses NEC for a code description that will direct the coder to the Tabular List showing an Other Specified code description.

Example:

ICD-10-CM	ICD-9-CM
H26.8 Other specified cataract	366.8 Other cataract
I25.89 Other forms of chronic ischemic heart disease	414.8 Other specified forms of chronic ischemic heart disease

---

Not Otherwise Specified (NOS) – The unspecified or Not Otherwise Specified (NOS) codes are available for use when the documentation of the condition identified by the provider is insufficient to assign a more specific code.

Example:

ICD-10-CM	ICD-9-CM
H40.9 Unspecified glaucoma	365.9 Unspecified glaucoma
J12.9 Viral pneumonia, unspecified	480.9 Viral pneumonia, unspecified

---

Punctuation

Similar to ICD-9-CM, punctuation is used in both the Alphabetic Index and the Tabular List. The types of punctuation included in ICD-10-CM are parentheses, brackets, and colons.

( ) Parentheses – Parentheses are used in both the Alphabetic Index and the Tabular List to enclose supplementary words that may be present or absent in the statement of a disease without affecting the code number to which it is assigned. The terms within the parentheses are referred to as *nonessential modifiers*.

Examples: Alphabetic Index
  ➢ **Anemia** (essential) (general) (hemoglobin deficiency) (infantile) (primary) (profound)
  ➢ **Diabetes, diabetic** (mellitus) (sugar)
  ➢ **Hemophilia** (classical) (familial) (hereditary)

Examples: Tabular List
  ➢ H44.611, Retained (old) magnetic foreign body in anterior chamber, right eye
  ➢ I10, Essential (primary) hypertension
  ➢ K51.011, Ulcerative (chronic) pancolitis with rectal bleeding

---

[ ] Brackets – The Tabular List uses square brackets to enclose synonyms, alternative wordings, or explanatory phrases. Brackets are used in the Alphabetic Index to identify manifestation codes.

Examples: Tabular List
> ➢ B06, Rubella [German measles]
> ➢ J00, Acute nasopharyngitis [common cold]

Examples: Alphabetic Index
☐ **Disease**, Alzheimer's G30.9 [F02.80]
☐ **Nephrosis**, in amyloidosis E85.4 [N08]

: Colon – Colons are used in the Tabular List after an incomplete term which needs one or more of the modifiers following the colon to make it assignable to a given category. The colon is used with both "includes" and "excludes" notes, in which the words that precede the colon are not considered complete terms and therefore must be appended by one of the modifiers indented under the statement before the condition can be assigned the correct code.

Example:
G73.7 Myopathy in diseases classified elsewhere
> *Excludes1:* myopathy in:
>> rheumatoid arthritis (M05.32)
>> sarcoidosis (D86.87)
>> scleroderma (M34.82)
>> sicca syndrome [Sjögren] (M35.03)
>> systemic lupus erythematosus (M32.19)

Note: Other ICD-10-CM format issues that are different from ICD-9-CM to make note of:
- Some symbols, that is, the lozenge, section mark, and braces are not included in ICD-10-CM.
- Dashes are used in both the ICD-10-CM Alphabetic Indexes and the Tabular List.
  - The indexes utilize the dash at the end of a code number to indicate the code is incomplete. To determine the additional character(s), locate the code in the Tabular List, review the options, and assign the appropriate code.

    - **Fracture, pathologic**
      ankle M84.47-
      carpus M84.44-
  - In the Tabular List, a dash preceded by a decimal point (.-) indicates an incomplete code. To determine the additional characters, locate the referenced category or subcategory elsewhere in the Tabular List, review the options, and assign the appropriate code.

    - **J43 Emphysema**
      Excludes1: emphysematous (obstructive) bronchitis (J44.-)

Instructional Notes

Similar to ICD-9-CM a variety of notes appear in both the Alphabetic Index and Tabular List of ICD-10-CM. The various types of notes are "includes" and "excludes" notes, "code first" notes, "use additional code" notes, and cross reference notes.

Inclusion Notes – Includes notes are used as conventions in the ICD-10-CM Tabular List to clarify the conditions included within a particular chapter, section, category, subcategory, or code. It is important to remember that the list of inclusions terms is not exhaustive and may include diagnoses not listed in the inclusion note. Inclusion notes are introduced by the word "includes" when appearing at the beginning of a chapter, section, or category.

Example:
K25   Gastric Ulcer
      Includes: erosion (acute) of stomach
                  pylorus ulcer (peptic)
                  stomach ulcer (peptic)

At the code level, the word "includes" does not precede the list of terms included in the code.

Example:
K31.5 Obstruction of duodenum
      Constriction of duodenum
      Duodenal ileus (chronic)
      Stenosis of duodenum
      Stricture of duodenum
      Volvulus of duodenum

Exclusion Notes – ICD-9-CM contains a single type of excludes note which has two different meanings leaving it to the coding professional to determine the correct meaning of the excludes note. In ICD-10-CM there are two types of excludes notes designated either as *Excludes1* or *Excludes2* in their title. Either or both may appear under a category, subcategory, or code.

The *Excludes1* note is a pure "excludes" note. It means *not coded here*. An *Excludes1* note indicates that the code excluded should never be used at the same time as the code above the *Excludes1* note. This note is used when two conditions cannot occur together, such as a congenital form versus an acquired form of the same condition.

Example:
K51.4 Inflammatory polyps of colon
      Excludes1: adenomatous polyp of colon (D12.6)
                  polyposis of colon (D12.6)
                  polyps of colon NOS (K63.5)

The *Excludes2* note means *not included here*. This type of "excludes" note indicates that the condition excluded is not part of the condition represented by the code, but a patient may have both conditions at the same time. When an *Excludes2* note appears under a code, it is acceptable to use both the code and the excluded code together if the patient has both conditions.

Example:
J37.1 Chronic laryngotracheitis
      Excludes2: acute laryngotracheitis (J04.2)
                  acute tracheitis (J04.1)

Code First and Use Additional Code Notes – "Code first" and "use additional code" notes are similar to their counterparts in ICD-9-CM. Certain conditions have both an underlying etiology and multiple body system manifestations due to the underlying etiology. For such conditions, ICD-10-CM, similar to ICD-9-CM, has a coding convention that requires the underlying condition be sequenced first followed by the manifestation. The "use additional code" note appears at the etiology code and a "code first" note at the manifestation code.

Example:

G30   **Alzheimer's disease**
Use additional code to identify:
      dementia with behavioral disturbance (F02.81)
      dementia without behavioral disturbance (F02.80)

F02   **Dementia in other diseases classified elsewhere**
Code first the underlying physiological condition, such as
      Alzheimer's (G30.-)

   F02.80 Dementia in other diseases classified elsewhere, without behavioral disturbance

   F02.81 Dementia in other diseases classified elsewhere, with behavioral disturbance

---

Cross Reference Notes – Cross reference notes are used in the ICD-10-CM Alphabetic Index to advise the coding professional to look elsewhere before assigning a code. The three cross reference notes (*see, see also,* and *see condition*) are the same as those found in ICD-9-CM.

Examples:

Pyocele
- mastoid – *see* Mastoiditis, acute
- sinus (accessory) – *see* Sinusitis
- turbinate (bone) J32.9
- urethra (*see also* Urethritis) N34.0

Mercurial – *see condition*

Mercurialism – *see* subcategory T56.1

Labyrinthitis (circumscribed) (destructive) (diffuse) (inner ear) (latent) (purulent) (suppurative) – *see also* subcategory H83.0

Activity 1 – Excludes Notes
Explain, in common terms, the complete meaning of this code description and its notations.

F06.1   Catatonic disorder due to known physiological condition

Excludes1:	catatonic stupor (R40.1)	
	stupor NOS (R40.1)	
Excludes2:	catatonic schizophrenia (F20.2)	
	dissociative stupor (F44.2)	

Activity 2 – Tabular Conventions
To gain skills in identifying the different types of notes, open the Tabular List and review the following, comparing the ICD-10-CM entries to the ICD-9-CM entries for the same terms. Identify their similarities and differences.

- Find the note for C25.4, Malignant neoplasms of endocrine pancreas, and compare it to the note found under code 157.4 in ICD-9-CM.
- Locate the note for subcategory H62.4, Otitis externa in other diseases classified elsewhere, and review it against the note found under codes 380.13 and 380.15 in ICD-9-CM.
- Find the note for category J44, Other chronic obstructive pulmonary disease, and compare it to the note found under code 496 in ICD-9-CM.
- Locate the note for code O94, Sequelae of complication of pregnancy, childbirth and the puerperium, and determine how it is similar to the note found under code 677 in ICD-9-CM.

Relational Terms

And – The term "and" is interpreted to mean "and/or" when it appears in a code title within the ICD-10-CM Tabular List.

With – The word "with" should be interpreted to mean "associated with" or "due to" when it appears in a code title, the Alphabetic Index, or an instructional note in the Tabular List. The term "with" in the Alphabetic Index is sequenced immediately following the main term, not in alphabetic order.

ICD-10-CM Guidelines

In 2013 the National Center for Health Statistics (NCHS) revised the draft *ICD-10-CM Official Guidelines for Coding and Reporting*. These guidelines have been approved by the four organizations referred to as the Cooperating Parties for ICD-10-CM: the American Hospital Association (AHA), the American Health Information Management Association (AHIMA), the Centers for Medicare and Medicaid Services (CMS), and NCHS. The guidelines are organized into four sections similar to the *ICD-9-CM Official Guidelines for Coding and Reporting*. Section I includes the structure and conventions of the classification and general guidelines that apply to the entire classification in addition to chapter-specific guidelines that correspond to the chapters as they are arranged in the classification. Section II includes guidelines for selection of principal diagnosis for non-outpatient settings. Section III includes guidelines for reporting additional diagnoses in non-outpatient settings. Section IV is for outpatient coding and reporting.

The General Coding Guidelines (Part B of Section I) for ICD-10-CM are similar to their ICD-9-CM General Coding Guidelines counterparts with one additional guideline – Laterality. The Laterality Guideline states, "Some ICD-10-CM codes indicate laterality, specifying whether the condition occurs on the left, right or is bilateral. If no bilateral code is provided and the condition is bilateral, assign separate codes for both the left and right side. If the side is not identified in the medical record, assign the code for the unspecified side."

The complete 2014 version of the ICD-10-CM guidelines can be located on the NCHS website (http://www.cdc.gov/nchs/icd/icd10cm.htm).

Activity – General Coding Guidelines
To gain an understanding of the ICD-10-CM General Coding Guidelines, open the ICD-10-CM Official Guidelines (http://www.cdc.gov/nchs/icd/icd10cm.htm). Study Section I.B.

The General Coding Guidelines for ICD-10-CM are similar to their ICD-9-CM General Coding Guidelines counterparts with a few exceptions, which are called out here:
- The Laterality (#13) Guideline states, "Some ICD-10-CM codes indicate laterality, specifying whether the condition occurs on the left, right or is bilateral. If no bilateral code is provided and the condition is bilateral, assign separate codes for both the left and right side. If the side is not identified in the medical record, assign the code for the unspecified side."
- Review the Documentation of Complications of Care (#16) Guidelines which states that "Code assignment is based on the provider's documentation of the relationship between the condition and the care or procedure." The guideline extends to any complications of care, regardless of the chapter the code is located in. It is important to note that not all conditions that occur during or following medical care or surgery are classified as complications. There must be a cause-and-effect relationship between the care provided and the condition and an indication in the documentation that it is a complication. If the complication is not clearly documented, query the provider for clarification.

Section 2 Review Questions

1. What is the purpose of the X in subcategory O45.8?
    a. Describes laterality
    b. To preserve the meaning of the sixth character
    c. To provide further specificity about the condition being coded
    d. To code to the highest level of specificity

2. Which of the following abbreviations is used in ICD-10-CM?
    a. NOC
    b. NES
    c. NEC
    d. NIC

3. True or false? ICD-10-CM uses inclusion terms in the same way that ICD-9-CM does.
    a. True
    b. False

4. What indicates synonyms, alternative wording, or explanatory phrases in the Tabular List?
    a. Parentheses
    b. Brackets
    c. Dash
    d. Colon

5. True or false? The seventh character is always a letter.
    a. True
    b. False

6. True or false? ICD-10-CM contains codes that specify laterality.
    a. True
    b. False

7. Which type of note is located under code H62.4?
    a. Use additional code for manifestation
    b. Code also external cause
    c. Code first underlying disease
    d. Includes

8. Which of the following is a convention found in the Alphabetic Index of ICD-10-CM?
    a. The colon
    b. The abbreviation NEC
    c. Use additional code notation
    d. Code first notation

9. True or false? For every code where ICD-10-CM provides codes for laterality, bilateral is listed as an option.
    a. True
    b. False

10. True or false? Similar to ICD-9-CM, the term "with" is sequenced immediately following the main term.
    a. True
    b. False

Section 3 – Organization and Classification of Diseases and Disorders – Chapters 1–7

This section is designed to present an overview of the changes to specific disorders and conditions classified to Chapters 1–7 of ICD-10-CM. Not every revision has been identified but certain conditions have been selected to point out concepts that represent organizational, terminology, and classification modifications.

Chapter 1: Certain infectious and parasitic diseases (A00-B99)

Chapter 1 of ICD-10-CM includes categories A00-B99 arranged in the following blocks:

A00-A09	Intestinal infectious diseases
A15-A19	Tuberculosis
A20-A28	Certain zoonotic bacterial diseases
A30-A49	Other bacterial diseases
A50-A64	Infections with a predominantly sexual mode of transmission
A65-A69	Other spirochetal diseases
A70-A74	Other diseases caused by chlamydia
A75-A79	Rickettsioses
A80-A89	Viral and prion infections of the central nervous system
A90-A99	Arthropod-borne viral fevers and viral hemorrhagic fevers
B00-B09	Viral infections characterized by skin and mucous membrane lesions
B10	Other human herpes viruses
B15-B19	Viral hepatitis
B20	Human immunodeficiency virus [HIV] disease
B25-B34	Other viral diseases
B35-B49	Mycoses
B50-B64	Protozoal diseases
B65-B83	Helminthiases
B85-B89	Pediculosis, acariasis and other infestations
B90-B94	Sequelae of infectious and parasitic diseases
B95-B97	Bacterial and viral infectious agents
B99	Other infectious diseases

While overall Chapter 1 of ICD-10-CM is organized similar to ICD-9-CM, some category and subcategory titles have been changed.

Examples:

ICD-9-CM	008, Intestinal infections due to other organisms
ICD-10-CM	A08, Viral and other specified intestinal infections
ICD-9-CM	024, Glanders
ICD-10-CM	025, Melioidosis
ICD-9-CM	A24, Glanders and melioidosis
ICD-9-CM	036.4, Meningococcal carditis
ICD-10-CM	A39.5, Meningococcal heart disease

Certain diseases have also been rearranged in Chapter 1 of ICD-10-CM. For example, a separate subchapter, or block, has been created and appropriate conditions grouped together for Infections with a predominantly sexual mode of transmission (A50-A64). Two additional examples of separate blocks being created with the appropriate conditions grouped together are Viral hepatitis (B15-B19) and Other viral diseases (B25-B34).

Some terminology changes and revisions to the classification of specific infectious and parasitic disease in ICD-10-CM have occurred as well. For instance, the term *sepsis* has replaced *septicemia* throughout Chapter 1. Additionally, *streptococcal sore throat* and its inclusion terms found in the Infectious and Parasitic Disease chapter of ICD-9-CM are reclassified in ICD-10-CM to Chapter 10: Diseases of the respiratory system.

Many of the codes in Chapter 1 of ICD-10-CM have been expanded to reflect manifestations of the disease with the use of fourth or fifth characters allowing the infectious disease and manifestation to be captured in one code instead of two.

Example:

A01.0 Typhoid fever
  Infection due to Salmonella typhi
  A01.00, Typhoid fever, unspecified
  A01.01, Typhoid meningitis
  A01.02, Typhoid fever with heart involvement
  A01.03, Typhoid pneumonia
  A01.04, Typhoid arthritis
  A01.05, Typhoid osteomyelitis
  A01.09, Typhoid fever with other complications

Activity – Chapter 1 Organization and Classification
To learn more about these changes to the organization, terminology, and classification of infectious and parasitic diseases in ICD-10-CM, open the Tabular List. Review and compare the following entries and identify their differences. You will need access to the ICD-9-CM Tabular List to complete this review.

ICD-10-CM	ICD-9-CM
B95-B97	041
B94.1	139.0
A48.1	482.84

Chapter 2: Neoplasms (C00-D49)

Chapter 2 of ICD-10-CM includes categories C00-D49 arranged in the following blocks:

C00-C75   Malignant neoplasms stated or presumed to be primary (of specific sites) and certain specified histologies, except neuroendocrine, and of lymphoid, hematopoietic and related tissues

         C00-C14   Malignant neoplasms of lip, oral cavity and pharynx

         C15-C26   Malignant neoplasms of digestive organs

         C30-C39   Malignant neoplasms of respiratory and intrathoracic organs

         C40-C41   Malignant neoplasms of bone and articular cartilage

         C43-C44   Malignant neoplasms of skin

         C45-C49   Malignant neoplasms mesothelial and soft tissue

         C50   Malignant neoplasms of breast

         C51-C58   Malignant neoplasms of female genital organs

         C60-C63   Malignant neoplasms of male genital organs

         C64-C68   Malignant neoplasms of urinary tract

         C69-C72   Malignant neoplasms of eye, brain and other parts of central nervous system

         C73-C75   Malignant neoplasms of thyroid and other endocrine glands

C7A   Malignant neuroendocrine tumors

C7B   Secondary neuroendocrine tumors

C76-C80   Malignant neoplasms of ill-defined, other secondary and unspecified sites

C81-C96   Malignant neoplasm of lymphoid, hematopoietic and related tissue

D00-D09   In situ neoplasms

D10-D36   Benign neoplasms except benign neuroendocrine tumors

D3A   Benign neuroendocrine tumors

D37-D48   Neoplasms of uncertain behavior, polycythemia vera and myelodysplastic syndromes

D49   Neoplasms of unspecified behavior

The neoplasm chapter has undergone some organizational changes, too. For example, in ICD-10-CM, the block of codes for *in situ neoplasms* is located before the block for *benign neoplasms*. An example of a classification improvement is the addition in ICD-10-CM of a separate fifth character for extranodal and solid organ sites for lymphomas and Hodgkin's. ICD-9-CM included these sites with the fifth digit for unspecified site in codes for Hodgkin's disease, non-Hodgkin's lymphoma, peripheral, and cutaneous T-cell lymphomas.

Activity – Chapter 2 Organization and Classification

In order to gain a better understanding of modifications to the organization, terminology, and classification of neoplasms in ICD-10-CM, open the Tabular List. Locate the following categories and compare the presentation of the codes in ICD-10-CM to the codes in ICD-9-CM.

ICD-10-CM	ICD-9-CM
C48	158
C54	182
C64-C68	189
C80	199

Chapter 3: Diseases of the blood and blood-forming organs and certain disorders involving the immune mechanism (D50-D89)

Chapter 3 of ICD-10-CM includes categories D50-D89 arranged in the following blocks:

D50-D53	Nutritional anemias
D55-D59	Hemolytic anemias
D60-D64	Aplastic and other anemias and other bone marrow failure syndromes
D65-D69	Coagulation defects, purpura and other hemorrhagic conditions
D70-D77	Other disorders of blood and blood-forming organs
D78	Intraoperative and postprocedural complications of spleen
D80-D89	Certain disorders involving the immune mechanism

Coding professionals will find the organizational structure of ICD-10-CM's Chapter 3 an improvement over ICD-9-CM's Chapter 4, Diseases of the Blood and Blood-forming Organs. Diseases and disorders have been grouped into subchapters or blocks making it easier to identify the type of conditions classified to Chapter 3. Modifications have also been made to specific categories that bring the terminology up-to-date with current medical practice. Other enhancements to Chapter 3 include classification changes that provide greater specificity than found in ICD-9-CM.

Example 1:

ICD-9-CM	281.2	Folate-deficiency anemia
ICD-10-CM	D52	Folate deficiency anemia

            D52.0, Dietary folate deficiency anemia
            D52.1, Drug-induced folate deficiency anemia
                    Code first (T36-T50) to identify drug
            D52.8, Other folate deficiency anemias
            D52.9, Folate deficiency anemia, unspecified

Example 2:

ICD-9-CM	282.4	Thalassemias
ICD-10-CM	D56	Thalassemia

            D56.0, Alpha thalassemia
            D56.1, Beta thalassemia
            D56.2, Delta-beta thalassemia
            D56.3, Thalassemia minor
            D56.4, Hereditary persistence of fetal hemoglobin [HPFH]
            D56.8, Other thalassemias
            D56.9, Thalassemia, unspecified

The last block in this chapter (D80-D89) groups disorders involving the immune mechanism. The immunodeficiency disorders have been reclassified from Chapter 4: Endocrine, Nutritional and Metabolic Diseases, and Immunity Disorders in ICD-9-CM to Chapter 3 in ICD-10-CM.

Activity – Chapter 3 Organization and Classification

To expand your knowledge of the alterations made to the organization, terminology, and classification of diseases of the blood and blood-forming organs and certain disorders involving the immune mechanism in ICD-10-CM, open the Tabular List. Find the following codes or categories and determine what changes were made between ICD revisions. You will need access to ICD-9-CM to complete this review.

ICD-10-CM	ICD-9-CM
D51.0	281.0
D73	289
D86	135

Chapter 4: Endocrine, nutritional and metabolic diseases (E00-E89)

Chapter 4 of ICD-10-CM includes categories E00-E90 arranged in the following blocks:

E00-E07	Disorders of thyroid gland
E08-E13	Diabetes mellitus
E15-E16	Other disorders of glucose regulation and pancreatic internal secretion
E20-E35	Disorders of other endocrine glands
E36	Intraoperative complications of endocrine system
E40-E46	Malnutrition
E50-E64	Other nutritional deficiencies
E65-E68	Overweight, obesity and other hyperalimentation
E70-E88	Metabolic disorders
E89	Postprocedural endocrine and metabolic complications and disorders, not elsewhere classified

A number of new subchapters have been added to the chapter for endocrine, nutritional, and metabolic diseases. For example, diabetes mellitus and malnutrition have their own subchapter while these conditions were grouped with diseases of other endocrine glands and nutritional deficiencies respectively. Code titles have been revised in a number of places in Chapter 4.

Note: Code descriptors for goiter are now consistent with present terminology.

A significant change to ICD-10-CM is the classification of diabetes mellitus. Instead of a single category (250) as in ICD-9-CM, there are five categories for diabetes mellitus in ICD-10-CM. Additionally, diabetes mellitus codes have been expanded to reflect manifestations and complications of the disease by using fourth or fifth characters rather than by using an additional code to identify the manifestation. ICD-10-CM classifies inadequately controlled, out of control, and poorly controlled diabetes mellitus to diabetes mellitus, by type with hyperglycemia.

Note: ICD-10-CM's five categories for diabetes mellitus:
- E08, Diabetes mellitus due to underlying condition
- E09, Drug or chemical induced diabetes mellitus
- E10, Type 1 diabetes mellitus
- E11, Type 2 diabetes mellitus
- E13, Other specified diabetes mellitus

Activity – Chapter 4 Organization and Classification
To increase your understanding of the revisions to the organization, terminology, and classification of endocrine, nutritional, and metabolic diseases in ICD-10-CM, open the Tabular List. Next, ascertain the modifications by evaluating the ICD-9-CM information against what was found for the ICD-10-CM category or code. You will need access to ICD-9-CM to complete this review.

ICD-10-CM	ICD-9-CM
E07.81	790.94
E28.310-E28.319	256.31
E32	254

Chapter 5: Mental, behavioral and neurodevelopmental disorders (F01-F99)

As explained earlier, Chapter 5 contains more subchapters, categories, subcategories, and codes than ICD-9-CM. Rather than grouping by psychotic, nonpsychotic disorders, or mental retardation as in ICD-9-CM, ICD-10-CM organizes mental and behavioral disorders in the following blocks:

F01-F09	Mental disorders due to known physiological conditions
F10-F19	Mental and behavioral disorders due to psychoactive substance use
F20-F29	Schizophrenia, schizotypal, delusional, and other non-mood psychotic disorders
F30-F39	Mood [affective] disorders
F40-F48	Anxiety, dissociative, stress-related, somatoform and other nonpsychotic mental disorders
F50-F59	Behavioral syndromes associated with physiological disturbances and physical factors
F60-F69	Disorders of adult personality and behavior
F70-F79	Intellectual disabilities
F80-F89	Pervasive and specific developmental disorders
F90-F98	Behavioral and emotional disorders with onset usually occurring in childhood and adolescence
F99	Unspecified mental disorder

Changes were necessary in many parts of Chapter 5 because of outdated terminology. For example, given what has been discovered in the past 20 years about the effects of nicotine, ICD-10-CM contains a separate category F17 for nicotine dependence with subcategories to identify the specific tobacco product and nicotine-induced disorders. ICD-9-CM has a single code, 305.1, for tobacco use disorder or tobacco dependence.

Note: A fairly substantial classification change was made to the codes for drug and alcohol abuse and dependence

---

The identification of the stage of the substance use, namely continuous or episodic, is not a part of ICD-10-CM. A single ICD-10-CM code identifies not only the substance but also the disorder the substance use induced. There continues to be codes for substance dependence "in remission."

Coding Tip: The codes in Chapter 5 of ICD-10-CM parallel the codes in DSM-IV TR in most cases.

Activity – Chapter 5 Organization and Classification
Refer to the Tabular List to find out more about the organization, terminology, and classification modifications to mental and behavioral disorders in ICD-10-CM. Locate the listed ICD-10-CM category or code. Then, evaluate the ICD-9-CM information against what was found and discern the variances.

ICD-10-CM	ICD-9-CM
F03	290.1
F10.1	305.0
F43.1	309.81

Chapter 6: Diseases of the nervous system (G00-G99)

Chapter 6 of ICD-10-CM includes categories G00-G99 arranged in the following blocks:

G00-G09	Inflammatory diseases of the central nervous system
G10-G14	Systemic atrophies primarily affecting the central nervous system
G20-G26	Extrapyramidal and movement disorders
G30-G32	Other degenerative diseases of the nervous system
G35-G37	Demyelinating diseases of the central nervous system
G40-G47	Episodic and paroxysmal disorders
G50-G59	Nerve, nerve root and plexus disorders
G60-G65	Polyneuropathies and other disorders of the peripheral nervous system
G70-G73	Diseases of myoneural junction and muscle
G80-G83	Cerebral palsy and other paralytic syndromes
G89-G99	Other disorders of the nervous system

The organization of Chapter 6 in ICD-10-CM is comparable to that in ICD-9-CM. One change to note is that only diseases of the nervous system are contained in Chapter 6 of ICD-10-CM. Diseases of the sense organs, namely eye/adnexa and ear/mastoid processes, each have their own chapter in ICD-10-CM while they are combined into a single chapter in ICD-9-CM. A few categories in Chapter 6 have rephrased titles and in some cases encompass a combination of conditions. Additionally, a number of codes for diseases of the nervous system have been expanded in ICD-10-CM.

> **Note:**
> - Category for Alzheimer's disease (G30) has been expanded to reflect onset (early versus late)
> - ICD-10-CM has two codes for phantom limb syndrome, differentiating whether pain is present or not

> **Note:** Classification of organic sleep disorders have undergone a significant change in ICD-10-CM:
> - First, these disorders are now included in Chapter 6 rather than the signs and symptoms chapter where ICD-9-CM had classified them
> - Second, sleep apnea has its own subcategory (G47.3) with fifth character specificity identifying the type

Activity – Chapter 6 Organization and Classification

To become more familiar with other revisions to the organization, terminology, and classification of diseases of the nervous system in ICD-10-CM, open the Tabular List. Find the ICD-10-CM category or code listed here and assess how it differs from the ICD-9-CM category or code.

ICD-10-CM	ICD-9-CM
G01	320.7
G40	345
G43	346

Chapter 7: Diseases of eyes and adnexa (H00-H59)

Chapter 7 of ICD-10-CM includes categories H00-H59 arranged in the following blocks:

H00-H05	Disorders of eyelid, lacrimal system and orbit
H10-H11	Disorders of conjunctiva
H15-H22	Disorders of sclera, cornea, iris and ciliary body
H25-H28	Disorders of lens
H30-H36	Disorders of choroid and retina
H40-H42	Glaucoma
H43-H44	Disorders of vitreous body and globe
H46-H47	Disorders of optic nerve and visual pathways
H49-H52	Disorders of ocular muscles, binocular movement, accommodation and refraction
H53-H54	Visual disturbances and blindness
H55-H57	Other disorders of eye and adnexa
H59	Intraoperative and postprocedural complications and disorders of eye and adnexa, not elsewhere classified

Chapter 7 is an entirely new chapter in ICD-10-CM. In ICD-9-CM, the conditions classified in this chapter are located in Chapter 6: Diseases of the Nervous System and Sense Organs. Chapter 7 in ICD-10-CM also has a different organization than what is found in ICD-9-CM. While the structure is still by "site" for diseases of the eye and adnexa, the order differs.

Some categories in Chapter 7 have undergone title changes to reflect the terminology used today. For example, ICD-9-CM uses *senile cataract* while ICD-10-CM utilizes the descriptor *age-related cataract*. Many of the classification changes in Chapter 7 have to do with the expansion of characters to provide for laterality. ICD-10-CM contains codes for right side, left side, and in some instances bilateral sides for diseases of the eye and adnexa.

Example:

H16.01 Central corneal ulcer

      H16.011, Central corneal ulcer, right eye

      H16.012, Central corneal ulcer, left eye

      H16.013, Central corneal ulcer, bilateral

      H16.019, Central corneal ulcer, unspecified eye

Activity – Chapter 7 Organization and Classification

For additional practice with learning the organization, terminology, and classification changes to the chapter of diseases of eyes and adnexa in ICD-10-CM, open the Tabular List. Review the ICD-10-CM category or code listed below and ascertain the modification.

ICD-10-CM	*ICD-9-CM*
H02.6	374.51
H40	365
H49	378.50

Section 4 – Chapters 1–7 Guidelines

This section is designed to highlight the revisions to the guidelines found in Chapters 1–7 of ICD-10-CM. All modifications have not been identified, but certain guiding principles have been selected to illustrate guideline variations from ICD-9-CM. Also included in this section is the review of chapter-specific coding guidelines published by NCHS.

Chapter 1: Certain infectious and parasitic diseases (A00-B99)

At the beginning of Chapter 1 is an instruction to use an additional code to identify resistance to antimicrobial drugs (Z16). This new guideline should be followed when assigning any code from this chapter.

Guidelines for code usage may also be category specific.

> **Note:** Under ICD-10-CM category B39, histoplasmosis, is a note to use an additional code for any associated manifestation. This differs from the note in ICD-9-CM in that the manifestation would be coded using a fifth-digit classification.

The NCHS has published chapter-specific guidelines for Chapter 1 of ICD-10-CM:
- Guideline I.C.1.a. Human immunodeficiency virus [HIV] infections
- Guideline I.C.1.b. Infectious agents as the cause of diseases classified to other chapters
- Guideline I.C.1.c. Infections resistant to antibiotics
- Guideline I.C.1.d. Sepsis, severe sepsis, and septic shock

Activity – Chapter 1 Guidelines

To gain an understanding of these rules, access the 2014 guidelines from the NCHS website (http://www.cdc.gov/nchs/icd/icd10cm.htm) and read Chapter 1: Certain infectious and parasitic diseases guidelines, I.C.1.a through I.C.1.e.1.d on pages 17–25.

Chapter 2: Neoplasms (C00-D49)

The NCHS has published chapter-specific guidelines for Chapter 2 of ICD-10-CM. Most of these guidelines are consistent with what we see in ICD-9-CM with a few exceptions. One guideline to take note of is I.C.2.c.1, Anemia associated with malignancy. This guideline states the following:

> When admission/encounter is for management of an anemia associated with the malignancy, and the treatment is only for anemia, the appropriate code for the malignancy is sequenced as the principal or first-listed diagnosis followed by the appropriate code for the anemia (such as code D63.0, Anemia in neoplastic disease).

The appropriate sequencing can be easily confused with the next guideline (I.C.2.c.2) for Anemia associated with chemotherapy, immunotherapy and radiation therapy, which states:

> When the admission/encounter is for management of an anemia associated with an adverse effect of the administration of chemotherapy or immunotherapy and the only treatment is for the anemia, the anemia code is sequenced first followed by the appropriate codes for the neoplasm and the adverse effect (T45.1X5, Adverse effect of antineoplastic and immunosuppressive drugs).

When the admission/encounter is for management of an anemia associated with an adverse effect of radiotherapy, the anemia code should be sequenced first, followed by the appropriate neoplasm code and code Y84.2, Radiological procedure and radiotherapy as the cause of abnormal reaction of the patient, or of later complication, without mention of misadventure at the time of the procedure.

Activity – Chapter 2 Guidelines

To gain an understanding of these rules, access the 2014 guidelines from the NCHS website (http://www.cdc.gov/nchs/icd/icd10cm.htm) and read Chapter 2: Neoplasm guidelines, I.C.2.a through I.C.2.r on pages 25–32.

Chapter 3: Diseases of the blood and blood-forming organs and certain disorders involving the immune mechanism (D50-D89)

At this time, there are no chapter-specific guidelines related to Chapter 3: Diseases of the blood and blood-forming organs and certain disorders involving the immune mechanism. There are important instructional notes throughout Chapter 3 that the coder should be aware of.

Examples:

D61.2 Aplastic anemia due to other external agents
> Code first, if applicable, toxic effects of substances chiefly nonmedicinal as to source (T51-T65)

D70.1 Agranulocytosis secondary to cancer chemotherapy
> Use additional code for adverse effect, if applicable, to identify drug (T45.1X5)
> Code also underlying neoplasm

Chapter 4: Endocrine, nutritional and metabolic diseases (E00-E89)

Instructions for coding "late effects" or sequelae have been expanded in Chapter 4 of ICD-10-CM. For example, *Excludes1* notes have been added to some categories between E50-E63 to indicate that the sequelae of the nutritional deficiency are assigned a code from category E64.

New guidelines that clarify code usage are also found under specific codes.

> **Note:** Under code E34.0, Carcinoid syndrome, is a note that states "May be used as an additional code to identify functional activity associated with a carcinoid tumor."
>
> No such note appears under the ICD-9-CM code 259.2 for this same condition.

The NCHS has published chapter-specific guidelines for Chapter 4 of ICD-10-CM:
- Guideline I.C.4.a. Diabetes mellitus

Activity – Chapter 4 Guidelines
To gain an understanding of these rules, access the 2014 guidelines from the NCHS website (http://www.cdc.gov/nchs/icd/icd10cm.htm) and read Chapter 4: Endocrine, nutritional and metabolic diseases guidelines I.C.4.a.1 through I.C.4.a.6 on pages 32–34.

Chapter 5: Mental and behavioral disorders (F01-F99)

Many changes were made to Chapter 5, including organization and terminology, which resulted in some guideline adjustments as well.

> *Example* In ICD-10-CM beneath code F54, Psychological and behavioral factors associated with disorders or diseases classified elsewhere, there is a note that states to "code first the associated physical disorder."
>
> The equivalent ICD-9-CM code, 316, has a note to "use additional code to identify the associated physical condition."

The NCHS has published chapter-specific guidelines for Chapter 5 of ICD-10-CM. Take note of Guideline I.C.5.c.2, which describes the hierarchy rules for coding psychoactive substance use, abuse, and dependence.

Activity – Chapter 5 Guidelines
To gain an understanding of these rules, access the 2014 guidelines from the NCHS website (http://www.cdc.gov/nchs/icd/icd10cm.htm) and read Chapter 5: Mental, behavioral, and neurodevelopmental disorders guidelines I.C.5.a through I.C.5.c on pages 34–35.

Chapter 6: Diseases of the nervous system (G00-G99)

In ICD-10-CM, there is a series of excluded conditions listed at the beginning of Chapter 6 that are applicable to all conditions within the nervous system chapter.

There are also additional guideline modifications made to specific codes.

Example: In ICD-10-CM beneath category G89, Pain, not elsewhere classified, there is a note that states "code also related psychological factors associated with pain."

However, below ICD-9-CM category 338, Pain, not elsewhere classified, the note instructs coding professionals to "use additional code to identify pain associated with psychological factors (307.89)."

The NCHS has published chapter-specific guidelines for Chapter 6 of ICD-10-CM that focus on dominant/nondominant side and pain.

Activity – Chapter 6 Guidelines
To gain an understanding of these rules, access the 2014 guidelines from the NCHS website (http://www.cdc.gov/nchs/icd/icd10cm.htm) and read Chapter 6: Diseases of the nervous system and sense organs guidelines I.C.6.a through I.C.6.b.6 on pages 35–39.

Chapter 7: Diseases of the eye and adnexa (H00-H59)

With the formation of a new chapter for diseases of the eye and adnexa, come new instructions on which conditions are excluded from Chapter 7 of ICD-10-CM. Since the placement of the note is at the beginning of Chapter 7, none of the listed conditions would be coded here.

Included in this chapter are a number of guidelines for code usage that are code specific.

Note: Under ICD-10-CM subcategory H47.5, Disorders of other visual pathways, is a note to code also the underlying condition. This differs from ICD-9-CM in that a single code is used to identify the visual pathway disorder and the associated condition.

Note: Under ICD-10-CM subcategory H54, Blindness and low vision, is a note to code first any associated underlying cause of the blindness. No such note appears under ICD-9-CM category 369, Blindness and low vision.

Activity – Chapter 7 Guidelines
To gain an understanding of these rules, access the 2014 guidelines from the NCHS website (http://www.cdc.gov/nchs/icd/icd10cm.htm) and read Chapter 7: Diseases of the eye and adnexa guidelines I.C.7.a.1 through I.C.7.a.5 on pages 39–40.

Sections 3 and 4 Review Questions

1. True or false? In ICD-10-CM, code B20 is used to report a diagnosis of symptomatic HIV disease.
    a. True
    b. False

2. What is the correct code(s) for bilateral acute conjunctivitis, unspecified?
    a. H10.31, H10.32
    b. H10.33
    c. H10.233
    d. H10.13

3. True or false? Bacteremia and septicemia NOS are coded to R65.2.
    a. True
    b. False

4. What is the correct ICD-10-CM code(s) for premature menopause with sleeplessness?
    a. N95.1
    b. E28.3, G47.0
    c. E28.310
    d. E28.319

5. True or false? In ICD-10-CM, all diabetes mellitus codes require documentation of whether the condition is under control.
    a. True
    b. False

6. True or false? A malignant neoplasm code should not be assigned as principal diagnosis if the care involved surgical removal of the neoplasm along with adjunct chemotherapy during the same episode of care.
    a. True
    b. False

7. The fifth character for category G43, Migraine, denotes what?
    a. Intractable or not intractable
    b. With or without mention of seizures
    c. With or without aura
    d. With or without prolonged aura

8. True or false? ICD-10-CM provides for greater specificity of diseases of the spleen than ICD-9-CM.
    a. True
    b. False

9. In cases where the affected side is documented, but not specified as dominant or nondominant, how should right side monoplegia be classified?
    a. Dominant
    b. Nondominant
    c. Unspecified
    d. Undetermined

10. When an encounter is for pain management due to the malignancy, what code should be sequenced first?
  a. Primary malignancy or appropriate metastatic site code
  b. The pain code
  c. Encounter for cancer staging
  d. Observation for suspected neoplasm

Section 5 – Organization and Classification of Diseases and Disorders – Chapters 8–14

This section is designed to present an overview of the changes to specific disorders classified to Chapters 8–14 of ICD-10-CM. Not every revision has been identified but certain conditions have been selected to point out concepts that represent organizational, terminology, and classification modifications.

Chapter 8: Diseases of the ear and mastoid process (H60-H95)

Chapter 8 of ICD-10-CM includes categories H60-H95 arranged in the following blocks:

H60-H62	Diseases of external ear
H65-H75	Diseases of middle ear and mastoid
H80-H83	Diseases of inner ear
H90-H94	Other disorders of ear
H95	Intraoperative and postprocedural complications and disorders of ear and mastoid process, not elsewhere classified

Chapter 8 is an entirely new chapter in ICD-10-CM. In ICD-9-CM, the conditions classified in this chapter are located in Chapter 6: Diseases of the Nervous System and Sense Organs. Diseases of the ear and mastoid process have been arranged into blocks making it easier to identify the types of conditions that would occur in the external ear (block 1), middle ear and mastoid (block 2), and inner ear (block 3). Block 4 is used for other disorders of the ear. Block 5 contains the codes for intraoperative and postprocedural complications. The intraoperative and postprocedural complications are grouped at the end of the chapter rather than scattered throughout different categories. Category and subcategory titles have been revised in a number of locations in Chapter 8.

Examples:

ICD-9-CM	381, Nonsuppurative otitis media and Eustachian tube disorders
ICD-10-CM	H65, Nonsuppurative otitis media
ICD-9-CM	380.10, Infective otitis externa, unspecified
ICD-10-CM	H60.0, Abscess of external ear
ICD-9-CM	386, Vertiginous syndromes and other disorders of vestibular system
ICD-10-CM	H81, Disorders of vestibular function

Although Chapter 8 in ICD-10-CM basically parallels the corresponding section in Chapter 6 of ICD-9-CM, there are quite a few changes. These changes include greater specificity added at the fourth-, fifth-, and sixth-character levels; the delineation of laterality; and the addition of many more "code first underlying disease" notes.

One last noted classification change in this chapter is that the ICD-9-CM category 381, Nonsuppurative otitis media and Eustachian tube disorders, has been split into two categories in ICD-10-CM; H65, Nonsuppurative otitis media and H68, Eustachian salpingitis and obstruction.

Activity – Chapter 8 Organization and Classification
To expand your knowledge of the alterations made to the organization, terminology, and classification of diseases of the ear and mastoid, refer to the Tabular List of ICD-10-CM, find the following codes or categories, and identify what changes were made between ICD revisions.

ICD-10-CM	ICD-9-CM
H65	381
H81.0	386.0
H83.2	386.5

Chapter 9: Diseases of the circulatory system (I00-I99)

Chapter 9 of ICD-10-CM includes categories I00-I99 arranged in the following blocks:

I00-I02	Acute rheumatic fever
I05-I09	Chronic rheumatic heart diseases
I10-I15	Hypertensive diseases
I20-I25	Ischemic heart diseases
I26-I28	Pulmonary heart disease and diseases of pulmonary circulation
I30-I52	Other forms of heart disease
I60-I69	Cerebrovascular diseases
I70-I79	Diseases of arteries, arterioles and capillaries
I80-I89	Diseases of veins, lymphatic vessels and lymph nodes, not elsewhere classified
I95-I99	Other and unspecified disorders of the circulatory system

The organization of Chapter 9 in ICD-10-CM is comparable to Chapter 7 in ICD-9-CM. One change to note is the order of conditions within the block for ischemic heart disease.

Note: In ICD-9-CM, the first condition is acute myocardial infarction. However, in ICD-10-CM angina pectoris begins the block for ischemic heart disease.

The terminology used to describe several cardiovascular conditions has been revised to reflect more current medical practice.

Examples:

ICD-9-CM	410, Acute myocardial infarction
ICD-10-CM	I21, ST elevation (STEMI) and non-ST elevation (NSTEMI) myocardial infarction
ICD-9-CM	411.1, Intermediate coronary syndrome
ICD-10-CM	I20.0, Unstable angina
ICD-9-CM	411.81, Acute coronary occlusion without myocardial infarction
ICD-10-CM	I24.0, Acute coronary thrombosis not resulting in myocardial infarction

---

Some revisions to the classification have occurred as well.

Note: In ICD-9-CM, the code for gangrene (785.4) is classified in Chapter 16: Symptoms, Signs and Ill-Defined Conditions whereas in ICD-10-CM this condition is classified in Chapter 9 and is coded as I96, Gangrene, NEC. Additionally, Binswanger's disease has been reclassified from Chapter 5, Mental Disorders, in ICD-9-CM to Chapter 9 in ICD-10-CM and is coded as I67.3.

One last noted change is with the classification of hypertension. In ICD-9-CM, hypertension codes classify the type of hypertension (benign, malignant, unspecified). In ICD-10-CM, hypertension codes no longer classify the type.

Activity – Chapter 9 Organization and Classification
To learn more about these changes to the organization, terminology, and classification of diseases of the circulatory system refer to the ICD-10-CM Tabular List, review and compare the following entries, and identify their differences.

ICD-10-CM	ICD-9-CM
I25.1	414.01
I40.0, I40.1	422.91, 422.92
I43	425.8

Chapter 10: Diseases of the respiratory system (J00-J99)

Chapter 10 of ICD-10-CM includes categories J00-J99 arranged in the following blocks:

J00-J06	Acute upper respiratory infections
J09-J18	Influenza and pneumonia
J20-J22	Other acute lower respiratory infections
J30-J39	Other diseases of upper respiratory tract
J40-J47	Chronic lower respiratory diseases
J60-J70	Lung diseases due to external agents
J80-J84	Other respiratory diseases principally affecting the interstitium
J85-J86	Suppurative and necrotic conditions of the lower respiratory tract
J90-J94	Other diseases of the pleura
J95	Intraoperative and postprocedural complications and disorders of respiratory system, not elsewhere classified
J96-J99	Other diseases of the respiratory system

While overall Chapter 10 of ICD-10-CM is organized similar to ICD-9-CM, diseases have been rearranged.

Modifications have also been made to specific categories that bring the terminology up-to-date with current medical practice.

Note:
- ICD-10-CM category J43, Emphysema, contains codes with panlobular emphysema and centrilobular emphysema in their titles
- ICD-10-CM category, J45, Asthma, classifies asthma as mild intermittent, mild persistent, moderate persistent, and severe persistent.

Other enhancements to Chapter 10 include classification changes that provide greater specificity than found in ICD-9-CM.

Note:
- ICD-10-CM has individual codes for acute recurrent sinusitis for each sinus whereas ICD-9-CM does not have a specific code for acute recurrent sinusitis
- ICD-10-CM subcategory J10.8, Influenza due to other identified influenza virus with other manifestations, has been expanded to reflect the manifestations of the influenza
- ICD-10-CM category J20, Acute bronchitis, has been expanded to reflect the manifestations of the acute bronchitis.

Activity – Chapter 10 Organization and Classification

To become more familiar with other revisions to the organization, terminology, and classification of diseases of the respiratory system refer to the ICD-10-CM Tabular List and find the ICD-10-CM category or code for those listed here. Assess how each differs from ICD-9-CM.

ICD-10-CM	*ICD-9-CM*
J18.1	481
J30-J39	470-478
J45	493

Chapter 11: Diseases of the digestive system (K00-K95)

Chapter 11 of ICD-10-CM includes categories K00-K95 arranged in the following blocks:

K00-K14	Diseases of oral cavity and salivary glands
K20-K31	Diseases of esophagus, stomach and duodenum
K35-K38	Diseases of appendix
K40-K46	Hernia
K50-K52	Noninfective enteritis and colitis
K55-K64	Other diseases of intestines
K65-K68	Diseases of peritoneum and retroperitoneum
K70-K77	Diseases of liver
K80-K87	Disorders of gallbladder, biliary tract and pancreas
K90-K95	Other diseases of digestive system

A number of new subchapters have been added to the chapter for diseases of the digestive system. For instance, in ICD-10-CM diseases of the liver have their own subchapter or block while these conditions were grouped with other diseases of the digestive system in ICD-9-CM. Some terminology changes and revisions to the classification of specific digestive conditions have occurred in ICD-10-CM as well.

Note: The term "hemorrhage" is used when referring to ulcers, and the term "bleeding" is used when classifying gastritis, duodenitis, diverticulosis, and diverticulitis
- K25.0, Acute gastric ulcer with hemorrhage
- K29.01, Acute gastritis with bleeding
- K57.31, Diverticulosis of large intestine without perforation or abscess with bleeding

---

ICD-10-CM category K50, Crohn's disease, has been expanded to the fourth, fifth, and sixth character in contrast to ICD-9-CM category 555, Regional enteritis. The expansion at the fourth character level specifies the site of the Crohn's disease, the fifth character indicates whether a complication was present, and the sixth character further classifies the specific complication.

In ICD-9-CM, the presence or absence of obstruction is used as an axis for classifying ulcers. In ICD-10-CM a fairly substantial classification change was made and the identification of obstruction is no longer a part of the ICD-10-CM ulcer code structure.

Activity – Chapter 11 Organization and Classification
To gain a better understanding of modifications to the organization, terminology, and classification of diseases of the digestive system, refer to the ICD-10-CM Tabular List, locate the following categories, and determine the revision.

ICD-10-CM	ICD-9-CM
K22	530
K37	541
K62	569

Chapter 12: Diseases of skin and subcutaneous tissue (L00-L99)

Chapter 12 of ICD-10-CM includes categories L00-L99 arranged in the following blocks:

L00-L08	Infections of the skin and subcutaneous tissue
L10-L14	Bullous disorders
L20-L30	Dermatitis and eczema
L40-L45	Papulosquamous disorders
L49-L54	Urticaria and erythema
L55-L59	Radiation-related disorders of the skin and subcutaneous tissue
L60-L75	Disorders of skin appendages
L76	Intraoperative and postprocedural complications of skin and subcutaneous tissue
L80-L99	Other disorders of the skin and subcutaneous tissue

ICD-10-CM Chapter 12 represents a complete restructuring to bring together groups of diseases that are related to one another in some way. Additionally, greater specificity has been added to many of the codes at either the fourth-, fifth-, and even sixth-character level. ICD-9-CM Chapter 12 has only three subchapters which have been expanded in ICD-10-CM to create the nine blocks listed above.

One example of an organizational change to Chapter 12 of ICD-10-CM is a subchapter or block for ICD-10-CM codes for radiation-related disorders of the skin and subcutaneous tissue. The conditions found in this block are not located together in ICD-9-CM.

Some categories in Chapter 12 have undergone title changes to reflect terminology in use today. For instance, ICD-10-CM uses "androgenic alopecia" but this term is not used at all in ICD-9-CM.

An example of a classification improvement is the addition of characters in ICD-10-CM to represent the site and severity of the decubitus ulcer.

Coding Tip: While ICD-9-CM did add a subcategory for pressure ulcer stages in FY2009, two codes are required to code this specificity. ICD-10-CM provides the site (including laterality) and the stage all in one code.

Activity – Chapter 12 Organization and Classification
For additional practice with learning the organization, terminology, and classification changes to the chapter on diseases of skin and subcutaneous tissue, refer to the ICD-10-CM Tabular List and locate the following categories or codes. Ascertain the modifications.

ICD-10-CM	*ICD-9-CM*
L03	681
L03.32	682.2
L98.4	707.1

Chapter 13: Diseases of the musculoskeletal system and connective tissue (M00-M99)

Chapter 13 contains many more subchapters, categories, and codes than ICD-9-CM. Rather than having just four subchapters grouping many conditions together, ICD-10-CM organizes the musculoskeletal system and connective tissue in the following blocks:

M00-M02	Infectious arthropathies
M05-M14	Inflammatory polyarthropathies
M15-M19	Osteoarthritis
M20-M25	Other joint disorders
M26-M27	Dentofacial anomalies [including malocclusion] and other disorders of jaw
M30-M36	Systemic connective tissue disorders
M40-M43	Deforming dorsopathies
M45-M49	Spondylopathies
M50-M54	Other dorsopathies
M60-M63	Disorders of muscles
M65-M67	Disorders of synovium and tendon
M70-M79	Other soft tissue disorders
M80-M85	Disorders of bone density and structure
M86-M90	Other osteopathies
M91-M94	Chondropathies
M95	Other disorders of the musculoskeletal system and connective tissue
M96	Intraoperative and postprocedural complications and disorders of musculoskeletal system, not elsewhere classified
M99	Biomechanical lesions, not elsewhere classified

Almost every code in Chapter 13 of ICD-10-CM has been expanded in some way with the expansion including very specific sites as well as laterality. Numerous codes have been moved from various chapters in ICD-9-CM to Chapter 13 in ICD-10-CM.

Examples:
- ➤ Category 274, Gout in ICD-9-CM, Chapter 3: Endocrine, Nutritional and Metabolic Diseases and Immunity Disorders, is classified as M10, Gout, in ICD-10-CM Chapter 13
- ➤ Code 268.2, Osteomalacia, unspecified in ICD-9-CM Chapter 3 is classified to category M83, Adult osteomalacia in ICD-10-CM Chapter 13
- ➤ Code 524.4, Malocclusion, unspecified, in ICD-9-CM Chapter 9: Diseases of the Digestive System, is classified to code M26.4, Malocclusion, unspecified in ICD-10-CM Chapter 13

Category M80 in ICD-10-CM classifies the type of osteoporosis in addition to the site of a current pathological fracture into one combination code.

Additionally, some categories and subcategories in Chapter 13 require the use of seventh characters.

Note: The seventh characters are	
A	initial encounter for fracture
B	subsequent encounter for fracture with routine healing
G	subsequent encounter for fracture with delayed healing
K	subsequent encounter for fracture with nonunion
P	subsequent encounter for fracture with malunion
S	sequelae

Activity – Chapter 13 Organization and Classification

To increase your understanding of the revisions to the organization, terminology, and classification of musculoskeletal system connective tissue diseases, refer to the ICD-10-CM Tabular List, locate the categories or codes listed below, and ascertain the modification by evaluating the ICD-9-CM information against the ICD-10-CM category or code.

ICD-10-CM	*ICD-9-CM*
M10	274.9
M15-M19	715
M48.4	733.95

Chapter 14: Diseases of the genitourinary system (N00-N99)

Chapter 14 of ICD-10-CM includes categories N00-N99 arranged in the following blocks:

N00-N08	Glomerular diseases
N10-N16	Renal tubulo-interstitial diseases
N17-N19	Acute kidney failure and chronic kidney disease
N20-N23	Urolithiasis
N25-N29	Other disorders of kidney and ureter
N30-N39	Other diseases of the urinary system
N40-N53	Diseases of male genital organs
N60-N65	Disorders of breast
N70-N77	Inflammatory diseases of female pelvic organs
N80-N98	Noninflammatory disorders of female genital tract
N99	Intraoperative and postprocedural complications and disorders of genitourinary system, not elsewhere classified

For the most part, those genitourinary disorders in diseases classified elsewhere have been placed in their own category at the end of each block of Chapter 14. This differs from ICD-9-CM in that these conditions were classified within different subcategories.

Note: One category, N08, Glomerular disorders in diseases classified elsewhere, is used to identify glomerulonephritis, nephritis, and nephropathy in diseases classified elsewhere.

Changes were necessary in some sections of Chapter 14 because of outdated terminology. For example, given what has been discovered since the last revision of ICD about male erectile dysfunction, ICD-10-CM includes category N52 for this condition with subcategories to identify the different causes of the dysfunction. ICD-9-CM has a single code, 607.84, for impotence of organic origin.

Coding Tip: To code to the highest level of specificity for post-traumatic urethral stricture, coding professionals will need to identify the patient's gender. This is not necessary for ICD-9-CM code selection for this disorder.

Activity – Chapter 14 Organization and Classification

To find out more about the organization, terminology, and classification modifications to diseases of the genitourinary system, refer to the ICD-10-CM Tabular list and locate the ICD-10-CM category or code listed here. Then evaluate the ICD-9-CM information against what was found and discern the variances.

ICD-10-CM	*ICD-9-CM*
N18	585
N30	595
N39.3	625.6/788.32

Section 6 – Chapters 8–14 Guidelines

This section is designed to highlight the revisions to the guidelines found in Chapters 8–14 of ICD-10-CM. All modifications have not been illustrated but certain guiding principles have been selected to show guideline variations from ICD-9-CM. Also included in this section is the review of chapter-specific coding guidelines published by NCHS.

Chapter 8: Diseases of the ear and mastoid process (H60-H95)

Guidelines on the use of codes may change from one revision to the next. For example, ICD-9-CM contains a note excluding otitis media with perforation of tympanic membrane from subcategory 384.2. In ICD-10-CM the note directly under H72, Perforation of tympanic membrane, states "code first any associated otitis media."

Example:

ICD-9-CM   **384.2, Perforation of Tympanic Membrane**
 Excludes: otitis media with perforation of tympanic membrane (382.00-382.9)

ICD-10-CM   **H72, Perforation of tympanic membrane**
 Code first any associated otitis media (H65.-, H66.1-, H66.2-, H66.3-, H66.4-, H66.9-,H67.-)
 Excludes1: acute suppurative otitis media with rupture of the tympanic
  membrane (H66.01-)
  traumatic rupture of ear drum (S09.2-)

Coding Tip: There is an instructional note in categories H65, H66, and H67 to use an additional code for any associated perforated tympanic membrane (H72.-)

Another new guideline is found under the categories for nonsuppurative otitis media (H65) and suppurative and unspecified otitis media (H66). The note instructs coding professionals to use an additional code to identify: exposure to environmental tobacco smoke (Z77.22), exposure to tobacco smoke in the perinatal period (P96.81), history of tobacco use (Z87.891), occupational exposure to environmental tobacco smoke (Z57.31), tobacco dependence (F17.-), or tobacco use (Z72.0).

At this time, there are no chapter-specific guidelines related to Chapter 8: Diseases of the ears and mastoid process.

Chapter 9: Diseases of the circulatory system (I00-I99)

There are guideline changes to a number of codes in this chapter. For example, ICD-10-CM Guideline I.C.9.e.4. states that a code from category I22, Subsequent STEMI and NSTEMI myocardial infarction, is to be used when a patient who has suffered an AMI has a new AMI within the 4 week time frame of the initial AMI. However, below category 410 in ICD-9-CM the note refers to 8 weeks or less time period.

Note: The instructional notes and guidelines are very important for these three categories to indicate correct code usage. A code from category I22, Subsequent acute myocardial infarction, must be used in conjunction with a code from category I21, ST elevation myocardial infarction (STEMI) and non-ST elevation myocardial infarction (NSTEMI). A code from category I23, certain current complications following ST elevation (STEMI) and non-ST elevation (NSTEMI) myocardial infarction must be used in conjunction with a code from category I21 or I22.

New guidelines that clarify code usage are also found under specific codes. Under code I05, rheumatic mitral valve diseases, is a note that states this category includes conditions classifiable to both I05.0 and I05.2-I05.9, whether specified as rheumatic or not.

The NCHS has published chapter-specific guidelines for Chapter 9 of ICD-10-CM:
- Guideline I.C.9.a. Hypertension
- Guideline I.C.9.b. Atherosclerotic coronary artery disease and angina
- Guideline I.C.9.c. Intraoperative and postprocedural cerebrovascular accident
- Guideline I.C.9.d. Sequelae of cerebrovascular disease
- Guideline I.C.9.e. Acute myocardial infarction

Activity – Chapter 9 Guidelines
To gain an understanding of these rules, access the 2014 guidelines from the NCHS website (http://www.cdc.gov/nchs/icd/icd10cm.htm) and read Chapter 9: Diseases of the circulatory system guidelines I.C.9.a through I.C.9.e.4 on pages 41–46.

Chapter 10: Diseases of the respiratory system (J00-J99)

At the beginning of Chapter 10 the following instructional guideline appears: "When a respiratory condition is described as occurring in more than one site and is not specifically indexed, it should be classified to the lower anatomic site."

Note: Tracheobronchitis is classified to bronchitis in J40, Bronchitis, not specified as acute or chronic.

An additional instructional guideline also appears at the beginning of Chapter 10 which instructs the coding professional to use an additional code, where applicable to identify: exposure to environmental tobacco smoke (Z77.22), exposure to tobacco smoke in the perinatal period (P96.81), history of tobacco use (Z87.891), occupational exposure to environmental tobacco smoke (Z57.31), tobacco dependence (F17.-), or tobacco use (Z72.0).

Coding Tip: Since these new guidelines appear at the beginning of the chapter, they should be followed when assigning any code from this chapter.

Guidelines for code usage may also be category specific. Under ICD-10-CM category J10, influenza, is a note to use an additional code to identify the virus. No such note appears under the ICD-9-CM category (487) for this same condition.

The NCHS has published chapter-specific guidelines for Chapter 10 of ICD-10-CM:
- Guideline I.C.10.a. Chronic obstructive pulmonary disease and asthma
- Guideline I.C.10.b. Acute respiratory failure
- Guideline I.C.10.c. Influenza due to certain identified influenza viruses
- Guideline I.C.10.d. Ventilator-associated pneumonia

Activity – Chapter 10 Guidelines
To gain an understanding of these rules, access the 2014 guidelines from the NCHS website (http://www.cdc.gov/nchs/icd/icd10cm.htm) and read Chapter 10: Diseases of the respiratory system guidelines I.C.10.a through I.C.10.d.2 on pages 46–48.

Chapter 11: Diseases of the digestive system (K00-K95)

Guideline modifications were made to specific codes in this chapter.

Note: For example, in ICD-9-CM ulcerative colitis does not have any instructions for code usage listed below category 556. In contrast, guidelines for category K51, Ulcerative colitis, state to use an additional code to identify manifestations.

No instructional note is found at the start of the subchapter for hernias in ICD-9-CM. However, this is not the case in ICD-10-CM. The note "Hernia with both gangrene and obstruction is classified to hernia with gangrene" applies to all conditions coded to categories K40–K46.

At this time, there are no chapter-specific guidelines related to Chapter 11: Diseases of the digestive system.

Chapter 12: Diseases of the skin and subcutaneous tissue (L00-L99)

Instructions for coding dermatitis and eczema have been expanded in Chapter 12. For example, the note "In this block, the terms dermatitis and eczema are used synonymously and interchangeably" has been added to categories L20-L30. Additionally, the "excludes" note has been expanded in ICD-10-CM for categories L20-L30 compared to categories 690-698 in ICD-9-CM.

Example:

ICD-9-CM   **Other Inflammatory Conditions of Skin and Subcutaneous Tissue (690-698)**
Excludes: panniculus (729.30-729.39)

ICD-10-CM   **Dermatitis and Eczema (L20-L30)**
Excludes2:   chronic (childhood) granulomatous disease (D71)
           dermatitis gangrenosa (L08.0)
           dermatitis herpetiformis (L13.0)
           dry skin dermatitis (L85.3)
           factitial dermatitis (L98.1)
           perioral dermatitis (L71.0)
           radiation-related disorders of skin and subcutaneous
             tissue (L55-L59)
           stasis dermatitis (I83.1-I83.2)

The NCHS has published chapter-specific guidelines for Chapter 12 of ICD-10-CM:
- Guideline I.C.12.a. Pressure ulcer stage codes

Activity – Chapter 12 Guidelines
To gain an understanding of these rules, access the 2014 guidelines from the NCHS website (http://www.cdc.gov/nchs/icd/icd10cm.htm) and read Chapter 12: Diseases of the skin and subcutaneous tissue guidelines I.C.12.a.1 through I.C.12.a.6 on pages 48–49.

Chapter 13: Diseases of the musculoskeletal system and connective tissue (M00-M99)

The first block of the chapter on diseases of the musculoskeletal system and connective tissue for infectious arthropathies includes arthropathies due to microbiological agents. To assist coding professionals on the correct usage of categories M00-M02, new guidelines provide definitions for direct and indirect infection.

Coding Tip: Distinction is made between the following types of etiological relationships:
- **Direct infection of joint**—where organisms invade synovial tissue and microbial antigen is present in the joint
- **Indirect infection**—which may be of two types: a reactive arthropathy, where microbial infection of the body is established but neither organisms nor antigens can be identified in the joint, and a postinfective arthropathy, where microbial antigen is present but recovery of an organism is inconstant and evidence of local multiplication is lacking

---

Instructional notes have also been added to different categories or subcategories to explain how codes should be assigned.

Examples:
M21.7   Unequal limb length (acquired)
   Note: The site used should correspond to the shorter limb
M50   Cervical disc disorders
   Note: Code to the most superior level of disorder

The NCHS has published chapter-specific guidelines for Chapter 13 of ICD-10-CM:
- Guideline I.C.13.a. Site and laterality
- Guideline I.C.13.b. Acute traumatic versus chronic or recurrent musculoskeletal conditions
- Guideline I.C.13.c. Coding of pathologic fractures
- Guideline I.C.13.d. Osteoporosis

Activity – Chapter 13 Guidelines
To gain an understanding of these rules, access the 2014 guidelines from the NCHS website (http://www.cdc.gov/nchs/icd/icd10cm.htm) and read Chapter 13: Diseases of the musculoskeletal system and connective tissue guidelines I.C.13.a through I.C.13.d.2 on pages 50–51.

Chapter 14: Diseases of the genitourinary system (N00-N99)

Throughout Chapter 14 are new includes notes that help to clarify the types of disorders that are classified to the various categories.

Example:

N00   Acute nephritis syndrome

      Includes: acute glomerular disease

                            acute glomerulonephritis

                            acute nephritis

N71   Inflammatory disease of uterus, except cervix

      Includes: endo (myo) metritis

                            metritis

                            myometritis

                            pyometra

                            uterine abscess

A similar change has occurred to the instruction for menopausal and other perimenopausal disorders. In ICD-9-CM, there is no guideline under category 627 to help coding professionals in their selection of a code for these disorders. However, ICD-10-CM includes a note stating menopausal and other perimenopausal disorders due to naturally occurring (age-related) menopause and perimenopause are classified to category N95.

The NCHS has published chapter-specific guidelines for Chapter 14 of ICD-10-CM:

- Guideline I.C.14.a. Chronic kidney disease

Activity – Chapter 14 Guidelines

To gain an understanding of these rules, access the 2014 guidelines from the NCHS website (http://www.cdc.gov/nchs/icd/icd10cm.htm) and read Chapter 14: Diseases of the genitourinary system guidelines I.C.14.a.1 through I.C.14.a.3 on pages 51–52.

Sections 5 and 6 Review Questions

1. True or false? If a patient with suppurative otitis media has a history of tobacco use, an additional code should be assigned.
    a. True
    b. False

2. According to NCHS Guidelines for Chapter 13 of ICD-10-CM, recurrent bone, joint, or muscle conditions are classified to which chapter?
    a. Chapter 13
    b. Chapter 18
    c. Chapter 19
    d. Chapter 20

3. True or false? The "code also" note found under ICD-10-CM category N17 should be interpreted to mean that the acute kidney failure should be assigned only as principal or first-listed.
    a. True
    b. False

4. True or false? If a patient has both acute systolic heart failure and hypertension, no causal condition relationship needs to be documented to use the combination code I11.0.
    a. True
    b. False

5. Review category I46. Which of the following is a false statement?
    a. Cardiac arrest is a non-specific principal diagnosis
    b. Code I46.8 is used as a secondary diagnosis code
    c. Code I46.2 is used as a secondary condition
    d. Cardiac arrest includes cardiogenic shock

6. True or false? The term "hemorrhage" is found in Chapter 11 in ICD-10-CM instead of the term "bleeding."
    a. True
    b. False

7. What is the correct ICD-10-CM code(s) for Crohn's disease of ileum with rectal bleeding and abscess?
    a. K50.011, K63.0
    b. K50.014
    c. K50.011, K50.014
    d. K50.014, K62.5

8. True or false? ICD-10-CM provides greater specificity than found in ICD-9-CM for acute recurrent sinusitis by providing an axis for recurrence.
    a. True
    b. False

9. Which of the following conditions is not classified to I40.1?
    a. Septic myocarditis
    b. Giant cell myocarditis
    c. Idiopathic myocarditis
    d. Fiedler's myocarditis

10.   The sixth character level for category L89 denotes what?
       a.   Site
       b.   Depth of the ulcer
       c.   Gangrene
       d.   Etiology

Section 7 – Organization and Classification of Diseases and Disorders – Chapters 15–21

This section is designed to present an overview of the changes to specific disorders classified to Chapters 15–21 of ICD-10-CM. Not every revision has been identified but certain conditions have been selected to point out concepts that represent organizational, terminology, and classification modifications.

Chapter 15: Pregnancy, childbirth and the puerperium (O00-O9A)

Chapter 15 of ICD-10-CM includes categories O00-O9A arranged in the following blocks:

O00-O08	Pregnancy with abortive outcome
O09	Supervision of high risk pregnancy
O10-O16	Edema, proteinuria and hypertensive disorders in pregnancy, childbirth and the puerperium
O20-O29	Other maternal disorders predominantly related to pregnancy
O30-O48	Maternal care related to the fetus and amniotic cavity and possible delivery problems
O60-O77	Complications of labor and delivery
O80, O82	Encounter for delivery
O85-O92	Complications predominantly related to the puerperium
O94-O9A	Other obstetric conditions, not elsewhere classified

With respect to classification changes, episode of care is no longer a secondary axis of classification for most conditions classified in Chapter 15. Instead ICD-10-CM identifies the trimester in which the condition occurred at the fifth- and sixth-character level.

Code titles have been revised in a number of locations in Chapter 15. For instance, ICD-9-CM's terminology states the indication for care such as inlet contraction of pelvis (653.2). ICD-10-CM terminology is much more descriptive of what the code represents, that is, maternal care for disproportion due to inlet contractions of pelvis (O33.2).

Other Examples of Title Changes:
ICD-9-CM   654, Abnormality of organs and soft tissues of pelvis
ICD-10-CM   O34, Maternal care for abnormality of pelvic organs

ICD-9-CM   664, Trauma to perineum and vulva during delivery
ICD-10-CM   O70, Perineal laceration during delivery

Codes for elective (legal or therapeutic) abortion are classified with the abortion codes in ICD-9-CM. In contrast, the elective abortion (without complication) code has been moved to code Z33.2, Encounter for elective termination of pregnancy, in Chapter 21 of ICD-10-CM. Complications of induced termination of pregnancy are found in category O04.

ICD-10-CM requires the use of a seventh character to identify the fetus to which certain complication codes apply.

Example:

O32   Maternal care for malpresentation of fetus

One of the following seventh characters is to be assigned to each code under category O32.

0	not applicable or unspecified
1	fetus 1
2	fetus 2
3	fetus 3
4	fetus 4
5	fetus 5
9	other fetus

The ICD-10-CM codes for obstructed labor incorporate the reason for the obstruction into the code; therefore, only one code is required rather than two as in ICD-9-CM. For example, to code obstructed labor due to face presentation the following two ICD-9-CM codes are required: 660.0X, Obstruction caused by malposition of fetus at onset of labor and 652.4X, Face or brow presentation. In ICD-10-CM, only code O64.2XX-, Obstructed labor due to face presentation, is coded.

Activity – Chapter 15 Organization and Classification

In order to gain a better understanding of modifications to the organization, terminology, and classification of pregnancy, childbirth, and the puerperium conditions in ICD-10-CM, open the Tabular List. Review and compare the following entries and identify their differences.

ICD-10-CM	*ICD-9-CM*
O12.1	646.2
O15	642.6
O80	650

Chapter 16: Certain conditions originating in the perinatal period (P00-P96)

Chapter 16 of ICD-10-CM includes categories P00-P96 arranged in the following blocks:

P00-P04	Newborn affected by maternal factors and by complications of pregnancy, labor and delivery
P05-P08	Disorders related to length of gestation and fetal growth
P09	Abnormal findings on neonatal screening
P10-P15	Birth trauma
P19-P29	Respiratory and cardiovascular disorders specific to the perinatal period
P35-P39	Infections specific to the perinatal period
P50-P61	Hemorrhagic and hematological disorders of newborn
P70-P74	Transitory endocrine and metabolic disorders specific to newborn
P76-P78	Digestive system disorders of newborn
P80-P83	Conditions involving the integument and temperature regulation of newborn
P84	Other problems with newborn
P90-P96	Other disorders originating in the perinatal period

A number of new subchapters have been added to Chapter 16 for certain conditions originating in the perinatal period.

Note: Codes for respiratory and cardiovascular disorders specific to the perinatal period are grouped together in block P19-P29.

Chapter 16 of ICD-10-CM also contains terminology updates. The first block in ICD-10-CM, newborns affected by maternal factors and by complications of pregnancy, labor, and delivery, the phrase "suspected to be" is included in the code title as a nonessential modifier to indicate that the codes are for use when the listed maternal condition is specified as the cause of confirmed or suspected newborn morbidity or potential morbidity.

Examples:
P00.3, Newborn (suspected to be) affected by other maternal circulatory and
    respiratory diseases
P00.4, Newborn (suspected to be) affected by maternal nutritional disorders
P00.5, Newborn (suspected to be) affected by maternal injury

Some revisions to the classification have occurred as well. For instance, the subclassification for 2,500 g and over for birth weight is no longer an option for category P05, Disorders of newborn related to slow growth and fetal malnutrition.

Activity – Chapter 16 Organization and Classification
In order to gain a better understanding of modifications to the organization, terminology, and classification of certain conditions originating in the perinatal period, reference the ICD-10-CM Tabular List, locate the following categories, and determine the revision.

ICD-10-CM	*ICD-9-CM*
P07.2	765.2
P36	771.81
P76.0	777.1

Chapter 17: Congenital malformations, deformations and chromosomal abnormalities (Q00-Q99)

Chapter 17 of ICD-10-CM includes categories Q00-Q99 arranged in the following blocks:

Q00-Q07	Congenital malformations of the nervous system
Q10-Q18	Congenital malformations of eye, ear, face and neck
Q20-Q28	Congenital malformations of the circulatory system
Q30-Q34	Congenital malformations of the respiratory system
Q35-Q37	Cleft lip and cleft palate
Q38-Q45	Other congenital malformations of the digestive system
Q50-Q56	Congenital malformations of genital organs
Q60-Q64	Congenital malformations of the urinary system
Q65-Q79	Congenital malformations and deformations of the musculoskeletal system
Q80-Q89	Other congenital malformations
Q90-Q99	Chromosomal abnormalities, not elsewhere classified

The arrangement of ICD-10-CM's Chapter 17 is an improvement over ICD-9-CM's Chapter 14. Congenital malformations, deformations, and chromosomal abnormalities have been grouped into subchapters or blocks making it easier to identify the type of conditions classified to Chapter 17.

Modifications have also been made to specific categories that bring the terminology up-to-date with current medical practice.

Example:

Q61   Cystic kidney disease
     Q61.0, Congenital renal cyst
     Q61.1, Polycystic kidney, infantile type
     Q61.2, Polycystic kidney, adult type

Other enhancements to Chapter 17 include classification changes that provide greater specificity than found in ICD-9-CM.

Examples:
Q35.1, Cleft hard palate
Q35.3, Cleft soft palate
Q35.5, Cleft hard palate with cleft soft palate
Q35.7, Cleft uvula
Q35.9, Cleft palate, unspecified

Activity – Chapter 17 Organization and Classification
To expand your knowledge of the alterations made to the organization, terminology, and classification of congenital malformations, deformations, and chromosomal abnormalities refer to the ICD-10-CM Tabular List, find the following codes or categories, and review the changes that were made between ICD revisions.

ICD-10-CM	ICD-9-CM
Q53/Q55.22	752.5
Q65-Q79	754
Q90/Q91	758

Chapter 18: Symptoms, signs and abnormal clinical and laboratory findings, not elsewhere classified (R00-R99)

Chapter 18 of ICD-10-CM includes categories R00-R99 arranged in the following blocks:

R00-R09	Symptoms and signs involving the circulatory and respiratory systems
R10-R19	Symptoms and signs involving the digestive system and abdomen
R20-R23	Symptoms and signs involving the skin and subcutaneous tissue
R25-R29	Symptoms and signs involving the nervous and musculoskeletal systems
R30-R39	Symptoms and signs involving the genitourinary system
R40-R46	Symptoms and signs involving cognition, perception, emotional state and behavior
R47-R49	Symptoms and signs involving speech and voice
R50-R69	General symptoms and signs
R70-R79	Abnormal findings on examination of blood, without diagnosis
R80-R82	Abnormal findings on examination of urine, without diagnosis
R83-R89	Abnormal findings on examination of other body fluids, substances and tissues, without diagnosis
R90-R94	Abnormal findings on diagnostic imaging and in function studies, without diagnosis
R97	Abnormal tumor markers
R99	Ill-defined and unknown cause of mortality

Chapter 18 of ICD-10-CM has undergone some organizational changes. For example, in ICD-10-CM codes for general symptoms and signs follow those related specifically to a body system or other relevant grouping.

In the comparison of Chapter 18 of ICD-10-CM to Chapter 16 of ICD-9-CM it is evident that some codes have been moved from one chapter to another.

Examples:

ICD-9-CM (Chapter 7)	427.89, Other specified cardiac dysrythmias
ICD-10-CM (Chapter 18)	R00.1, Bradycardia, unspecified
ICD-9-CM (Chapter 8)	511.0, Pleurisy without mention of effusion or current tuberculosis
ICD-10-CM (Chapter 18)	R09.1, Pleurisy
ICD-9-CM (Chapter 9)	527.7, Disturbance of salivary secretion
ICD-10-CM (Chapter 18)	R68.2, Dry mouth, unspecified

A fairly substantial classification change was made to hematuria. Various types of hematuria are coded in Chapter 18 unless included with the underlying condition such as acute cystitis with hematuria. In those cases, the code is found in Chapter 14, Diseases of the genitourinary system.

Activity – Chapter 18 Organization and Classification
To increase your understanding of the revisions to the organization, terminology, and classification of symptoms, signs, and abnormal clinical and laboratory findings, refer to the ICD-10-CM Tabular List, review the listed categories or codes, and determine the modification by evaluating the ICD-9-CM information against what was found for the ICD-10-CM category or code.

ICD-10-CM	ICD-9-CM
R10	789.0
R41.81	797
R90-R94	793/794

Chapter 19: Injury, poisoning and certain other consequences of external causes (S00-T88)

As previously mentioned, a significant modification was made to the organization of Chapter 19. Type of injury is the first axis of classification for the injuries in ICD-9-CM whereas specific types of injuries found in categories S00-S99 of Chapter 19 are arranged by body region beginning with the head and concluding with the ankle and foot. This results in the grouping of injury types together under the site where it occurred.

S00-S09	Injuries to the head
S10-S19	Injuries to the neck
S20-S29	Injuries to the thorax
S30-S39	Injuries to the abdomen, lower back, lumbar spine, pelvis and external genitals
S40-S49	Injuries to the shoulder and upper arm
S50-S59	Injuries to the elbow and forearm
S60-S69	Injuries to the wrist, hand and fingers
S70-S79	Injuries to the hip and thigh
S80-S89	Injuries to the knee and lower leg
S90-S99	Injuries to the ankle and foot
T07	Injuries involving multiple body regions
T14	Injury of unspecified body region
T15-T19	Effects of foreign body entering through natural orifice
T20-T32	Burns and corrosions
T20-T25	Burns and corrosions of external body surface, specified by site
T26-T28	Burns and corrosions confined to eye and internal organs
T30-T32	Burns and corrosions of multiple and unspecified body regions
T33-T34	Frostbite
T36-T50	Poisoning by, adverse effect of and underdosing of drugs, medicaments and biological substances
T51-T65	Toxic effects of substances chiefly nonmedicinal as to source
T66-T78	Other and unspecified effects of external causes
T79	Certain early complications of trauma
T80-T88	Complications of surgical and medical care, not elsewhere classified

In addition, generally the listings of conditions that follow the site are as follows:
- Superficial injury
- Open wound
- Fracture
- Dislocation and sprain
- Injury of nerves
- Injury of blood vessels
- Injury of muscle and tendon
- Crushing injury
- Traumatic amputation
- Other and unspecified injuries

Some categories in Chapter 19 have undergone title changes to reflect terminology in use today.

Note: ICD-10-CM uses the terms "displaced" and "nondisplaced" in the code descriptors while these terms were not used in ICD-9-CM.

In ICD-10-CM, codes from blocks T20-T32 classify burns and corrosions. The addition of the term "corrosion" is new in ICD-10-CM. The burn codes identify thermal burns, except for sunburns, that come from a heat source. The burn codes are also for burns resulting from electricity and radiation. Corrosions are burns due to chemicals.

A significant classification change was made to poisonings by and adverse effects of drugs, medicaments, and biological substances (T36-T50). ICD-10-CM does not provide different category codes to identify poisonings versus adverse effect. Instead under a single category for a specific drug are codes for poisonings, adverse effects, and underdosing of drugs, medicaments and biological substances. "Underdosing" is a new term in ICD-10-CM and is defined as taking less of a medication than is prescribed by a provider or the manufacturer's instructions with a resulting negative health consequence.

Example:

T46.1 Poisoning by, adverse effect of, and underdosing of calcium-channel blockers
       T46.1X1, Poisoning by calcium-channel blocker, accidental (unintentional)
       T46.1X2, Poisoning by calcium-channel blocker, intentional self-harm
       T46.1X3, Poisoning by calcium-channel blocker, assault
       T46.1X4, Poisoning by calcium-channel blocker, undetermined
       T46.1X5, Adverse effect of calcium-channel blocker
       T46.1X6, Underdosing of calcium-channel blocker

Coding Tip: Sequencing issues and problems are eliminated because poisonings, adverse effects, and underdosing are combination codes.

Activity – Chapter 19 Organization and Classification
For additional practice with learning the organizational, terminology, and classification changes to the chapter on injury, poisoning, and certain other consequences of external causes, refer to the ICD-10-CM Tabular List, refer to the below category or code, and ascertain the modification.

ICD-10-CM	ICD-9-CM
S12.0	805.01
S41	880
S43.50	840.0

Chapter 20: External causes of morbidity (V00-Y99)

Chapter 20 of ICD-10-CM includes categories V00-Y99 arranged in the following blocks:

V00-X58	Accidents
V00-V99	Transport accidents
V00-V09	Pedestrian injured in transport accident
V10-V19	Pedal cycle rider injured in transport accident
V20-V29	Motorcycle rider injured in transport accident
V30-V39	Occupant of three-wheeled motor vehicle injured in transport accident
V40-V49	Car occupant injured in transport accident
V50-V59	Occupant of pick-up truck or van injured in transport accident
V60-V69	Occupant of heavy transport vehicle injured in transport accident
V70-V79	Bus occupant injured in transport accident
V80-V89	Other land transport accidents
V90-V94	Water transport accidents
V95-V97	Air and space transport accidents
V98-V99	Other and unspecified transport accidents
W00-X58	Other external causes of accidental injury
W00-W19	Slipping, tripping, stumbling and falls
W20-W49	Exposure to inanimate mechanical forces
W50-W64	Exposure to animate mechanical forces
W65-W74	Accidental non-transport drowning and submersion
W85-W99	Exposure to electric current, radiation and extreme ambient air temperature and pressure
X00-X08	Exposure to smoke, fire and flames
X10-X19	Contact with heat and hot substances
X30-X39	Exposure to forces of nature
X52-X58	Accidental exposure to other specified factors
X71-X83	Intentional self-harm
X92-Y08	Assault
Y21-Y33	Event of undetermined intent
Y35-Y38	Legal intervention, operations of war, military operations and terrorism
Y62-Y84	Complications of medical and surgical care
Y62-Y69	Misadventures to patients during surgical and medical care
Y70-Y82	Medical devices associated with adverse incidents in diagnostic and therapeutic use
Y83-Y84	Surgical and other medical procedures as the cause of abnormal reaction of the patient, or of later complication, without mention of misadventure at the time of the procedure
Y90-Y99	Supplementary factors related to causes of morbidity classified elsewhere

As previously noted, codes for external causes are no longer found in a supplemental classification in ICD-10-CM. The causes currently located in the ICD-9-CM E code chapter have been disseminated to Chapter 19: Injury, poisoning and certain other consequences of external causes, or Chapter 20: External causes of morbidity. Codes in Chapter 20 capture the cause of the injury or health condition, the intent (unintentional or accidental; or intentional, such as suicide or assault), the place where the event occurred, the activity of the patient at the time of the event, and the person's status (namely civilian, military).

Changes in terminology were also necessary due to the revisions made overall to this chapter.

> **Note:** ICD-10-CM category V45 is titled "Car occupant injured in collision with railway train or railway vehicle" while the title of ICD-9-CM category E810 is "Motor vehicle traffic accident involving collision with train."

In numerous instances, conditions included as subcategory codes in ICD-9-CM have been given a specific category code in ICD-10-CM allowing expansion of the codes at the fourth-, fifth-, or sixth-character level.

> *Example:*
> ICD-9-CM   E884.0, Fall from playground equipment
> ICD-10-CM   W09,   Fall on and from playground equipment
>   W09.0, Fall on or from playground slide
>   W09.1, Fall from playground swing
>   W09.2, Fall on or from jungle gym
>   W09.8, Fall on or from other playground equipment

Activity – Chapter 20 Organization and Classification
To find out more about the organization, terminology, and classification modifications to external causes of morbidity, refer to the ICD-10-CM Tabular List, locate the listed ICD-10-CM category or code, evaluate the ICD-9-CM information against what was found, and discern the variances.

ICD-10-CM	*ICD-9-CM*
W00-W19	E880-E888
W54-W64	E905-E906
Y38	E979

Chapter 21: Factors influencing health status and contact with health services (Z00-Z99)

Coding professionals will find the listing of codes for factors influencing health status and contact with health services a bit different in ICD-10-CM than what is currently found in ICD-9-CM. The following blocks represent the ICD-10-CM arrangement:

Z00-Z13	Persons encountering health services for examinations
Z14-Z15	Genetic carrier and genetic susceptibility to disease
Z16	Resistance to antimicrobial drugs
Z17	Estrogen receptor status
Z18	Retained foreign body fragment
Z20-Z28	Persons with potential health hazards related to communicable diseases
Z30-Z39	Persons encountering health services in circumstances related to reproduction
Z40-Z53	Encounters for other specific health care
Z55-Z65	Persons with potential health hazards related to socioeconomic and psychosocial circumstances
Z66	Do not resuscitate status
Z67	Blood type
Z68	Body mass index (BMI)
Z69-Z76	Persons encountering health services in other circumstances
Z77-Z99	Persons with potential health hazards related to family and personal history and certain conditions influencing health status

Some categories in Chapter 21 have rephrased titles to better reflect the situations the codes classify.

Note: The description for Z08 is "Encounter for follow-up examination after completed treatment for malignant neoplasm" compared to ICD-9-CM code title for V67.2 "Follow-up examination following chemotherapy."

An example of decreased specificity in ICD-10-CM is code Z23, Encounter for immunization. This code is not further classified. In ICD-9-CM, category codes V03, V04, V05, and V06 are used to identify the types of immunizations.

Activity – Chapter 21 Organization and Classification

To become more familiar with other revisions to the organization, terminology, and classifications of factors influencing health status and contact with health services, refer to the ICD-10-CM Tabular list, find the ICD-10-CM category or code for those listed here, and assess how it differs from ICD-9-CM.

ICD-10-CM	ICD-9-CM
Z33.2	635
Z91.010	V15.01
Z96	V43

Section 8 – Chapter 15–21 Guidelines

This section is designed to highlight the revisions to the guidelines found in Chapters 15–21 of ICD-10-CM. All modifications have not been illustrated but certain guiding principles have been selected to show guideline variations from ICD-9-CM. Also included in this section is the review of chapter-specific coding guidelines published by NCHS.

Chapter 15: Pregnancy, childbirth and the puerperium (O00-O9A)

At the beginning of Chapter 15 are guidelines that provide instructions for coding professionals.

> **Note:** Codes from this chapter are for use only on maternal records, never on newborn records.

> **Note:** Trimesters are counted from the first day of the last menstrual period. They are defined as follows:
> - 1st trimester – less than 14 weeks 0 days
> - 2nd trimester – 14 weeks 0 days to less than 28 weeks 0 days
> - 3rd trimester – 28 weeks 0 days until delivery

These guidelines should be followed when selecting a code from this chapter.

There are guideline changes to a number of codes in this chapter as well.

> *Examples:*
>
> | | |
> |---|---|
> | ICD-9-CM | For category 643, Excessive vomiting in pregnancy, early vomiting and late vomiting are differentiated by 22 completed weeks |
> | ICD-10-CM | For category O21, Excessive vomiting in pregnancy, early vomiting and late vomiting are differentiated by 20 completed weeks |
> | | |
> | ICD-9-CM | For category 640, hemorrhage in early pregnancy is defined as hemorrhage before completion of 22 weeks gestation |
> | ICD-10-CM | For category O20, hemorrhage in early pregnancy is defined as hemorrhage before completion of 20 weeks of gestation |

The NCHS has published chapter-specific guidelines for Chapter 15 of ICD-10-CM:
- Guideline I.C.15.a. General rules for obstetric cases
- Guideline I.C.15.b. Selection of OB principal or first-listed diagnosis
- Guideline I.C.15.c. Pre-existing conditions versus conditions due to the pregnancy
- Guideline I.C.15.d. Pre-existing hypertension in pregnancy
- Guideline I.C.15.e. Fetal conditions affecting the management of the mother
- Guideline I.C.15.f. HIV infection in pregnancy, childbirth and the puerperium
- Guideline I.C.15.g. Diabetes mellitus in pregnancy
- Guideline I.C.15.h. Long-term use of insulin
- Guideline I.C.15.i. Gestational (pregnancy induced) diabetes
- Guideline I.C.15.j. Sepsis and septic shock complicating abortion, pregnancy, childbirth and the puerperium
- Guideline I.C.15.k. Puerperal sepsis
- Guideline I.C.15.l. Alcohol and tobacco use during pregnancy, childbirth and the puerperium

- Guideline I.C.15.m. Poisoning, toxic effects, adverse effects and underdosing in a pregnant patient
- Guideline I.C.15.n. Normal delivery, code O80
- Guideline I.C.15.o. The peripartum and postpartum periods
- Guideline I.C.15.p. Code O94, sequelae of complications of pregnancy, childbirth and the puerperium
- Guideline I.C.15.q. Abortions
- Guideline I.C.15.r. Abuse in pregnant patient

Activity – Chapter 15 Guidelines
To gain an understanding of these rules, access the 2014 guidelines from the NCHS website (http://www.cdc.gov/nchs/icd/icd10cm.htm) and read Chapter 15: Pregnancy, childbirth and the puerperium guidelines I.C.15.a.1 through I.C.15.r on pages 52–60.

Chapter 16: Certain conditions originating in the perinatal period (P00-P96)

Throughout Chapter 16 are new notes that help to clarify how codes are to be used.

Examples:

The following note appears under P07: When both birth weight and gestational age of the newborn are available, both should be coded with birth weight sequenced before gestational age.

The following note appears under P08.21: Newborn with gestation period over 40 completed weeks to 42 completed weeks.

Codes from this chapter are only for use on the newborn or infant record, never on the maternal record as indicated by a note that appears at the beginning of Chapter 16. Codes from this chapter are also only applicable for liveborn infants. Further, should a condition originate in the perinatal period and continue throughout the life of the child, the perinatal code should continue to be used regardless of the age of the patient as explained by an introductory note to Chapter 16.

The NCHS has published chapter-specific guidelines for Chapter 16 of ICD-10-CM:
- Guideline I.C.16.a. General perinatal rules
- Guideline I.C.16.b. Observation and evaluation of newborns for suspected conditions not found
- Guideline I.C.16.c. Coding additional perinatal diagnoses
- Guideline I.C.16.d. Prematurity and fetal growth retardation
- Guideline I.C.16.e. Low birth weight and immaturity status
- Guideline I.C.16.f. Bacterial sepsis of newborn
- Guideline I.C.16.g. Stillbirth

Activity – Chapter 16 Guidelines
To gain an understanding of these rules, access the 2014 guidelines from the NCHS website (http://www.cdc.gov/nchs/icd/icd10cm.htm) and read Chapter 16: Newborn (perinatal) guidelines I.C.16.a through I.C.16.g on pages 61–63.

Chapter 17: Congenital malformations, deformations and chromosomal abnormalities (Q00-Q99)

Additional guideline modifications were made to specific codes. For example, in ICD-9-CM certain congenital malformations of the anterior segment of the eye do not have any instructions for code usage listed below codes 743.44 or 743.45. In contrast, guidelines for code Q13.1 and Q13.81 state to use an additional code for associated glaucoma.

Congenital anomalies or syndromes may occur as a set of symptoms or multiple malformations. If there is no specific code, a code should be assigned for each manifestation of the syndrome, from any chapter in the classification. For syndromes with specific codes, additional codes may be assigned to identify manifestations not included in the specific code.

The NCHS has published chapter-specific guidelines for Chapter 17 of ICD-10-CM:
- Guideline I.C.17. Congenital malformations, deformations and chromosomal abnormalities (Q00-Q99)

Activity – Chapter 17 Guidelines
To gain an understanding of these rules, access the 2014 guidelines from the NCHS website (http://www.cdc.gov/nchs/icd/icd10cm.htm) and read Chapter 17: Congenital malformations, deformations and chromosomal abnormalities guideline I.C.17 on pages 63–64.

Chapter 18: Symptoms, signs and abnormal clinical and laboratory findings, not elsewhere classified (R00-R99)

A lengthy guideline appears at the beginning of Chapter 18 in ICD-10-CM outlining the conditions classified to this chapter. Additionally, guidelines for code usage appear at the subchapter level.

> **Note:** Many of the new blocks and categories in chapter 18 have extensive *Excludes1* notes such as the one found under R09, Other symptoms and signs involving the circulatory and respiratory system.

New guidelines that clarify code usage are also found under specific codes. Code R52, Pain unspecified, includes inclusive terms and *Excludes1* notes.

The NCHS has published chapter-specific guidelines for Chapter 18 of ICD-10-CM:
- Guideline I.C.18.a. Use of symptom codes
- Guideline I.C.18.b. Use of a symptom code with a definitive diagnosis code
- Guideline I.C.18.c. Combination codes that include symptoms
- Guideline I.C.18.d. Repeated falls
- Guideline I.C.18.e. Coma scale
- Guideline I.C.18.f. Functional quadriplegia
- Guideline I.C.18.g. SIRS due to non-infectious process
- Guideline I.C.18.h. Death NOS

> **Activity – Chapter 18 Guidelines**
> To gain an understanding of these rules, access the 2014 guidelines from the NCHS website (http://www.cdc.gov/nchs/icd/icd10cm.htm) and read Chapter 18: Symptoms, signs and abnormal clinical and laboratory findings, not elsewhere classified guidelines I.C.18.a through I.C.18.h on pages 64–66.

Chapter 19: Injury, poisoning and certain other consequences of external causes (S00-T88)

The following guideline appears at the beginning of Chapter 19: Use secondary code(s) from Chapter 20, External causes of morbidity, to indicate cause of injury. Codes within the T section that include the external cause do not require an additional external cause code.

Instructions for coding open wounds have changed in ICD-10-CM. The note in ICD-9-CM defines "complicated" used in the fourth-digit subdivisions to mean those open wounds with infection. ICD-10-CM contains a note under the different categories for open wounds and directs the coding professional to code also any associated wound infection.

A similar change has occurred to the instruction for complications of surgical and medical care, not elsewhere classified (T80-T88). In ICD-9-CM, there is no guideline under this subchapter. However, ICD-10-CM includes a note stating to use an additional code (Y62-Y82) to identify devices involved and details of circumstances.

Note: Most categories in Chapter 19 have seventh characters that identify the encounter:
A   initial encounter
D   subsequent encounter
S   sequela

Additional seventh characters are available to identify specific encounters for fracture coding. Seventh characters for fractures are unique to each type of bone and type of fracture.

Coding Tip: It is necessary to review the fracture seventh characters carefully before assigning a seventh character.

The NCHS has published chapter-specific guidelines for Chapter 19 of ICD-10-CM:
- Guideline I.C.19.a. Seventh characters
- Guideline I.C.19.b. Coding of injuries
- Guideline I.C.19.c. Coding of traumatic fractures
- Guideline I.C.19.d. Coding of burns and corrosions
- Guideline I.C.19.e. Adverse effects, poisoning, underdosing and toxic effects
- Guideline I.C.19.f. Adult and child abuse, neglect and other maltreatment
- Guideline I.C.19.g. Complications of care

Activity – Chapter 19 Guidelines
To gain an understanding of these rules, access the 2014 guidelines from the NCHS website (http://www.cdc.gov/nchs/icd/icd10cm.htm) and read Chapter 19: Injury, poisoning and certain other consequences of external causes guidelines I.C.19.a through I.C.19.g.5 on pages 66–75.

Chapter 20: External causes of morbidity (V00-Y99)

New notes have been added in Chapter 20 to indicate which categories require the seventh character to indicate whether the episode of care being identified was the initial, subsequent, or a secondary consequence or result (sequelae).

While there is an instructional note found at the start of category E849, place of occurrence, in ICD-9-CM, it has been expanded in ICD-10-CM. The new guidelines state to use Y92 in conjunction with the activity code and the place of occurrence should be recorded only at the initial encounter for treatment.

> **Coding Tip:** Use an activity code from category Y93 in addition to the place of occurrence code from category Y92.

The NCHS has published chapter-specific guidelines for Chapter 20 of ICD-10-CM:
- Guideline I.C.20.a. General external cause coding guidelines
- Guideline I.C.20.b. Place of occurrence guideline
- Guideline I.C.20.c. Activity code
- Guideline I.C.20.d. Place of occurrence, activity, and status codes used with other external cause code
- Guideline I.C.20.e. If the reporting format limits the number of external cause codes
- Guideline I.C.20.f. Multiple external cause coding guidelines
- Guideline I.C.20.g. Child and adult abuse guideline
- Guideline I.C.20.h. Unknown or undetermined intent guideline
- Guideline I.C.20.i. Sequela (late effects) of external cause guidelines
- Guideline I.C.20.j. Terrorism guidelines
- Guideline I.C.20.k. External cause status

Activity – Chapter 20 Guidelines
To gain an understanding of these rules, access the 2014 guidelines from the NCHS website (http://www.cdc.gov/nchs/icd/icd10cm.htm) and read Chapter 20: External causes of morbidity guidelines I.C.20.a through I.C.20.k on pages 76–81.

Chapter 21: Factors influencing health status and contact with health services (Z00-Z99)

The note at the beginning of this chapter has been modified from what it states in ICD-9-CM. All codes in Chapter 21 are affected by these revised guidelines. Here is the note:

> Z codes represent reasons for encounters. A corresponding procedure code must accompany a Z code if a procedure is performed. Categories Z00-Z99 are provided for occasions when circumstances other than a disease, injury or external cause classifiable to categories A00-Y89 are recorded as 'diagnoses' or 'problems'. This can arise in two main ways:
>
> a) When a person who may or may not be sick encounters the health services for some specific purpose, such as to receive limited care or service for a current condition, to donate an organ or tissue, to receive prophylactic vaccination (immunization), or to discuss a problem which is in itself not a disease or injury.
> b) When some circumstance or problem is present which influences the person's health status but is not in itself a current illness or injury.

Instructional notes also have been added to different categories to explain how codes should be assigned.

Examples:
Under category Z01, Encounter for other special examination without complaint, suspected or reported diagnosis, is the following note: Codes from category Z01 represent the reason for the encounter. A separate procedure code is required to identify any examination or procedure performed.

Under category Z85, Personal history of malignant neoplasm, is the following note: Code first any follow-up examination after treatment of malignant neoplasm (Z08).

The NCHS has published chapter-specific guidelines for Chapter 21 of ICD-10-CM:
- Guideline I.C.21.a. Use of Z codes in any healthcare setting
- Guideline I.C.21.b. Z codes indicate a reason for an encounter
- Guideline I.C.21.c. Categories of Z codes

Activity – Chapter 21 Guidelines
To gain an understanding of these rules, access the 2014 guidelines from the NCHS website (http://www.cdc.gov/nchs/icd/icd10cm.htm) and read Chapter 21: Factors influencing health status and contact with health services guidelines I.C.21.a through I.C.21.c on pages 81–97.

Sections 7 and 8 Review Questions

1. True or false? An injury code with the seventh character D for subsequent encounter may be used for as long as a patient is receiving treatment for an injury.
   a. True
   b. False

2. True or false? If a patient has both an open wound of the shoulder and an associated wound infection, only one code is assigned in both ICD-9-CM and ICD-10-CM.
   a. True
   b. False

3. ICD-10-CM contains codes for all but one of the following conditions:
   a. Eclampsia in labor
   b. Eclampsia in the puerperium
   c. Eclampsia in the first trimester
   d. Eclampsia in the second trimester

4. What is the correct ICD-10-CM code(s) for severe generalized abdominal pain with abdominal rigidity?
   a. R19.3
   b. R10.0
   c. R10.84
   d. R19.3, R10.0

5. What is the purpose of the fifth character for category Y38, Terrorism?
   a. A placeholder
   b. To identify the person injured
   c. As a way to indicate place of occurrence
   d. To classify the encounter

6. True or false? Before assigning codes from the ICD-10-CM chapter on pregnancy, childbirth and the puerperium, coding professionals need to determine if a condition was pre-existing prior to pregnancy or developed during the pregnancy in order to select the correct code.
   a. True
   b. False

7. Codes for bacterial sepsis of newborn are found in which block in Chapter 16?
   a. P90-P96, Other disorders originating in the perinatal period
   b. P50-P61, Hemorrhagic and hematological disorders of newborn
   c. P84, Other problems with newborn
   d. P35-P39, Infections specific to the perinatal period

8. True or false? Codes from the ICD-10-CM chapter on congenital malformations, deformations and chromosomal abnormalities may be used only up until the 28th day following birth.
   a. True
   b. False

9. If a condition is discovered during a screening, the screening code is:
    a. Not assigned
    b. Assigned but coded secondary to the condition discovered
    c. Assigned with the condition discovered coded secondary
    d. Assigned without a code for the discovered condition

10. True or false? ICD-10-CM placed a single category of codes for poisonings, adverse effects of and underdosing of drugs, medicaments, and biological substances.
    a. True
    b. False

Final Review Questions

1. The final rule to adopt ICD-10-CM and ICD-10-PCS states the compliance date for ICD-10-CM is:
    a. October 1, 2013
    b. January 16, 2009
    c. October 1, 2014
    d. January 1, 2014

2. All of the following are new features of ICD-10-CM, *except:*
    a. Injuries are grouped by body part rather than by categories of injuries
    b. The concept of laterality has been added
    c. Newly recognized conditions and conditions that are not uniquely identified in ICD-9-CM have been given codes
    d. Codes for intraoperative complications and postprocedural disorders have been combined

3. According to the note under Chapter 18: Symptoms, signs and abnormal clinical and laboratory findings, not elsewhere classified, categories in this chapter include signs and symptoms that point rather definitely to a given diagnosis.
    a. True
    b. False

4. ICD-10-CM and ICD-9-CM have similar structures in which of the following?
    a. Hypertension table
    b. Note placement
    c. Morphology appendix
    d. All of the above

5. What is the purpose of the X placeholder in category X78?
    a. To code to the highest level of specificity
    b. As a placeholder for future expansion
    c. As filler so a seventh character may be assigned
    d. To provide further specificity about the condition being coded

6. ICD-10-CM code N30.01, Acute cystitis with hematuria, represents which use of a combination code?
    a. Two diagnoses
    b. A diagnosis with an associated sign or symptom
    c. A diagnosis with an associated complication
    d. All of the above

7. Codes in Chapter 20, External causes of morbidity, identify all of the following *except:*
    a. Intent (unintentional/accidental, intentional self-harm or assault)
    b. Place where the event occurred
    c. Activity of the patient at the time of the event
    d. Poisoning by medicaments and biological substances

8. A patient with a diagnosis of interstitial cystitis due to E coli with hematuria is coded:
    a. N30.11, N02.9
    b. N30.10, N02.9, B96.20
    c. N30.11, B96.20
    d. N30.91, B96.20

9. ICD-10-CM category J44 is used to classify all but the following:
    a. Chronic asthmatic (obstructive) bronchitis
    b. Asthmatic bronchitis
    c. Chronic obstructive asthma
    d. Chronic obstructive pulmonary disease

10. What is the correct ICD-10-CM code for acute nonsuppurative otitis media, right ear?
    a. H65.91
    b. H65.111
    c. H65.199
    d. H65.191

11. A patient with a diagnosis of fatigue fracture of vertebra, lumbar region, and subsequent encounter for fracture with delayed healing is coded:
    a. M48.46G
    b. M48.46XG
    c. M48.45XG
    d. M48.47XG

12. True or false? Uncontrolled hypertension and controlled hypertension have different codes in ICD-10-CM.
    a. True
    b. False

13. According to NCHS Guidelines, which of the following is the default for a patient with a diagnosis of right-side hemiplegia, ICD-10-CM category G81?
    a. Dominant side
    b. Nondominant side
    c. Unspecified side
    d. Right side

14. ICD-10-CM code H40.0 is used to classify:
    a. Glaucoma suspect
    b. Ocular hypertension
    c. Borderline glaucoma
    d. All of the above

15. ICD-10-CM category Q35 does not contain a specific code for which of the following conditions in which ICD-9-CM does?
    a. Bilateral cleft palate
    b. Cleft soft palate
    c. Cleft uvula
    d. Cleft hard palate

16. True or false? Codes from categories P00-P04 may be assigned if testing or treatment is done and no problem with the infant is determined.
    a. True
    b. False

17. What documentation is necessary in order to choose the correct fifth character for post-traumatic urethral stricture?
    a. Gender
    b. Severity
    c. Cause
    d. Manifestation

18. For ICD-10-CM categories V00-V99, the type of vehicle the victim is an occupant in is identified in the:
    a. First two characters
    b. Last two characters
    c. Seventh character
    d. The placeholder X

19. True or false? If the abnormal test finding corresponds to a confirmed diagnosis, the abnormal test findings code should not be coded in addition to the confirmed diagnosis.
    a. True
    b. False

20. Codes from which category/categories is/are assigned for a patient who has suffered from an AMI and has a new AMI within the four-week time frame of the initial AMI?
    a. I21
    b. I22
    c. I21, I22
    d. I21, I25

Part I: ICD-10-CM Diagnostic Coding

ICD-10-CM Resources – References

2014 ICD-10-CM is available at http://www.cdc.gov/nchs/icd/icd10cm.htm or http://www.cms.hhs.gov/ICD10

- 2014 ICD-10-CM Index to Diseases and Injuries
- 2014 ICD-10-CM Tabular List of Diseases and Injuries
  - Instructional Notations
- 2014 Official Guidelines for Coding and Reporting
- 2014 Table of Drugs and Chemicals
- 2014 Neoplasm Table
- 2014 Index to External Causes
- 2014 Mapping "ICD-9-CM to ICD-10-CM" and "ICD-10-CM to ICD-9-CM"

ICD-10-CM Coding Conventions and Coding Guidelines Review

ICD-10-CM Coding Conventions

1. The ICD-10-CM code for electrocution is T75.4 and requires the use of a seventh
    character to identify the encounter. Which of the following is the correct code for an initial
    encounter to treat the electrocution?
    a.   T75.4A
    b.   T75.4XA
    c.   T75.4XXA
    d.   T75.4

2. Nonessential modifiers are enclosed in:
    a.   Boxes
    b.   Brackets
    c.   Parentheses
    d.   Colons

3. True or false? When an *Excludes2* note appears under a code, it is acceptable to use
    both the code and the excluded code together.
    a.   True
    b.   False

4. The first character of an ICD-10-CM code is:
    a.   Always a number
    b.   Always a letter
    c.   Can be either a number or letter
    d.   None of the above

5. A(n) _____ note means "not coded here."
    a.   *Includes*
    b.   *Excludes2*
    c.   *Excludes1*
    d.   None of the above

6. Codes titled "other" or "other specified" are to be used:
    a.   When the record itself is not available for review
    b.   When the information in the medical record provides detail for which a specific
         code does not exist
    c.   When only outpatient diagnostic records are being coded
    d.   When the information in the medical record is insufficient to assign a more
         specific code

7. True or false? Similar to ICD-9-CM, in ICD-10-CM all categories are three characters.
    a.   True
    b.   False

8. True or false? When the term "and" is used in a narrative statement it is interpreted to
    mean only "and."
    a.   True
    b.   False

9.   True or false? In ICD-10-CM all inclusion notes contain all conditions for which a particular code number is to be used and are considered to be "exhaustive."
      a.   True
      b.   False

10.   True or false? In ICD-10-CM a "code also" note provides sequencing guidance to the coding professional.
      a.   True
      b.   False

ICD-10-CM Coding Guidelines

11.   If an encounter is solely for chemotherapy, immunotherapy, or radiation therapy for a neoplastic condition, the first reported diagnosis is:
      a.   The diagnosis toward which the treatment is directed
      b.   The appropriate Z51 code
      c.   Either a or b
      d.   The diagnosis that the physician lists first on the order

12.   True or false? When assigning the principal diagnosis for a patient with AIDS, the AIDS code would always be sequenced before any other conditions.
      a.   True
      b.   False

13.   A patient has liver metastasis due to adenocarcinoma of the rectum which was resected two years ago. The patient has been receiving radiotherapy to the liver with some relief of pain. The patient is being admitted at this time for management of severe anemia due to the malignancy. The principal diagnosis listed on this admission is:
      a.   Liver metastasis
      b.   Adenocarcinoma of the rectum
      c.   Anemia
      d.   Admission for radiotherapy

14.   True or false? Code P95, Stillbirth, is only for use for institutions that maintain separate records for stillborns and should never be used on the mother's record.
      a.   True
      b.   False

15.   True or false? A fracture not described as "displaced" or "not displaced" by default should be coded as "not displaced."
      a.   True
      b.   False

16.   A patient is admitted six weeks post-acute anterolateral myocardial infarction with a subsequent posterior acute MI. Which is the appropriate coding and sequencing for the encounter for the posterior acute MI in ICD-10-CM?
      a.   I21.09, STEMI involving other coronary artery of anterior wall,
            I22.8, Subsequent STEMI of other sites
      b.   I21.29, STEMI of other sites,
            I25.2, Old myocardial infarction
      c.   I22.8, Subsequent STEMI of other sites;
            I21.09, STEMI involving other coronary artery of anterior wall
      d.   I22.8, Subsequent STEMI of other sites,
            I25.2, Old myocardial infarction

17. When multiple burns are present, the first sequenced diagnosis is the:
    a. Burn that is treated surgically
    b. Burn that is closest to the head
    c. Highest-degree burn
    d. Any of the above

18. True or false? A place of occurrence code should be used only at the initial encounter for treatment.
    a. True
    b. False

19. In ICD-10-CM diabetes mellitus codes include:
    a. The type of diabetes mellitus
    b. The body system affected
    c. The complication affecting that body system
    d. All of the above

20. True or false? A causal relationship can be assumed in a patient with both coronary atherosclerosis and angina pectoris and thus, the appropriate combination code should be assigned.
    a. True
    b. False

21. True or false? Patients with a prior diagnosis of an HIV-related illness should be assigned the code for AIDS (B20) on every subsequent admission.
    a. True
    b. False

22. Which of the following would be assigned to code I11.0, Hypertensive heart disease with heart failure?
    a. Left heart failure with benign hypertension
    b. Hypertensive cardiomegaly
    c. Congestive heart failure due to hypertension
    d. All of the above would be assigned to code I11.0

23. When an OB patient enters the hospital for complications of pregnancy during one trimester and remains in the hospital into a subsequent trimester, the final character selected for the antepartum conditions should be:
    a. For the trimester in which the complication developed
    b. For the trimester in which the patient delivered
    c. For the trimester in which the patient was discharged
    d. Any trimester as long as the same character is used for all complications

24. True or false? In the case where a 20-day-old baby has a condition that may be either due to the birth process or community-acquired and there is no documentation to support either one, the default should be community-acquired rather than birth process.
    a. True
    b. False

25. True or false? Regardless of the number of external cause codes assigned on a particular record, there should be only one place of occurrence code and one activity code assigned to a record.
    a. True
    b. False

26.   True or false? A noncompliance code or complication of care code is to be used with an underdosing code to indicate intent.
        a.   True
        b.   False

27.   When reporting an encounter for a patient who is HIV positive but has never had any symptoms, the following code is assigned:
        a.   B20, Human immunodeficiency virus [HIV] disease
        b.   Z21, Asymptomatic HIV infection status
        c.   R75, Inconclusive laboratory evidence of human immunodeficiency virus (HIV)
        d.   Z20.6, Contact with and (suspected) exposure to HIV

28.   In reviewing the medical record of a patient admitted for a left herniorrhaphy, the coder notes an extremely low potassium level on the laboratory report. In examining the physician's order, the coder notices that intravenous potassium was ordered. The physician has not listed any indication of an abnormal potassium level or any related condition within the medical record. The best course of action for the coder to take is to:
        a.   Confer with the physician and ask if the condition should be listed as a final diagnosis
        b.   Code the record as is
        c.   Code the condition as an abnormal blood chemistry
        d.   Code the abnormal potassium level as a complication following surgery

29.   True or false? When coding severe sepsis a minimum of three codes is required.
        a.   True
        b.   False

30.   When a patient seeks medical attention for an injury that occurred several days prior to the medical encounter, which is the appropriate seventh character?
        a.   A, initial encounter
        b.   D, subsequent encounter
        c.   S, sequela
        d.   No seventh character is used when there is delayed treatment

Coding in ICD-10-CM

ICD-10-CM differs from ICD-9-CM in its organization and structure, code composition, and level of detail; however, many components stay the same. ICD-10-CM has the same hierarchical structure as ICD-9-CM, and all codes with the same first three characters have common traits. Each character beyond the first three adds more specificity. Even though ICD-10-CM has more characters (up to seven) and uses alpha characters, each code must be at least three characters, with a decimal point used after the third character. Most, but not all, three-character categories have been subdivided. Up to four characters may follow the decimal. However, not every code will have four characters after the decimal; the concept is the same as ICD-9-CM.

The first character of the ICD-10-CM code is an alpha character, and each letter is associated with a particular chapter, except for the letters **D** and **H**. The letter D is used in both Chapter 2: Neoplasms, and Chapter 3: Diseases of the blood and blood-forming organs and certain disorders involving the immune mechanism. The letter H is used in both Chapter 7: Diseases of the eye and adnexa, and Chapter 8: Diseases of the ear and mastoid process. To allow for future revisions or expansions of the classification, every available code is not used.

The letters I and O are used in ICD-10-CM, but they shouldn't be confused with the numbers 1 and 0 because the letters I and O are only used in the first character position and this character is always a letter.

ICD-9-CM	ICD-10-CM
• Consists of three to five characters • First digit is numeric but occasionally can be alpha (E or V) • Second, third, fourth, and fifth digits are numeric • Always at least three digits • Decimal placed after the first three characters (or with E codes, placed after the first four characters) • Alpha characters are not case-sensitive	• Consists of three to seven characters • First character is always alpha • All letters used except U • Character 2 always numeric • Characters 3 through 7 can be alpha or numeric • Always at least three digits • Decimal placed after the first three characters • Alpha characters are not case-sensitive

A few important changes to ICD-10-CM are listed here:
- ICD-10-CM consists of 21 chapters.
- The order of some chapters has been rearranged, with reclassification of some conditions.
- The addition of a sixth character in some chapters.
- A seventh character added in some chapters (primarily pregnancy, injury, and external cause chapters).
- ICD-10-CM includes full code titles for all codes (no references back to common fourth and fifth digits).
- No supplementary classifications, with all codes incorporated into main classification.
- Expansion of postoperative complications and a distinction made between intraoperative complications and postprocedural disorders.

- Category restructuring and code reorganization.
- A placeholder X is used in some codes to allow for future expansion and also to fill out empty characters when a code contains fewer than six characters and a seventh character applies.
- Instructional note, guideline, and time frame changes.
- Combination codes for conditions and common symptoms or manifestations have been added.
- Laterality (meaning left or right side) has been added where applicable.
- Seventh characters added for type of encounter (initial, subsequent, and sequela) for injuries and external causes.

Coding and Use of Seventh Characters

While more detailed information will be provided later in this training, certain basic information is provided here so that correct seventh characters can be assigned throughout this training course when encountered.

Seventh characters have been added in some chapters, primarily in the obstetrics, injury, and external cause chapters. They may be either alpha or numeric and are added to the end of the code in the seventh position when applicable. They provide additional information about the characteristics of the encounter. Seventh characters have different meanings depending on the section, and the applicable values are available in the Tabular section of ICD-10-CM. The category will identify the necessity to use the seventh character. The applicable seventh character is required for all codes within that category, or as the notes in the Tabular List instruct. A code that has an applicable seventh character is considered invalid without the seventh character. The seventh character must always be the seventh character in the data field, and if the code is not six characters, a placeholder of X is required to fill empty characters.

The meanings of the seventh character vary across chapters and categories. In the Injury and External Cause chapters the seventh character identifies the encounter (initial, subsequent, sequela). Fracture codes include additional information that can be provided by the seventh character. See the Tabular List for the exact seventh characters available for fracture coding.

The seventh characters for "initial encounter" are used while the patient is receiving active treatment of the condition. Examples of active treatment are: surgical treatment, emergency department encounter, and evaluation and treatment by a new physician.

The seventh characters for "subsequent encounter" are used for encounters after the patient has received active treatment of the condition and is receiving routine care for the condition during the healing or recovery phase. Examples of subsequent care are: cast change or removal, removal of external or internal fixation device, medication adjustment, other aftercare and follow-up visits following treatment of the injury or condition.

Seventh character S, sequela, is for use for complications or conditions that arise as a direct result of a condition, such as scar formation after a burn. The scars are a sequela of the burn. When using seventh character S, it is necessary to use both the injury code that precipitated the sequela and the code for the sequela itself. The S is added only to the injury code, not the sequela code. The seventh character S identifies the injury responsible for the sequela. The specific type of sequela (e.g., scar) is sequenced first, followed by the injury code.

The aftercare Z codes should not be used for aftercare for conditions such as injuries or poisonings, where seventh characters are provided to identify subsequent care. For example, for aftercare of an injury, assign the acute injury code with the seventh character D, subsequent encounter.

There are combination codes for poisonings and the associated external cause (accidental, intentional self-harm, assault, undetermined).

The seventh character in Chapter 15 represents the fetus in a multiple gestation that is affected by the condition being coded. These are discussed in more detail in the Pregnancy, Childbirth and the Puerperium lesson.

Chapter 1: Certain infectious and parasitic diseases (A00-B99)

This chapter of ICD-10-CM covers two alpha-characters, A and B. The following notes are available at the beginning of the chapter:

Includes: Diseases generally recognized as communicable or transmissible

Use additional code to identify resistance to antimicrobial drugs (Z16-)

Excludes1:   Certain localized Infections - see body system-related chapters

Excludes2:   carrier or suspected carrier of infectious disease (Z22.-)
infectious and parasitic diseases complicating pregnancy, childbirth and the puerperium (O98.-)
infectious and parasitic diseases specific to the perinatal period (P35-P39)
influenza and other acute respiratory infections (J00-J22)

Chapter 1 of ICD-10-CM includes a new section called infections with a predominantly sexual mode of transmission (A50-A64). Many codes have been moved from other places in the classification to this section.

When coding sepsis or AIDS, it is important to review the coding guidelines and the notes at the category level of ICD-10-CM.

There is an important note in the Sequelae of Infectious and Parasitic Diseases (B90-B94) section. Note: Categories B90-B94 are to be used to indicate conditions in categories A00-B89 as the cause of sequelae, which are themselves classified elsewhere. The "sequelae" include conditions specified as such; they also include residuals of diseases classifiable to the above categories if there is evidence that the disease itself is no longer present. Codes from these categories are not to be used for chronic infections. Code chronic current infections to active infectious disease as appropriate.

Code first condition resulting from (sequela) the infectious or parasitic disease.

Bacterial and viral infectious agents (B95-B97) also have a note that specifies that these categories are provided for use as supplementary or additional codes to identify the infectious agent(s) in diseases classified elsewhere. The following are examples of how to index these conditions:
- Infection, infected, infective; bacterial as cause of disease classified elsewhere; Streptococcus group A – B95.0
- Streptococcus, streptococcal; group A, as cause of disease classified elsewhere – B95.0

Chapter 1 Coding Cases

1.1. This 80-year-old female patient was seen with fever, malaise, and left flank pain. A urinalysis was performed and showed bacteria more than 100,000/ml. This was followed by a culture, showing E. coli growth as the cause of the UTI. What **diagnosis** codes are assigned?

Code(s): _____

Coding Guideline I.C.1.c. Infections Resistant to Antibiotics
Many bacterial infections are resistant to current antibiotics. It is necessary to identify all infections documented as antibiotic resistant. Assign a code from category Z16, Resistance to antimicrobial drugs, following the infection code only if the infection codes does not identify drug resistance.

1.2. This 78-year-old gentleman is seen for continued follow-up for C. diff colitis. Cultures of the organism have found this infection to be resistant to flagyl. A new drug regimen will be started at this time. What is the correct **diagnosis** code assignment?

Code(s): _____

Coding Guideline I.B.10. Sequela (Late Effects)
A *sequela* is the residual effect (condition produced) after the acute phase of an illness or injury has terminated. There is no time limit on when a sequela code can be used. The residual may be apparent early, such as in cerebral infarction, or it may occur months or years later, such as that due to a previous injury. Coding of sequela generally requires two codes sequenced in the following order: The condition or nature of the sequela is sequenced first. The sequela code is sequenced second.

1.3. This patient is seen for right lower leg muscle atrophy as a result of a previous bout of polio. What **diagnosis** codes are assigned?

Code(s): _____

1.4. This patient is seen for an acute case of bacterial food poisoning due to Salmonella. No complications are present at this time and the patient will be treated appropriately. What **diagnosis** codes are assigned?

Code(s): _____

Coding Note: ICD-10-CM has created a range of codes to identify infections with a predominantly sexual mode of transmission (A50-A64). It is important to note that human immunodeficiency virus [HIV] disease is excluded from this range of codes.

1.5.   This young woman is seen for pelvic pain due to pelvic inflammatory disease. The source of the PID is a result of sexually transmitted chlamydia. What **diagnosis** codes are assigned?

Code(s): _____

Coding Guideline I.C.1.a.2.a. Patient Admitted for HIV-related Condition
If a patient is admitted with an HIV-related condition, the principal diagnosis should be B20, Human immunodeficiency virus [HIV] disease followed by additional diagnosis codes for all reported HIV-related conditions.

1.6.   This 42-year-old HIV positive male has a fever and shortness of breath. The diagnostic workup, including chest x-ray and sputum culture, resulted in a diagnosis of Pneumocystis pneumonia. This was documented as Pneumocystis pneumonia due to AIDS. What **diagnosis** codes are assigned?

Code(s): _____

Coding Guideline I.C.1.d.1.a. Sepsis
For a diagnosis of sepsis, assign the appropriate code for the underlying systemic infection. If the type of infection or causal organism is not further specified, assign code A41.9, Sepsis, unspecified organism.

A code from subcategory R65.2, Severe sepsis, should not be assigned unless severe sepsis or an associated acute organ dysfunction is documented.

1.7.   This 87-year-old nursing home patient is being treated with IV antibiotics for E. coli sepsis. What **diagnosis** codes are assigned?

Code(s): _____

Coding Guideline I.C.1.d.1.b. Severe Sepsis
The coding of severe sepsis requires a minimum of two codes: first a code for the underlying systemic infection, followed by a code from subcategory R65.2, Severe sepsis. If the causal organism is not documented, assign code A41.9, Sepsis, unspecified organism, for the infection. Additional code(s) for the associated organ dysfunction are also required.

1.8.   This 75-year-old woman was taken to the emergency department after being found semi-conscious with markedly abnormal vital signs, a fever of over 39 degrees C, a heart rate of 100, and a respiratory rate of 22/min. On admission to the ICU the physician documented her condition as severe sepsis with acute respiratory failure. The final diagnosis, provided by the physician, was gram-negative sepsis with acute respiratory failure. What **diagnosis** codes are assigned?

Code(s): _____

Coding Guideline I.C.1.d.2. Septic Shock

Septic shock generally refers to circulatory failure associated with severe sepsis and, therefore, it represents a type of acute organ dysfunction.

For cases of septic shock, the code for the systemic infection should be sequenced first, followed by code R65.21, Severe sepsis with septic shock or code T81.12, Postprocedural septic shock. Any additional codes for the other acute organ dysfunctions should also be assigned. As noted in the sequencing instructions in the Tabular List, the code for septic shock cannot be assigned as a principal diagnosis.

1.9. This 25-year-old woman was transferred from an outside facility for treatment of septic shock and acute meningococcal sepsis. The outside facility was unable to manage her severe illness. What **diagnosis** codes are assigned?

Code(s): _____

1.10. This 28-year-old man was admitted with flank pain and renal colic. After diagnostic workup, he was found to have nephrolithiasis. He wanted to avoid surgery and was treated conservatively with fluids and straining of the urine. Two days after admission he developed a cough and fever and was diagnosed with hospital-acquired Pseudomonas pneumonia and was treated appropriately with antibiotics. What **diagnosis** codes are assigned?

Code(s): _____

1.11. This 40-year-old woman with known chronic viral hepatitis resulting from hepatitis B is seen for initiation of antiviral therapy. What **diagnosis** codes are assigned?

Code(s): _____

Chapter 2: Neoplasms (C00-D49)

All neoplasms are classified in this chapter, whether they are functionally active or not. An additional code from Chapter 4 may be used to identify functional activity associated with any neoplasm.

There have been some changes in the classification system regarding neoplasm coding. A few are listed here:

- Codes moved from other chapters to Chapter 2, for example, Waldenström's macroglobulinemia
- Heading changes, for example, Malignant neoplasm of retroperitoneum and peritoneum moved from Malignant neoplasms of digestive organs and peritoneum to Malignant neoplasms of mesothelial and soft tissue
- Melanoma in situ has a unique category, D03 (previously included in ICD-9-CM category 172, Malignant melanoma of skin)

Neoplasms of uncertain behavior are defined as those whose histologic confirmation whether the neoplasm is malignant or benign cannot be made. Neoplasms of unspecified behavior includes terms such as "growth" NOS, neoplasm NOS, new growth NOS, or tumor NOS. The term "mass," unless otherwise stated, is not to be regarded as a neoplastic growth.

Malignant neoplasms of ectopic tissue are to be coded to the site mentioned; for example, ectopic pancreatic malignant neoplasms are coded to pancreas, unspecified (C25.9).

In addition, notes and coding guidelines govern the correct assignment of codes in this chapter, and should be reviewed.

Morphology [Histology]

Chapter 2 classifies neoplasms primarily by site (topography), with broad groupings for behavior (malignant, in situ, benign, and so on). The Neoplasm Table should be used to identify the correct topography code. In a few cases, such as for malignant melanoma and certain neuroendocrine tumors, the morphology (histologic type) is included in the category and codes.

Coding Guideline I.C.2. General Neoplasm Guidelines
The neoplasm table in the Alphabetic Index should be referenced first. However, if the "histological" is documented, that term should be referenced first, rather than going immediately to the Neoplasm Table, in order to determine which column in the Neoplasm Table is appropriate.

Primary Malignant Neoplasms Overlapping Site Boundaries

A primary malignant neoplasm that overlaps two or more contiguous (next to each other) sites should be classified to the subcategory/code .8 (overlapping lesion), unless the combination is specifically indexed elsewhere. For multiple neoplasms of the same site that are not contiguous, such as tumors in different quadrants of the same breast, codes for each site should be assigned.

Malignant Neoplasm of Ectopic Tissue

Malignant neoplasms of ectopic tissue are to be coded to the site mentioned; for example, ectopic pancreatic malignant neoplasms are coded to pancreas, unspecified (C25.9).

Chapter 2 Coding Cases

1.12. The diagnosis for this 61-year-old female patient is small cell carcinoma of the right lower lobe of the lung with metastasis to the intrathoracic lymph nodes, brain, and right rib. What **diagnosis** codes are assigned?

Code(s): _____

1.13. Assign the code(s) for the following diagnosis: Benign carcinoid of the cecum.

Code(s): _____

1.14. Assign the code(s) for the following diagnosis: Subacute monocytic leukemia in remission.

Code(s): _____

1.15. This 25-year-old female is treated for melanoma of the left breast and left arm. What **diagnosis** codes are assigned?

Code(s): _____

Coding Guideline I.C.2.c.3. Management of Dehydration Due to the Malignancy
When the admission/encounter is for management of dehydration due to the malignancy or the therapy, or a combination of both, and only the dehydration is being treated (Intravenous rehydration), the dehydration is sequenced first, followed by the code(s) for the malignancy.

Coding Guideline I.C.6.b.5. Neoplasm-Related Pain
Code G89.3 is assigned to pain documented as being related, associated, or due to cancer, primary or secondary malignancy, or tumor. The code is assigned regardless of whether the pain is acute or chronic.

This code may be assigned as the principal or first-listed code when the stated reason for the admission/encounter is documented as pain control/pain management. The underlying neoplasm should be reported as an additional diagnosis.

When the reason for the admission/encounter is management of the neoplasm and the pain associated with the neoplasm is also documented, code G89.3 may be assigned as an additional diagnosis. It is not necessary to assign an additional code for the site of the pain.

1.16. This female patient with terminal carcinoma of the central portion of the right breast, metastatic to the liver and brain, was seen for dehydration and chronic intractable neoplasm-related pain. Patient was rehydrated with IVs and given IV pain medication with no treatment directed toward the cancer. What **diagnosis** codes are assigned?

Code(s): _____

1.17. This 50-year-old female was diagnosed with left breast carcinoma four years ago, at which time she had a left mastectomy performed with chemotherapy administration. She has been well since that time with no further treatment except for yearly checkups. The patient is now being seen with visual disturbances, dizziness, headaches, and blurred vision. Workup was completed which revealed metastasis to the brain, accounting for these symptoms. This was identified as being metastatic from the breast, not a new primary. What **diagnosis** codes are assigned?

Code(s): _____

Coding Guideline I.C.2.e.2. Patient Admission/Encounter Solely for Administration of Chemotherapy, Immunotherapy, and Radiation Therapy

If a patient admission/encounter is solely for the administration of chemotherapy, immunotherapy, or radiation therapy assign code Z51.0, Encounter for antineoplastic radiation therapy; Z51.11, Encounter for antineoplastic chemotherapy; or Z51.12, Encounter of antineoplastic immunotherapy as the first-listed or principal diagnosis. If a patient receives more than one of these therapies during the same admission more than one of these codes may be assigned, in any sequence.

1.18. The encounter is to receive chemotherapy following the recent diagnosis of carcinoma of the small intestines. The tumor was in the area where the duodenum and jejunum join. The cancer was resected two months ago and the patient has been receiving chemotherapy. What **diagnosis** codes are assigned?

Code(s): _____

Chapter 3: Diseases of the blood and blood-forming organs and certain disorders involving the immune mechanism (D50-D89)

Chapter 3 of ICD-10-CM includes codes primarily from ICD-9-CM Chapter 4, Diseases of the Blood and Blood-Forming Organs, but also includes many codes from ICD-9-CM Chapter 3, Endocrine, Nutritional and Metabolic Diseases and Immunity Disorders. It also includes some codes from ICD-9-CM Chapter 1, Infectious and Parasitic Diseases (for example, sarcoidosis).

Chapter 3 Coding Cases

> **Coding Guideline I.C.2.c.1. Anemia Associated with Malignancy**
> When admission/encounter is for management of an anemia associated with the malignancy, and the treatment is only for anemia, the appropriate code for the malignancy is sequenced as the principal or first-listed diagnosis followed by the appropriate code for the anemia (such as D63.0, Anemia in neoplastic disease).

1.19. This elderly woman is receiving a blood transfusion for severe anemia due to her left breast carcinoma. Assign the correct **diagnosis** code(s).

Code(s): _____

1.20. Code the following: Congenital red cell aplastic anemia.

Code(s): _____

1.21. This patient is seen for continued follow-up regarding his periodic neutropenia. Assign the correct **diagnosis** code(s).

Code(s): _____

1.22. Code the following: Thalassemia, minor.

Code(s): _____

1.23. This 48-year-old female is seen for sickle-cell crisis with acute chest syndrome. Assign the correct **diagnosis** code(s).

Code(s): _____

1.24. Code the following diagnosis: Severe combined immunodeficiency [SCID] with low T- and B-cell numbers.

Code(s): _____

Chapter 4: Endocrine, nutritional and metabolic diseases (E00-E89)

All neoplasms, whether functionally active or not, are classified in Chapter 2. Appropriate codes in Chapter 4 (namely, E05.8, E07.0, E16-E31, E34.-) may be used as additional codes to indicate either functional activity by neoplasms and ectopic endocrine tissue or hyperfunction and hypofunction of endocrine glands associated with neoplasms and other conditions classified elsewhere. Excluded in this chapter are transitory endocrine and metabolic disorders specific to the newborn (P70-P74).

Diabetes Mellitus

The diabetes mellitus codes are now combination codes that include the type of diabetes, the body system affected, and the complications affecting that body system. As many diabetes codes as are necessary to describe all of the complications of the disease may be used, and should be sequenced based on the reason for a particular encounter. The diabetes mellitus codes are no longer classified as controlled or uncontrolled. There is a note in the Index that inadequately controlled, out of control, and poorly controlled are coded to Diabetes, by type, with hyperglycemia.

The categories for diabetes in ICD-10-CM are
- Diabetes mellitus due to underlying condition (E08)
- Drug or chemical induced diabetes mellitus (E09)
- Type 1 diabetes mellitus (E10)
- Type 2 diabetes mellitus (E11)
- Other specified diabetes mellitus (E13)

It is important to review the coding guidelines and the notes in each category when coding diabetes mellitus. There is one particular note available in each category except for diabetes mellitus type 1. This note states "Use additional code to identify any insulin use (Z79.4)." This code would not be assigned with type 1 cases because insulin is required to sustain life.

Chapter 4 Coding Cases

> **Coding Guideline I.C.4.a. Diabetes Mellitus**
> The diabetes mellitus codes are combination codes that include the type of diabetes mellitus, the body system affected, and the complications affecting that body system. As many codes within a particular category as are necessary to describe all of the complications of the disease may be used. They should be sequenced based on the reason for a particular encounter. Assign as many codes from categories E08-E13 as needed to identify all of the associated conditions that the patient has.

1.25. This 62-year-old male is being seen for mild nonproliferative diabetic retinopathy with macular edema. He has type 2 DM and takes insulin on a daily basis. He also has diabetic cataract in his right eye. What **diagnosis** codes are assigned?

Code(s): _____

1.26. The patient, a type 1 diabetic with diabetic chronic kidney disease, stage 3, is being seen for regulation of insulin dosage. The patient has an abscessed right molar, which was determined, in part, to be responsible for elevation of the patient's blood sugar. What **diagnosis** codes are assigned?

Code(s): _____

> **Coding Guideline I.C.4.a.6. Secondary Diabetes Mellitus**
> Codes under categories E08, Diabetes mellitus due to underlying condition, and E09, Drug or chemical induced diabetes mellitus, identify complications/manifestations associated with secondary diabetes mellitus. Secondary diabetes is always caused by another condition or event (e.g., cystic fibrosis, malignant neoplasm of pancreas, pancreatectomy, adverse effect of drug, poisoning).

> **Coding Guideline I.C.4.a.6.b. Assigning and Sequencing Secondary Diabetes Codes and Its Causes**
> The sequencing of the secondary diabetes codes in relationship to codes for the cause of the diabetes is based on the Tabular List instructions for categories E08 and E09.

1.27. Assign the codes for a 32-year-old female with secondary diabetes mellitus due to acute idiopathic pancreatitis. She has diabetic hyperglycemia and takes insulin.

Code(s): _____

1.28. Assign the code(s) for the following diagnosis: Morbid obesity with a BMI of 42 in an adult.

Code(s): _____

1.29. Assign the code(s) for the following diagnosis: Bulimia with moderate protein–calorie malnutrition.

Code(s): _____

1.30. The patient was seen with severe abdominal cramping, nausea and vomiting, and diarrhea. She states that she ate turkey salad several hours before these symptoms developed. The patient has had the symptoms for about 15 hours. Lab tests show dehydration. The patient was treated with IV therapy. Diagnosis: Dehydration. Salmonella gastroenteritis, abdominal cramping, nausea, vomiting, and diarrhea. What **diagnosis** codes are assigned?

Code(s): _____

1.31. The patient is a 31-year-old male with a history of type 1 diabetes mellitus and is on 15 units of NPH and 10 units of Regular in the morning, and 10 units of NPH and 5 of Regular in the evening. The patient is currently having symptoms of nausea with severe vomiting. The patient at the same time has had increased frequency of urination and polydipsia. The patient is also severely dehydrated. The patient was hydrated, and, as a result, his blood sugar decreased from more than 600 to normal levels. The patient was diagnosed with diabetic ketoacidosis, type 1. What **diagnosis** codes are assigned?

Code(s): _____

Coding Guideline I.C.19.e.5.a. Adverse Effect
When coding an adverse effect of a drug that has been correctly prescribed and properly administered, assign the appropriate code for the nature of the adverse effect followed by the appropriate code for the adverse effect of the drug (T36-T50). The code for the drug should have a fifth or sixth character 5.

Coding Note: A note appears in the Tabular, under category E09, instructing to "Use additional code for adverse effect, if applicable, to identify drug (T36-T50 with fifth or sixth character 5)." **Use the Drugs and Chemical Table to locate this code**.

An additional note appears in the Tabular under category E09 instructing to "Use additional code to identify any insulin use (Z79.4)."

1.32. The 34-year-old patient is being seen for ongoing management of steroid-induced diabetes mellitus which was due to the prolonged use of corticosteroids, which have been discontinued. The patient's diabetes is managed with insulin which he has been taking for the last two years. What **diagnosis** codes are assigned?

Code(s): _____

1.33. The patient is being seen because of increasingly irritating symptomatology, including nervousness, irritability, increased perspiration, shakiness and increased appetite with unexplained weight loss, increased heart rate, palpitations, and sleeping difficulties. A thyroid stimulating hormone test revealed elevated levels and a thyroid nuclear medicine scan revealed hyperactivity of the entire thyroid gland. Based on the diagnostic findings the patient was diagnosed with hyperthyroidism with multinodular goiter. The patient was started on oral anti-thyroid medication. Arrangements were also made for patient to see a cardiologist due to the fact that her palpitations were more pronounced than seen in other patients with hyperthyroidism. What **diagnosis** codes are assigned?

Code(s): _____

1.34. This type 1 diabetic patient has a severe chronic diabetic left foot ulcer with diabetic peripheral angiopathy. He also has diabetic stage 2 chronic kidney disease. He is being evaluated to see if debridement is required for this ulcer with breakdown of the skin. What **diagnosis** codes are assigned?

Code(s): _____

Chapter 5: Mental, behavioral and neurodevelopmental disorders (F01-F99)

The codes in this chapter include disorders of psychological development, but exclude symptoms, signs, and abnormal clinical laboratory finding (R00-R99). The arrangement of the codes within the various sections of ICD-10-CM is significantly different.

A number of changes to category and subcategory titles have been made; for example, ICD-9-CM subcategory 296.0 is Bipolar I disorder, single manic episode, but the ICD-10-CM counterpart, category F30, is Manic episode.

There are unique codes for alcohol and drug use (not specified as abuse or dependence), and abuse and dependence, so careful review of the documentation is required. And there are changes to the codes for drug and alcohol abuse and dependence as they no longer identify continuous or episodic use. A history of drug or alcohol dependence is coded as "in remission." Further, there are combination codes for drug and alcohol use and associated conditions, such as withdrawal, sleep disorders, or psychosis. There is a code for blood alcohol level (Y90.-) that can be assigned as an additional code when documentation indicates its use.

There is a change in sequencing involving the intellectual disability codes (F70-F79). In ICD-9-CM, an additional code for any associated psychiatric or physical condition(s) should be sequenced after the intellectual disability code. In ICD-10-CM, any associated physical or developmental disorder should be coded first.

Chapter 5 Coding Cases

1.35. Code the following diagnosis: Alcohol abuse with intoxication.

Code(s): _____

1.36. This young man is seen for continued follow-up for treatment of his dependence on amphetamines. How should this diagnosis be coded?

Code(s): _____

1.37. This 25-year-old male presents to the clinic requesting assistance for cessation of chewing tobacco use. He has been a chronic user of chewing tobacco since age 13 and is now motivated to quit. Counseling on the options for chewing tobacco cessation was provided to the patient. Diagnosis: Counseling for cessation of tobacco dependence. What **diagnosis** codes are assigned?

Code(s): _____

Coding Note: The ICD-10-CM classification system does not provide separate "history" codes for alcohol and drug abuse. These conditions are identified as "in remission" in ICD-10-CM.

Coding Guideline I.C.5.b.1. In Remission
Selection of codes for "in remission" for categories F10-F19, Mental and behavioral disorders due to psychoactive substance use (categories F10-F19 with -.21) requires the provider's clinical judgment. The appropriate codes for "in remission" are assigned only on the basis of provider documentation (as defined in the Official Guidelines for Coding and Reporting).

1.38.   Joe, a 43-year-old male, is currently receiving treatment for alcohol dependence. As a result of Joe's drinking he is also on medication for chronic alcoholic gastritis. He also has a history of cocaine dependence. What **diagnosis** codes are assigned?

Code(s): _____

1.39.   The patient is seen for individual psychotherapy as part of his long-term treatment for borderline personality disorder. His condition is described as "cluster B personality disorder." The patient has been taking his monoamine oxidase inhibitor (MAOI) medication and reports he feels it has helped him manage his impulsive, overly emotional, and erratic behavior. The patient is also a recovering alcoholic which the therapist describes as being "in remission." The patient will return next week for his scheduled appointment. What **diagnosis** codes are assigned?

Code(s): _____

Coding Note: ICD-10-CM provides a code to indicate blood alcohol level. Under the category F10, there is a "use additional code" note for blood alcohol level. Blood alcohol level can be indexed in the Index to External Causes.

1.40.   This 18-year-old male has been drinking since he was 13. He was brought to the ER and then admitted because of acute alcohol inebriation. Blood alcohol level shows 22 mg/100 ml. The discharge diagnosis is acute alcohol intoxication with chronic alcohol dependence, continuous. What **diagnosis** codes are assigned?

Code(s): _____

Chapter 6: Diseases of the nervous system (G00-G99)

Sense organs have been separated from nervous system disorders, creating two new chapters for diseases of eye and adnexa (Chapter 7) and diseases of the ear and mastoid process (Chapter 8).

The following conditions have been moved from ICD-9-CM Chapter 7: Diseases of the Circulatory System, to ICD-10-CM Chapter 6: Basilar and carotid artery syndromes, transient global amnesia, and transient cerebral ischemic attack.

A note at categories G81 (Hemiplegia and hemiparesis), G82 (Paraplegia and quadriplegia) and G83 (Other paralytic syndromes) provides this information: This category is to be used only when the listed conditions are reported without further specification, or are stated to be old or longstanding but of unspecified cause. The category is also for use in multiple coding to identify these conditions resulting from any cause. Paralytic sequelae of cerebral infarct/stroke are in Chapter 9: Diseases of the circulatory system.

The terminology for epilepsy has been updated, with terms to classify the disorder such as: localization-related idiopathic epilepsy, generalized idiopathic epilepsy, and special epileptic syndromes. Within those various categories, more specificity is possible, such as identifying seizures of localized onset, complex partial seizures, intractable, and status epilepticus. A note with category G40, Epilepsy and recurrent seizures and G43, Migraine provides the following terms to be considered equivalent to intractable: pharmacoresistent (pharmacologically resistant), treatment resistant, refractory (medically), and poorly controlled.

Chapter 6 Coding Cases

1.41. This 52-year-old male has been having increasing dementia and forgetfulness. He has been wandering off and leaving his home and forgetting where he is or where he is going. The diagnosis of dementia due to early-onset Alzheimer's was established. What **diagnosis** codes are assigned?

Code(s): _____

1.42. This patient, a 15-year-old female, is being seen for management of juvenile myoclonic epilepsy. The patient did not respond to treatment and was diagnosed with an intractable seizure. What **diagnosis** codes are assigned?

Code(s): _____

> **Coding Guideline I.C.6.a. Dominant/Nondominant Side**
> Codes from category G81, Hemiplegia and hemiparesis, and subcategories, G83.1, Monoplegia of lower limb, G83.2, Monoplegia of upper limb, and G83.3, Monoplegia, unspecified, identify whether the dominant or nondominant side is affected. Should the affected side be documented, but not specified as dominant or nondominant and the classification system does not indicate a default, code selection is as follows:
> - For ambidextrous patients, the default should be dominant
> - If the left side is affected the default is nondominant
> - If the right side is affected the default is dominant

1.43. Assign the code(s) for the following diagnosis: Left-sided hemiplegia.

Code(s): _____

> **Coding Guideline II.C. Two or More Diagnoses that Equally Meet the Definition of Principal Diagnosis**
> In the unusual instance when two or more diagnoses equally meet the criteria for principal diagnosis as determined by the circumstances of admission, diagnostic workup, and/or therapy provided, and the Alphabetic Index, Tabular List, or another coding guideline does not provide sequencing direction, any one of the diagnoses may be sequenced first.

1.44. The patient was admitted with high fever, stiff neck, chest pain, and nausea. A lumbar puncture was performed and results were positive for meningitis. Chest x-ray revealed pneumonia. Sputum cultures grew pneumococcus. Patient was treated with IV antibiotics. The established diagnoses were pneumococcal meningitis and pneumococcal pneumonia. Code the **diagnoses** for this case only.

Code(s): _____

1.45. This patient has been taking Haloperidol as prescribed for paranoid schizophrenia. He is being seen for change in facial expressions and stiffness in the arms and legs. Diagnosis: Secondary Parkinsonism due to Haloperidol. The drug will be discontinued. What **diagnosis** codes are assigned?

Code(s): _____

1.46. This 45-year-old female patient has breast cancer of the right breast with multiple metastases to the liver. She is seen to control the severe acute pain of the liver metastases. What **diagnosis** codes are assigned?

Code(s): _____

1.47. The patient, a type 2 diabetic with neuropathy, developed weakness of the left arm and leg. The patient was brought to the emergency room where he could speak but was unable to use his left arm and leg. Diagnostic radiographic procedures were scheduled; however, the patient completely recovered and was able to ambulate with no neurological deficits within 24 hours. Due to the complete recovery, it was determined that the patient had experienced a TIA. During this encounter the patient also was treated for an intractable classical migraine. What **diagnosis** codes are assigned?

Code(s): _____

Chapter 7: Diseases of the eye and adnexa (H00-H59)

Chapter 7 is a new chapter in ICD-10-CM, and these conditions were previously included with Diseases of the Nervous System and Sense Organs.

Codes have been expanded to increase anatomic specificity and add the concept of laterality. Many of the codes include right, left, bilateral, and unspecified eye. If the option of bilateral is not available (e.g., eczematous dermatitis of eyelid), and the condition is present in both eyes, it is correct to assign the code for right and left. If, however, a code exists for bilateral, that should be assigned, not right and left eye.

Chapter 7 Coding Cases

1.48. This 40-year-old woman presents to her physician with bilateral eye pain. Her condition is diagnosed as nonulcerative bilateral blepharitis of the upper eyelids. What is the correct **diagnosis** coding for this case?

Code(s): _____

1.49. Code the following diagnosis: Recurrent pterygium, bilateral.

Code(s): _____

1.50. This elderly woman is seen in the clinic for follow-up of her age-related nuclear cataract. At this time, it is only in her left eye. Code the **diagnosis** for this case.

Code(s): _____

> **Coding Note:** Multiple codes in the H40 category require a seventh character to designate the stage of the glaucoma. These stages are as follows:
>   0 – stage unspecified
>   1 – mild stage
>   2 – moderate stage
>   3 – severe stage
>   4 – indeterminate stage

> **Coding Guideline I.C.7.a.5. Indeterminate Stage Glaucoma**
> Assignment of the seventh character 4, Indeterminate stage, should be based on the clinical documentation. The seventh character 4 is used for glaucomas whose stage cannot be clinically determined. This seventh character should not be confused with the seventh character 0, unspecified, which should be assigned when there is no documentation regarding the stage of the glaucoma.

1.51. This is a visit for this patient with moderate primary open-angle glaucoma of the left eye. What is the correct **diagnosis** code for this case?

Code(s): _____

1.52. This patient presents to his physician with continued eye problems following cataract surgery. Ultimately, this is diagnosed as bullous keratopathy, left eye, due to cataract surgery. What is the correct **diagnosis** codes?

Code(s): _____

1.53. This elderly woman was being treated for her right eye age-related cortical cataract at this day-surgery center. After the procedure was completed, the patient suffered a postoperative hemorrhage of the eye. This was addressed by the surgeon. What is the correct **diagnosis** code(s)?

Code(s): _____

Chapter 8: Diseases of the ear and mastoid process (H60-H95)

Chapter 8 is also a new chapter in ICD-10-CM and includes conditions previously found in the Nervous System and Sense Organs chapter.

Codes have also been expanded to increase anatomic specificity and add the concept of laterality.

A number of new instructional notes have been added. The note at the beginning of the chapter states to use an external cause code following the code for the ear condition, if applicable, to identify the cause of the ear condition.

The following note addresses otitis media categories H65, H66:
> Use additional code for any associated perforated tympanic membrane (H72.-)
> Use additional code to identify:
>> exposure to environmental tobacco smoke (Z77.22)
>> exposure to tobacco smoke in the perinatal period (P96.81)
>> history of tobacco use (Z87.891)
>> occupational exposure to environmental tobacco smoke (Z57.31)
>> tobacco dependence (F17.-)
>> tobacco use (Z72.0)

Notes indicating that the underlying disease should be coded first have been added; for example, there is a note under the ICD-10-CM category for perforation of tympanic membrane indicating that any associated otitis media should be coded first.

Chapter 8 Coding Cases

1.54. A five-year-old female is seen for acute ear pain. Examination reveals left acute serous otitis media. Further examination revealed a total perforated tympanic membrane of the right ear due to chronic otitis media. What **diagnoses** codes are assigned?

Code(s): _____

1.55. Assign the code for the following diagnosis: Ménière's vertigo of left ear.

Code(s): _____

1.56. This 50-year-old female, admitted to the hospital for surgery, has bilateral conductive hearing loss due to nonobliterative otosclerosis of the stapes at the oval window. She is unable to hear with hearing aids and has decided to undergo left stapedectomy. During the surgery an inadvertent laceration was made to the tympanic meatal flap, which was repaired. What **diagnosis** codes are assigned?

Code(s): _____

Chapter 9: Diseases of the circulatory system (I00-I99)

Some codes have been moved to Chapter 9 from other chapters in ICD-9-CM, for example, Binswanger's disease; chronic and mesenteric lymphadenitis; and gangrene.

The type of hypertension (benign, malignant, unspecified) is not used as an axis for the ICD-10-CM hypertension codes; there is only one code for essential hypertension (I10).

The category for late effects of cerebrovascular disease has been retitled "Sequelae of cerebrovascular disease," and it has been restructured by expanding all subcategory codes. This expansion involves specifying laterality, changing subcategory titles, making terminology changes, adding sixth characters, and providing greater specificity in general. Late effects of cerebrovascular disease are differentiated by type of stroke (hemorrhage, infarction).

The terminology has changed for some cardiovascular conditions; for example, "intermediate coronary syndrome" has been retitled "unstable angina."

Acute Myocardial Infarction (AMI)

The time frame for acute myocardial infarction (AMI) codes has changed from eight weeks or less in ICD-9-CM to four weeks or less in ICD-10-CM.

In the acute myocardial infarction codes, ST elevation (STEMI) and non-ST elevation (NSTEMI) are in the ICD-10-CM code titles instead of just being inclusion terms.

Chapter 9 contains codes for initial AMIs (I21) and subsequent AMIs (I22). A code from category I22, Subsequent ST elevation (STEMI) and non-ST elevation (NSTEMI) myocardial infarction is to be used when a patient who has suffered an AMI has a new AMI within the four-week time frame of the initial AMI. A code from category I22 must be used in conjunction with a code from category I21. The sequencing of the I22 and I21 codes depends on the circumstances of the encounter.

It is important to review the use additional code related to tobacco use or exposure.

Chapter 9 Coding Cases

1.57.   This patient is seen today for follow-up for his benign hypertension. What is the correct **diagnosis** code?

   Code(s): _____

Coding Guideline I.C.9.a.3. Hypertensive Heart and Chronic Kidney Disease
Assign codes from combination category I13, Hypertensive heart and chronic kidney disease, when both hypertensive kidney disease and hypertensive heart disease are stated in the diagnosis. Assume a relationship between the hypertension and the chronic kidney disease, whether or not the condition is so designated. If heart failure is present, assign an additional code from category I50 to identify the type of heart failure.

The appropriate code from category N18, Chronic kidney disease, should be used as a secondary code with a code from I13 to identify the stage of chronic kidney disease.

1.58. Code the following diagnoses: Stage 3 chronic kidney disease with congestive heart failure (CHF) due to hypertension.

Code(s): _____

Coding Guideline I.C.9.e.3. AMI Documented as Nontransmural or Subendocardial but Site Provided
If an AMI is documented as nontransmural or subendocardial, but the site is provided, it is still coded as subendocardial AMI.

Coding Guideline I.C.9.e.1. ST Elevation Myocardial Infarction (STEMI) and Non-ST Elevation Myocardial Infarction (NSTEMI)
If NSTEMI evolves to STEMI, assign the STEMI code. If STEMI converts to NSTEMI due to thrombolytic therapy, it is still coded as a STEMI.

1.59. This 54-year-old female is being treated for an acute non-ST anterior wall myocardial infarction which she suffered 5 days ago. She also has atrial fibrillation. What is the correct **diagnosis** code(s)?

Code(s): _____

Coding Guideline I.C.9.e.4. Subsequent Myocardial Infarction
A code from category I22, Subsequent ST elevation (STEMI) and non-ST elevation (NSTEMI) myocardial infarction is to be used when a patient who has suffered an AMI has a new AMI within the 4 week time frame of the initial AMI. A code from category I22 must be used in conjunction with a code from category I21. The sequencing of the I22 and I21 codes depends on the circumstances of the encounter.

1.60. This same patient (from problem #1.59) presented to the emergency department two weeks later and was diagnosed with an acute inferior wall myocardial infarction. She is still being monitored following her initial heart attack two weeks earlier and continues to have atrial fibrillation. She will be transferred to a larger facility for cardiac catheterization and possible further intervention. What **diagnosis** codes are assigned?

Code(s): _____

> **Coding Note:** A code from category I23 must be used in conjunction with a code from category I21 or category I22. The I23 code should be sequenced first, if it is the reason for encounter, or, it should be sequenced after the I21 or I22 code if the complication of the MI occurs during the encounter for the MI.

1.61. This patient is seen in consultation after readmission for postinfarction angina. She was discharged two days ago after treatment for an anterior wall ST elevation myocardial infarction. What is the correct **diagnosis** code assignment?

Code(s): _____

> **Coding Guideline I.C.9.b. Atherosclerotic Coronary Artery Disease and Angina**
> ICD-10-CM has combination codes for atherosclerotic heart disease with angina pectoris. The subcategories for these codes are I25.11, Atherosclerotic heart disease of native coronary artery with angina pectoris and I25.7, Atherosclerosis of coronary artery bypass graft(s) and coronary artery of transplanted heart with angina pectoris.
>
> When using one of these combination codes it is not necessary to use an additional code for angina pectoris. A causal relationship can be assumed in a patient with both atherosclerosis and angina pectoris, unless the documentation indicates the angina is due to something other than the atherosclerosis.

1.62. What is the correct **diagnosis** coding for a patient with coronary artery disease (CAD) with angina? This patient has no previous history of CABG.

Code(s): _____

1.63. This 63-year-old male is being seen for treatment of his unstable angina. This gentleman has a history of 2-vessel coronary artery bypass approximately 18 months ago. A recent cardiac catheterization shows continued evidence of coronary arteriosclerosis but both of the bypass grafts are patent. Also, of note, is that this patient suffered a cerebrovascular infarction three years ago which resulted in right-side (dominant) hemiparesis. What is the correct diagnosis code(s)?

Code(s): _____

1.64. This 75-year-old man is seen today for treatment of his congestive heart failure. After study, the final **diagnosis** was documented as acute on chronic diastolic congestive heart failure. What is the correct diagnosis code assignment?

Code(s): _____

1.65. Code the following case: Acute cerebral infarction, thrombosis of the left anterior cerebral artery with residual right-sided hemiplegia.

Code(s): _____

Coding Guideline I.C.9.d.1. Category I69, Sequelae of Cerebrovascular Disease
Category I69 is used to indicate conditions classifiable to categories I60-I67 as the causes of sequela (neurologic deficits), themselves classified elsewhere. These "late effects" include neurologic deficits that persist after the initial onset of conditions classifiable to categories I60-I67. The neurologic deficits caused by cerebrovascular disease may be present from the onset or may arise at any time after the onset of the condition classifiable to categories I60-I67.

Codes from category I69, Sequelae of cerebrovascular disease, that specify hemiplegia, hemiparesis and monoplegia identify whether the dominant or nondominant side is affected. Should the affected side be documented, but not specified as dominant or nondominant, and the classification system does not indicate a default, code selection is as follows:
    For ambidextrous patients, the default should be dominant
    If the left side is affected, the default is non-dominant
    If the right side is affected, the default is dominant

Coding Guideline I.C.9.d.2. Codes from Category I69 with Codes from I60-I67
Codes from category I69 may be assigned on a health care record with codes from I60-I67, if the patient has a current cerebrovascular disease and deficits from an old cerebrovascular disease.

1.66. This pleasant gentleman is seen in the clinic to follow up from a previous stroke. He suffered a cerebrovascular infarction 6 months ago which left him with aphasia and left-sided hemiparesis on his nondominant side. The patient will be referred to outpatient rehabilitation for speech, physical, and occupational therapy. What is the correct **diagnosis** code(s)?

    Code(s): _____

1.67. This 62-year-old male patient was admitted to the hospital with progressive episodes of chest pain determined to be crescendo angina. The patient has no previous history of CABG. He had myocardial infarction five years ago and was diagnosed with coronary artery disease and progressively has been having more frequent episodes of chest pain. During the hospital stay, he was given IV nitroglycerin and was subsequently placed on Cardizem for further treatment of his angina. He was scheduled for cardiac catheterization next week. No other complications arose during the hospitalization. What is the correct **diagnosis** code(s)?

    Code(s): _____

1.68. This patient is seen for evaluation of his continuing unstable angina. After significant evaluation, his symptoms were found to be due to atherosclerosis of his bypassed graft. This is an autologous arterial graft. Final diagnosis: CAD of bypass graft with unstable angina and hypertensive congestive heart failure. The patient will be scheduled for surgery. What is the correct **diagnosis** code(s)?

    Code(s): _____

1.69. This patient is being treated for a current inferolateral ST elevation myocardial infarction. This case is complicated by the development a hemopericardium as a result of the infarction. What is the correct **diagnosis** code(s)?

Code(s): _____

1.70. Assign the correct **diagnosis** code(s): Acute cerebrovascular infarction—embolism of the left cerebellar artery with dysphagia and right hemiplegia.

Code(s): _____

Chapter 10: Diseases of the respiratory system (J00-J99)

Certain codes have moved to Chapter 10 from other locations, for example, streptococcal sore throat.

Lobar pneumonia has a unique code in a category for pneumonia, unspecified organism, rather than being classified to the code for pneumococcal pneumonia.

The terminology used to describe asthma has been updated to reflect the current clinical classification of asthma. The following terms have been added to describe asthma: mild intermittent and three degrees of persistent—mild persistent, moderate persistent, and severe persistent. Intrinsic asthma (nonallergic) and extrinsic (allergic) are both classified to J45.909, Unspecified asthma, uncomplicated.

A note at the beginning of the chapter states: When a respiratory condition is described as occurring in more than one site and is not specifically indexed, it should be classified to the lower anatomic site (for example, tracheobronchitis to bronchitis in J40).

Some of the codes in Chapter 10 have been expanded to include notes indicating that an additional code should be assigned or an associated condition should be sequenced first. The following are examples of the notations:
- Use additional code to identify the infectious agent
- Use additional code to identify the virus
- Code first any associated lung abscess
- Code first the underlying disease
- Use additional code to identify other conditions such as tobacco use or exposure

Chapter 10 Coding Cases

1.71.   A four-year-old child was seen with a high fever, cough, and chest pain. Diagnosis of diffuse bronchopneumonia was made. Gram stain of the sputum showed numerous small gram-negative coccobacilli. Diagnosis: H. influenza pneumonia. What **diagnosis** codes are assigned?

Code(s): _____

1.72.   The patient has increasing shortness of breath, weakness, and ineffective cough. Treatment included oxygen therapy and advice for smoking cessation. Diagnoses listed as acute respiratory insufficiency due to acute exacerbation of COPD and tobacco dependence. What **diagnosis** codes are assigned?

Code(s): _____

1.73. This 10-year-old female child is being seen because of severe persistent asthma with acute exacerbation. What **diagnosis** codes are assigned?

Code(s): _____

1.74. This 75-year-old female was brought to the ER with severe difficulty in breathing. She was intubated and started on mechanical ventilation and admitted. Diagnoses for this patient: Acute respiratory failure, acute infectious bronchitis with acute exacerbation of COPD. What **diagnosis** codes are assigned?

Code(s): _____

1.75. This 60-year-old male was admitted to the hospital with chest rales, dyspnea, cyanosis, and hypotension. He has severe gastroesophageal reflux causing him to aspirate food. He was treated for his aspiration pneumonia with respiratory therapy and antibiotics. What **diagnosis** codes are assigned?

Code(s): _____

1.76. A 17-year-old college student was treated for cough, fever, body aches, and headache. Diagnosis: Upper respiratory tract infection due to novel influenza A virus. What **diagnosis** codes are assigned?

Code(s): _____

1.77. The physician has documented the following diagnoses for this elderly patient: COPD with emphysema, CHF, hypertension, and atrial fibrillation. What **diagnosis** codes are assigned?

Code(s): _____

> **Coding Note:** In the Tabular, there is a note under category J44 to code also type of asthma, if applicable (J45.-).

> **Coding Note:** In the Tabular there is an *Excludes2* note under category J45 for asthma with chronic obstructive pulmonary disease.
>
> By definition, when an *Excludes2* note appears under a code, it is acceptable to use both the code and the excluded code together if the patient has both conditions at the same time.

1.78. **Discharge Diagnosis:** Moderate persistent asthma with status asthmaticus
Acute exacerbation of chronic obstructive pulmonary disease

Hospital Course: The patient presented with gradual increase in shortness of breath, which was unresponsive to home nebulizer treatments. In the emergency room, he received more respiratory treatments; however, he failed to improve. Therefore, the patient was admitted to the hospital. At the time of admission, the theophylline level was 5.9. Chest x-ray showed no evidence of active infiltrates. The patient was bolused with intravenous steroids and started on frequent respiratory therapy treatments. IV aminophylline boluses and drip were used to increase his theophylline level to therapeutic range. The patient gradually cleared and by the next day was much better. His IV aminophylline was changed to p.o. The Ventolin treatments were decreased to q 4 hr. and his steroids were rapidly tapered back to 10 mg of Prednisone. What **diagnosis** codes are assigned?

Code(s): _____

1.79. A ventilator-dependent patient (due to COPD with emphysema) is admitted to the hospital for dehydration. IV fluids are started for hydration and the patient is placed on the hospital's ventilator. What is the appropriate **diagnosis** code assignment?

Code(s): _____

> **Coding Note:** A note appears in the Tabular under code I69.391 to use an additional code to identify the type of dysphagia, if known (R13.1-).

1.80. An elderly nursing home patient was seen for pneumonia. The patient has frequent aspiration pneumonia because of his difficulty in swallowing (neurogenic) due to a previous cerebral infarction. In addition to the aspiration-type pneumonia, the patient also has stage 1 decubitus ulcers on both his left and right hip. What **diagnosis** codes are assigned?

Code(s): _____

Chapter 11: Diseases of the digestive system (K00-K95)

Some of the disease categories in Chapter 11 have been restructured to bring together those groups that are in some way related. For example, Chapter 11 contains two new sections: Diseases of liver (K70-K77) and Disorders of gallbladder, biliary tract, and pancreas (K80-K87). And in some cases, headings of subcategories have been changed; for example, angiodysplasia of intestine is in a subcategory for "other specified disorders of intestine" in ICD-9-CM, whereas it is in a subcategory for "vascular disorders of intestine" in ICD-10-CM.

Instructional notes indicating that an additional code should be assigned for associated conditions and external causes or that an underlying condition should be coded first have been expanded.

Chapter 11 Coding Cases

> **Coding Note:** Hernia with both gangrene and obstruction is classified to hernia with gangrene.

1.81. This patient is seen for treatment of a recurrent right inguinal hernia with gangrene and obstruction. What is the correct code assignment for this case?

Code(s): _____

1.82. Assign the **diagnosis** code(s) for Acute gastric ulcer with hemorrhage.

Code(s): _____

1.83. This patient has been diagnosed with choledocholithiasis with acute cholangitis and obstruction. What is the correct **diagnosis** code(s)?

Code(s): _____

> **Coding Note:** ICD-10-CM provides combination codes for complications commonly associated with Crohn's disease. These combination codes can be found under subcategory K50.0.

1.84. This 30-year-old woman has been treated for Crohn's disease of the small intestine since she was 18-years-old. She has had several exacerbations of the disease in the past years. At this time, small bowel x-ray shows a small bowel obstruction. The obstruction was found to be a result of an exacerbation of her Crohn's disease. What is the correct diagnosis code(s)?

Code(s): _____

1.85. A 70-year-old female was visiting relatives in the area and was brought to the emergency department, complaining of vomiting blood and having very dark stools that appeared to be bloody. The patient had gone out to dinner with relatives and shortly after returning home, started vomiting and having diarrhea and blamed it on the large meal. She continued to have these symptoms overnight and her family members insisted she come to the hospital. The patient is taking Prinivil, Lanoxin, and Lasix for congestive heart failure and atrial fibrillation and these medications were continued. The gastroenterologist was called to consult and found a past history of gastric ulcer. The patient had EGD 5 months earlier showing chronic bleeding ulcer in the antrum of the stomach. She was placed on medication and warned that this may be a recurrent problem. The patient refused a follow-up EGD and requested to be released to return home and receive treatment from her regular physician. It should be noted that serial blood counts did not find any significant anemia. The patient was discharged with a diagnosis of chronic bleeding gastric ulcer and copies of her medical records to take home for review by her private physician. What is the correct **diagnosis** code(s)?

Code(s): _____

1.86. A 68-year-old man was admitted to the hospital for bilateral inguinal hernia repair that could not be done on an outpatient basis because of anticipated extended recovery time required due to his COPD, chronic low back pain, and hypertension. After being prepared for surgery, the patient complained of precordial chest pain. The surgery was canceled and the patient was returned to his room. Cardiac studies failed to find a reason for the chest pain which resolved later that day. What are the correct **diagnosis** codes?

Code(s): _____

1.87. This nursing home patient has extensive cellulitis of the abdominal wall. The examination performed reveals that his existing gastrostomy site is infected. He had a feeding tube inserted four months ago because of carcinoma of the middle esophagus. The physician confirmed that the responsible organism for the infection is methicillin resistant *Staph. aureus* (MRSA). What **diagnosis** codes are assigned?

Code(s): _____

Chapter 12: Diseases of the skin and subcutaneous tissue (L00-L99)

Chapter 12 has been restructured to bring together groups of diseases that are related to one another in some way, moving from three subsections in ICD-9-CM to nine subsections in ICD-10-CM. In ICD-10-CM, these are referred to as blocks.

Instructional notes have been expanded and have several uses in this chapter. They indicate an additional code should be used to identify the organism or infectious agent. Notes also indicate that the underlying disease or associated underlying condition should be coded first. Examples are listed here:

- L14, Bullous disorders in diseases classified elsewhere, Code first underlying disease
- L97, Non-pressure chronic ulcer of lower limb, not elsewhere classified, Code first any associated underlying condition

A note under block L20-L30, Dermatitis and eczema, indicates that in this block, the terms "dermatitis" and "eczema" are used synonymously and interchangeably.

For pressure ulcers (L89), the site, laterality, and severity are specified in a single code in ICD-10-CM. The severity identified is stage 1 through stage 4. Any associated gangrene should be sequenced first.

Non-pressure chronic ulcers of lower limbs NEC (L97) are also specified by site, laterality, and severity. Code first any associated underlying condition such as:

> Any associated gangrene (I96)
> Atherosclerosis of the lower extremities (I70.23-, I70.24-, I70.33-, I70.34-, I70.43-, I70.44-, I70.53-, I70.54-, I70.63-, I70.64-, I70.73-, I70.74-)
> Chronic venous hypertension (I87.31-, I87.33-)
> Diabetic ulcers (E08.621, E08.622, E09.621, E09.622, E10.621, E10.622, E11.621, E11.622, E13.621, E13.622)
> Postphlebitic syndrome (I87.01-, I87.03-)
> Postthrombotic syndrome (I87.01-, I87.03-)
> Varicose ulcer (I83.0-, I83.2-)

Chapter 12 Coding Cases

Coding Guideline I.C.19.e. Adverse Effects, Poisoning, Underdosing and Toxic Effects
Codes in categories T36-T65 are combination codes that include the substance that was taken as well as the intent.

No additional external cause code is required for poisonings, toxic effects, adverse effects, and underdosing codes.

Coding Guideline I.C.19.e.5.a. Adverse Effect
When coding an adverse effect of a drug that has been correctly prescribed and properly administered, assign the appropriate code for the nature of the adverse effect followed by the appropriate code for the adverse effect of the drug (T36-T50). The code for the drug should have a fifth or sixth character of 5.

Coding Note: An instructional note appears in the Tabular, under codes L27.0 and L27.1, stating to use additional code for adverse effect, if applicable, to identify drug (T36-T50 with fifth or sixth character 5).

1.88. Assign the code(s) for the following diagnosis: Dermatitis covering entire body due to antibiotics (penicillin) taken correctly as prescribed.

Code(s): _____

Coding Guideline I.B.14. Documentation for BMI and Pressure Ulcer Stages
For the body mass index (BMI) and pressure ulcer stage codes, code assignment may be based on medical record documentation from clinicians who are not the patient's provider (i.e., physician or other qualified healthcare practitioner legally accountable for establishing the patient's diagnosis), since this information is typically documented by other clinicians involved in the care of the patient (e.g., a dietitian often documents the BMI and nurses often documents the pressure ulcer stages). However, the associated diagnosis (such as overweight, obesity, or pressure ulcer) must be documented by the patient's provider. If there is conflicting medical record documentation, either from the same clinician or different clinicians, the patient's attending provider should be queried for clarification.

Coding Guideline I.C.12.a.1. Pressure Ulcer Stages
Codes from category L89, Pressure ulcer, are combination codes that identify the site of the pressure ulcer as well as the stage of the ulcer. ICD-10-CM classifies pressure ulcer stages based on severity, which is designated by stages 1-4, unspecified stage, and unstageable. Assign as many codes from category L89 as needed to identify all the pressure ulcers the patient has, if applicable.

1.89. This patient has a gangrenous pressure ulcer of the right hip and a pressure ulcer of the sacrum documented by the physician. The nursing assessment indicates a stage 2 pressure ulcer of the sacrum with a stage 3 decubitus ulcer of the right hip. What **diagnosis** codes are assigned?

Code(s): _____

> **Coding Guideline I.B.14 Documentation for BMI, Non-Pressure ulcers and Pressure Ulcer Stages**
> For the body mass index (BMI), depth of non-pressure chronic ulcers and pressure ulcer stage codes, code assignment may be based on medical record documentation from clinicians who are not the patient's provider, since this information is typically documented by other clinicians involved in the care of the patient (e.g., a dietitian often documents the BMI and nurses often document the pressure ulcer stages). However, the associated diagnosis (such as overweight, obesity, or pressure ulcer) must be documented by the patient's provider. If there is conflicting medical record documentation, either from the same clinician or different clinicians, the patient's attending provider should be queried for clarification.

1.90. Assign the code(s) for the following diagnosis: Atherosclerosis of the right ankle (native artery), with non-healing ulcer, with breakdown of the skin. The breakdown of the skin was documented only by the nurse.

Code(s): _____

1.91. This 35-year-old male patient presents with edema, redness, and pain of the left big toe. He did not seek treatment because he thought it would improve on its own. He does not remember any injury, but the pain has gotten progressively worse for the past week. Diagnosis: Gangrenous abscess of the entire left big toe. What **diagnosis** codes are assigned?

Code(s): _____

1.92. This elderly patient was seen for treatment of cellulitis in the right lower extremity. The cultures grew streptococcus B, and this was documented by the physician as the cause of the cellulitis. Patient also has stage 1 decubitus ulcer of the left buttock and stage 2 decubitus ulcer in the right gluteal region. What **diagnosis** codes are assigned?

Code(s): _____

1.93. The patient was seen for treatment of a fine rash that had developed on the patient's trunk and upper extremities over the last three to four days. The patient was diagnosed with hypertension seven days ago and started on Ramipril 10 mg daily. The physician determined the rash to be dermatitis due to the Ramipril. The Ramipril was discontinued and the patient was prescribed a new antihypertensive medication, Captopril. In addition, the physician prescribed a topical cream for the localized dermatitis. What **diagnosis** codes are assigned?

Code(s): _____

1.94. The patient was seen with extensive inflammation and irritation of the skin of both upper eyelids and under her eyebrows that was spreading to her temples and forehead. Upon questioning the patient, the physician learned that she had recently used new eye cosmetics. The physician had examined the patient during a prior visit for cystic acne. During this visit, the physician also examined the patient's cystic acne on her forehead and jawline. The patient was advised to continue using the medication previously prescribed. Diagnosis was irritant contact dermatitis due to cosmetics and cystic acne. The patient was also advised to immediately discontinue use of any make-up on the face and was given a topical medication to resolve the inflammation. What **diagnosis** codes are assigned?

Code(s): _____

1.95. The patient was seen for intravenous antibiotic treatment of cellulitis of the right anterior neck. The patient is also a known morphine drug abuser and exhibited considerable drug-seeking behavior and continuously requested morphine. All narcotics were discontinued and the patient exhibited no drug withdrawal symptoms.

Diagnoses: Cellulitis, right anterior neck; morphine drug abuse

What **diagnosis** codes are assigned?

Code(s): _____

Chapter 13: Diseases of the musculoskeletal system and connective tissue (M00-M99)

A number of block, category, and subcategory title changes have been made in Chapter 13, for example, subsection 710-719 in ICD-9-CM, Arthropathies and Related Disorders, is called Infectious arthropathies in section M00-M25 in ICD-10-CM. Also a number of conditions have moved to this chapter from other chapters in ICD-9-CM; for example, gout moved from Chapter 3; polyarteritis nodosa moved from Chapter 7; and categories 524, Dentofacial anomalies, including malocclusion, and 526, Diseases of the jaw, moved from Chapter 9.

Bone, joint, or muscle conditions that are the result of a healed injury and recurrent bone, joint, or muscle conditions are also usually found in Chapter 13. Any current, acute injury should be coded to the appropriate injury code from Chapter 19, Injury, poisoning and certain other consequences of external causes; chronic or recurrent conditions should generally be coded with a code from Chapter 13.

The following seventh characters are required for codes in Chapter 13 that represent pathological or stress fractures in category M84.3-M84.6:

A – initial encounter for fracture
D – subsequent encounter for fracture with routine healing
G – subsequent encounter for fracture with delayed healing
K – subsequent encounter for fracture with nonunion
P – subsequent encounter for fracture with malunion
S – sequela

Seventh character A is for use as long as the patient is receiving active treatment for the fracture. Examples of active treatment are: surgical treatment, emergency department encounter, and evaluation and treatment by a new physician. Seventh character D is to be used for encounters after the patient has completed active treatment. Examples of subsequent treatment are: cast change or removal, removal of external or internal fixation device, medication adjustment, other aftercare and follow-up visits following treatment for the fracture.

As with many of the other chapters, codes have been greatly expanded to include greater anatomic specificity and laterality, and instructional notes have been expanded indicating that additional codes should be assigned for associated conditions or an underlying condition should be coded first.

Some terms have been defined in the classification. In category M66, Spontaneous rupture of synovium and tendon a spontaneous rupture is defined as one that occurs when a normal force is applied to tissues that are inferred to have less than normal strength. At category M80, Osteoporosis with current pathological fracture, a fragility fracture is defined as a fracture sustained with trauma no more than a fall from a standing height or less that occurs under circumstances that would not cause a fracture in a normal healthy bone.

Chapter 13 Coding Cases

1.96. Assign the correct diagnosis code: Bacterial septic arthritis, right knee.

Code(s): _____

1.97. This young man is being treated for his ongoing juvenile rheumatoid arthritis. This condition is found only in both ankles. What **diagnosis** codes are assigned?

Code(s): _____

Coding Guideline I.C.13.a. Site and Laterality
Most of the codes within Chapter 13 have site and laterality designations. The site represents either the bone, joint, or muscle involved.

Coding Note: ICD-10-CM has three different categories for pathologic fractures: due to neoplastic disease, due to osteoporosis, and due to other specified disease.

1.98. This 76-year-old man, originally diagnosed with left upper lobe lung carcinoma 5 years ago, is seen for a fracture of the shaft of the right femur. Eight months ago, he was diagnosed with metastatic bone cancer (from the lung) and this fracture is a result of the metastatic disease. This patient's lung cancer was treated with radiation and there is no longer evidence of an existing primary malignancy. What **diagnosis** codes are assigned for this case?

Code(s): _____

Coding Guideline I.C.13.d.2. Osteoporosis with Current Pathological Fracture
Category M80, Osteoporosis with current pathological fracture, is for patients who have a current pathologic fracture at the time of an encounter. The codes under M80 identify the site of the fracture. A code from category M80, not a traumatic fracture code, should be used for any patient with known osteoporosis who suffers a fracture, even if that patient had a minor fall or trauma, if that fall or trauma would not usually break a normal, healthy bone.

1.99. Julia is an 80-year-old female with senile osteoporosis. She complains of severe back pain with no history of trauma. X-rays revealed pathological compression fractures of several lumbar vertebrae. What **diagnosis** codes are assigned?

Code(s): _____

Chapter 14: Diseases of the genitourinary system (N00-N99)

Several block and category title changes have been made in Chapter 14; for example, subsection 617-629 in ICD-9-CM is Other Disorders of Female Genital Tract, whereas the corresponding section in ICD-10-CM, N80-N98, is Noninflammatory disorders of the female genital tract.

Codes have also moved to Chapter 14 from other chapters in ICD-9-CM; for example, ICD-9-CM code 099.40, Other nongonococcal urethritis, unspecified, moved from Chapter 1, but its ICD-10-CM counterpart, code N34.1, Nonspecific urethritis, is in Chapter 14.

Several notes are available to indicate that an additional code should be used. Some examples follow:

- N17, Acute Kidney failure – Code also associated underlying condition
- N18, Chronic kidney disease (CKD) – Code first any associated:
    - diabetic chronic kidney disease (E08.22, E09.22, E10.22, E11.22, E13.22)
    - hypertensive chronic kidney disease (I12.-, I13.-)
    - Use additional code to identify kidney transplant status, if applicable (Z94.0)
- N30, Cystitis – Use additional code to identify infectious agent (B95-B97)
- N31, Neuromuscular dysfunction of bladder, NEC – Use additional code to identify any associated urinary incontinence (N39.3-N39.4-)
- N33, Bladder disorders in diseases classified elsewhere – Code first underlying disease, such as: schistosomiasis (B65.0-B65.9)
- N40.1, Enlarged prostate with lower urinary tract symptoms (LUTS) – Use additional code for associated symptoms, when specified:
    - incomplete bladder emptying (R39.14)
    - nocturia (R35.1)
    - straining on urination (R39.16)
    - urinary frequency (R35.0)
    - urinary hesitancy (R39.11)
    - urinary incontinence (N39.4-)
    - urinary obstruction (N13.8)
    - urinary retention (R33.8)
    - urinary urgency (R39.15)
    - weak urinary stream (R39.12)

Chapter 14 Coding Cases

1.100. This 40-year-old male presents with proteinuria and hematuria. Diagnosis established is chronic nephritic syndrome with diffuse membranous glomerulonephritis. What **diagnosis** code is assigned?

Code(s): _____

1.101. This 30-year-old female was seen with frequent urination with pain. Diagnosis: Acute suppurative cystitis, with hematuria due to E coli. What **diagnosis** codes are assigned?

Code(s): _____

1.102. Assign the code(s) for the following diagnosis: Premenopausal menorrhagia.

Code(s): _____

1.103. An 80-year-old man presented with complaints of lower abdominal pain and the inability to urinate over the past 24 hours, diagnosed as acute kidney failure due to acute tubular necrosis, caused by a urinary obstruction. The urinary obstruction was a result of the patient's benign prostatic hypertrophy. The patient was treated with medications and the acute kidney failure was resolved prior to discharge. The patient will require resection of the prostate but will return at a later date for surgery. What **diagnosis** codes are assigned?

Code(s): _____

Coding Guideline I.C.14.a.2. Chronic Kidney disease and Kidney Transplant Status
Patients who have undergone kidney transplant may still have some form of CKD, because the kidney transplant may not fully restore kidney function. Therefore, the presence of CKD alone does not constitute a transplant complication. Assign the appropriate N18 code for the patient's stage of CKD and code Z94.0, Kidney transplant status. If a transplant complication such as failure or rejection or other transplant complication is documented, see Section I.C.19.g for information on coding complications of a kidney transplant. If the documentation is unclear as to whether the patient has a complication of the transplant, query the physician.

1.104. This 45-year-old female is currently being treated for chronic kidney disease, stage 3. She has previously undergone a kidney transplant but still continues to suffer from chronic kidney disease. This patient is also treated for hypothyroidism following removal of the thyroid for thyroid carcinoma. At this time, there is no longer evidence of an existing thyroid malignancy. What **diagnosis** codes are assigned?

Code(s): _____

1.105. A 78-year-old female is seen with fever, malaise, and left flank pain. A urinalysis shows bacteria of more than 100,000/ml present in the urine and subsequent urine culture shows Proteus growth as the cause of the urinary tract infection. The patient was treated with intravenous antibiotics. The patient also has a history of repeated UTIs over the past several years. What **diagnosis** codes are assigned?

Code(s): _____

Chapter 15: Pregnancy, childbirth and the puerperium (O00-O9A)

Codes have been moved from other chapters in ICD-9-CM to Chapter 15 in ICD-10-CM, for example, encounter for supervision of high-risk pregnancy has been moved from the Supplementary Classification of Factors Influencing Health Status and Contact with Health Services to ICD-10-CM Chapter 15, to category O09.

The episode of care (delivered, antepartum, postpartum) is no longer the axis of classification, but rather the trimester in which the condition occurred. Because certain obstetric conditions or complications occur during certain trimesters, not all conditions include codes for all three trimesters. And some codes do not include the trimester classification at all because the condition always occurs in a specific trimester, or the concept of trimester of pregnancy is not applicable.

The note at the beginning of the chapter defines trimesters: Trimesters are counted from the first day of the last menstrual period. They are defined as follows:
- 1st trimester - less than 14 weeks 0 days
- 2nd trimester - 14 weeks 0 days to less than 28 weeks 0 days
- 3rd trimester - 28 weeks 0 days until delivery

Chapter notes apply to the entire chapter. Note: Codes from this chapter are for use only on maternal records, never on newborn records. A code from category Z3A, Weeks of gestation, should be coded to identify the specific week of the pregnancy. The date of admission should be used to determine weeks of gestation for inpatient admissions that encompass more than one gestational week.

Codes from this chapter are for use for conditions related to or aggravated by the pregnancy, childbirth, or by the puerperium (maternal causes or obstetric causes).

The time frame for differentiating the abortion and fetal death codes has changed from 22 to 20 weeks (see subcategory O36.4). The time frame for differentiating early and late vomiting in pregnancy has changed from 22 to 20 weeks (see category O21). Preterm labor is defined as before 37 completed weeks of gestation (see category O60).

Certain codes in Chapter 15 require a seventh character to identify the fetus in a multiple gestation that is affected by the condition being coded. These are the applicable seventh characters:

> 0 – not applicable or unspecified
> 1 – fetus 1
> 2 – fetus 2
> 3 – fetus 3
> 4 – fetus 4
> 5 – fetus 5
> 9 – other fetus

The seventh character 0 is for single gestations and multiple gestations where the affected fetus is unspecified. Seventh characters 1 through 9 are for cases of multiple gestations to identify the fetus for which the code applies. A code from category O30, Multiple gestation must also be assigned when assigning these codes.

Multiple notes and coding guidelines apply to this chapter, so a very careful review is indicated to become proficient at coding these conditions.

One of the blocks in Chapter 21, Factors influencing health status and contact with health services is Z30-Z39, Persons encountering health services in circumstances related to reproduction. Several categories relate to the pregnant female and will be discussed in this chapter of the training. They are

Z32	Encounter for pregnancy test and childbirth and childcare instruction
Z33	Pregnant state
Z34	Encounter for supervision of normal pregnancy
Z36	Encounter for antenatal screening of mother
Z3A	Weeks of gestation
Z37	Outcome of delivery
Z39	Encounter for maternal postpartum care and examination

Outcome of delivery codes (Z37.0–Z37.9) are intended for use as an additional code to identify the outcome of delivery on the mother's record. It is not for use on the newborn record. These codes exclude stillbirth (P95).

Chapter 15 Coding Cases

Coding Note: The note at the beginning of chapter 15 specifies the use of an additional code from category Z3A, Weeks of gestation, to identify the specific week of the pregnancy. This is found in the Alphabetic Index under Pregnancy, weeks of gestation.

1.106. This 36-year-old G2 P1 woman is 26-weeks pregnant and being seen for gestational hypertension. At this time, she is not having any other problems. What is the correct **diagnosis** code(s)?

Code(s): _____

1.107. Code the following: 16-week pregnancy with mild hyperemesis and urinary tract infection which grew out E. coli.

Code(s): _____

1.108. This 24-year-old woman is 3 weeks postpartum and seen today for breast pain. Final diagnosis documented as nonpurulent postpartum mastitis. What is the correct code?

Code(s): _____

Coding Guideline I.C.15.a.6. Seventh Character for Fetus Identification
Where applicable, a seventh character is to be assigned for certain categories (O31, O32, O33.3-, O33.6, O35, O36, O40, O41, O60.1, O60.2, O64, and O69) to identify the fetus for which the complication code applies.

Coding Guideline I.C.15.b.5. Outcome of Delivery
A code from category Z37, Outcome of delivery, should be included on every maternal record when a delivery has occurred. These codes are not to be used on subsequent records or on the newborn record.

1.109. This woman is G1P0 at 39 weeks with twin gestation. The delivery was complicated by nuchal cord, without compression, of fetus 2. Both infants were liveborn and healthy. What is the correct **diagnosis** code(s)?

Code(s): _____

1.110. This 34-year-old woman, who is G4, P3, 28 weeks, is seen today for continued follow-up of her gestational diabetes. Her diabetes has been well controlled on oral medications. What is the correct **diagnosis** code?

Code(s): _____

Coding Guideline I.C.15.a.3. Final Character for Trimester
The majority of codes in Chapter 15 have a final character indicating the trimester of pregnancy. The time frames for the trimesters are indicated at the beginning of the chapter. If trimester is not a component of a code it is because the condition always occurs in a specific trimester, or the concept of trimester of pregnancy is not applicable. Certain codes have characters for only certain trimesters because the condition does not occur in all trimesters, but it may occur in more than just one.

Assignment of the final character for trimester should be based on the provider's documentation of the trimester (or number of weeks) for the current admission/encounter. This applies to the assignment of trimester for pre-existing conditions as well as those that develop during or are due to the pregnancy. The provider's documentation of the number of weeks may be used to assign the appropriate code identifying the trimester.

Whenever delivery occurs during the current admission, and there is an "in childbirth" option for the obstetric complication being coded, the "in childbirth" code should be assigned.

1.111. Code the following **diagnosis** code(s): 20-week pregnancy with low weight gain and pre-existing essential hypertension complicating the pregnancy.

Code(s): _____

> **Coding Guideline I.C.15.n.1. Encounter for Full-term Uncomplicated Delivery**
> Code O80 should be assigned when a woman is admitted for a full-term normal delivery and delivers a single, healthy infant without any complications antepartum, during the delivery, or postpartum during the delivery episode. Code O80 is always the principal diagnosis. It is not to be used if any other code from Chapter 15 is needed to describe a current complication of the antenatal, delivery, or perinatal period. Additional codes from other chapters may be used with code O80 if they are not related to or are in any way complicating the pregnancy.

> **Coding Guideline I.C.15.n.3. Outcome of Delivery for O80**
> Z37.0, Single live birth, is the only outcome of delivery code appropriate for use with O80.

1.112. The patient is admitted in active labor during week 39 of pregnancy. The patient experienced no complications during her pregnancy. The patient labored for 8 hours and delivered a liveborn male over an intact perineum. Code the **diagnosis** codes only.

Code(s): _____

1.113. The patient, G1P0, was admitted in active labor at 38 completed weeks of gestation. She is a type 2 diabetic who has been monitored during this pregnancy with no complications and no use of insulin. The patient was dilated to 6 cm approximately 7 hours following admission. Pitocin augmentation was started and she progressed to complete dilation. A second degree perineal laceration occurred during delivery and was repaired. A female infant was delivered with Apgar scores of 9 and 9. Code the **diagnosis** codes only.

Code(s): _____

> **Coding Guideline I.C.15.f HIV. Infection in Pregnancy, Childbirth, and the Puerperium**
> During pregnancy, childbirth, or the puerperium, a patient admitted because of an HIV-related illness should receive a principal diagnosis from subcategory O98.7-, Human immunodeficiency [HIV] disease complicating pregnancy, childbirth, and the puerperium, followed by the code(s) for the HIV-related illness(es).

1.114. This 25-year-old patient has admitted with difficulty breathing. She has AIDS and is 21 weeks pregnant. Workup reveals Pneumocystis carinii pneumonia. What is the correct **diagnosis** code(s)?

Code(s): _____

> **Coding Guideline I.C.15.b.4. When a Delivery Occurs**
> When a delivery occurs, the principal diagnosis should correspond to the main circumstances or complication of the delivery.

> **Coding Note:** Third trimester is defined as 28 weeks 0 days until delivery.

1.115. The patient, G3P2, was admitted at approximately 34 weeks' gestation with a history of contractions for the last 24 hours. She was experiencing contractions every 5 to 8 minutes. An ultrasound showed an intrauterine fetal death of triplet 2 but the other two were progressing normally. The contractions stopped for approximately 24 hours and then started again. It was noted by the physician that the continued contractions were due to fetus 2. The patient was given magnesium sulfate for tocolysis which was unsuccessful. The patient also developed a fever with an infection of the amniotic sac. The patient continued to be in active labor and due to the infection was allowed to spontaneously deliver the three infants, two liveborn and one fetal death. The patient experienced no postpartum complications. Code the **diagnoses** codes only.

Code(s): _____

> **Coding Guideline I.C.15.o.1. Postpartum Period**
> The postpartum period begins immediately after delivery and continues for six weeks following delivery.

> **Coding Guideline I.C.15.o.2. Postpartum Complication**
> A postpartum complication is any complication occurring within the six-week period.

1.116. The patient presented three weeks after undergoing a cesarean section. The patient has a temperature of 102 degrees Fahrenheit and the cesarean section wound (operative wound) is red with minimal drainage of the incision. A wound culture grew Streptococcus group B. Discharge diagnosis: Postoperative obstetric cesarean surgical wound infection, Streptococcus, group B. Assign the correct **diagnosis** code(s). (Do not assign external cause codes.)

Code(s): _____

> **Coding Guideline I.C.15.b.4. When a Delivery Occurs**
> In cases of cesarean delivery, the selection of the principal diagnosis should be the condition established after study that was responsible for the patient's admission. If the patient was admitted with a condition that resulted in the performance of a cesarean procedure that condition should be selected as the principal diagnosis. If the reason for the admission/encounter was unrelated to the condition resulting in the cesarean delivery, the condition related to the reason for the admission/encounter should be selected as the principal diagnosis, even if a cesarean was performed.

> **Coding Note:** ICD-10-CM provides a combination code for obstructed labor incorporating the obstructed labor with the reason for the obstruction into one code.

1.117. The patient, G2P1, in the 39th week of gestation was admitted with contractions occurring every 4–6 minutes. The cervix was 30% effaced with 5 cm dilation. The patient expressed her wishes for a trial vaginal delivery despite the fact that she had delivered her first child via cesarean delivery. The membranes spontaneously ruptured shortly after admission. Four hours later, the patient was given Pitocin augmentation and within 90 minutes she progressed to complete dilation and began pushing. The patient pushed for two hours and was unable to progress satisfactorily. She was taken to surgery, where a repeat low cervical cesarean section was performed for obstruction due to brow presentation. The outcome was a liveborn male infant weighing 6 pounds and 7 ounces with Apgar scores of 8 and 9. What **diagnoses** codes are coded?

Code(s): _____

> **Coding Note:** The first trimester of pregnancy is defined as less than 14 weeks 0 days.

1.118. The patient, G2P1, in her 12th week of pregnancy developed severe cramping and vaginal bleeding. The patient was subsequently taken to the emergency department and was admitted to the hospital. After examination, the physician documented that the patient had an incomplete early spontaneous abortion. During this pregnancy the patient had been treated for gestational hypertension of pregnancy, for which she was monitored during this hospital stay. The patient was taken to surgery where a dilation and curettage was performed. There were no complications following surgery. Code the **diagnoses** codes only.

Code(s): _____

Chapter 16: Certain conditions originating in the perinatal period (P00-P96)

Again block and category title changes have been made in this chapter; for example, ICD-9-CM subsection 760-763 is titled "Maternal Causes of Perinatal Morbidity and Mortality," whereas the ICD-10-CM counterpart, P00-P04, is titled "Newborn affected by maternal factors and by complications of pregnancy, labor, and delivery."

While conditions originating in the perinatal period and congenital anomalies each had a specific chapter in ICD-9-CM, they are listed in a different order in ICD-10-CM. Certain conditions originating in the perinatal period is Chapter 16 and Congenital malformations, deformations, and chromosomal abnormalities is Chapter 17 in ICD-10-CM.

The phrase "fetus or newborn" used in many ICD-9-CM codes is not used in ICD-10-CM. The term "newborn" is consistently used in code titles in Chapter 16 to clarify that these codes are for use on newborn records only, never on maternal records.

The introductory notes at the beginning of the chapter provide clarification. Note: Codes from this chapter are for use on newborn records only, never on maternal records and include conditions that have their origin in the fetal or perinatal period (before birth through the first 28 days after birth) even if morbidity occurs later. Coding Guideline I.C.16.a.1 further states that Chapter 16 codes may be used throughout the life of the patient if the condition is still present. Coding Guideline i.c.16.a.4 clarifies that conditions originating in the perinatal period, and continuing throughout the life of the patient, would have perinatal codes assigned regardless of the patient's age.

A note at block P00-P04, Newborn affected by maternal factors and by complications of pregnancy, labor, and delivery also provides guidance. Note: These codes are for use when the listed maternal conditions are specified as the cause of confirmed morbidity or potential morbidity that have their origin in the perinatal period (before birth through the first 28 days after birth). Codes from these categories are also for use for newborns who are suspected of having an abnormal condition resulting from exposure from the mother or the birth process, but without signs or symptoms, and which after examination and observation, is found not to exist. These codes may be used even if treatment is begun for a suspected condition that is ruled out.

A note provides direction for coding birth weight and gestational age at categories P07 and P08 for disorders related to short gestation/low birth weight and long gestation/high birth weight. Note: When both birth weight and gestational age of the newborn are available, both should be coded with birth weight sequenced before gestational age.

Category Z38 in Chapter 21, Factors influencing health status and contact with health services classifies liveborn infants according to place of birth and type of delivery. This category is for use as the principal code on the initial record of a newborn baby. It is not to be used on the mother's record.

Chapter 16 Coding Cases

> **Coding Guideline I.C.16.f. Bacterial Sepsis of Newborn**
> Category P36, Bacterial sepsis of newborn, includes congenital sepsis. If a perinate is documented as having sepsis without documentation of congenital or community acquired, the default is congenital and a code from category P36 should be assigned. If the P36 code includes the causal organism, an additional code from category B95, Streptococcus, Staphylococcus, and Enterococcus as the cause of diseases classified elsewhere, or B96, Other bacterial agents as the cause of diseases classified elsewhere, should **not** be assigned. If the P36 code does not include the causal organism, assign an additional code from category B96. If applicable, use additional codes to identify severe sepsis (R65.2-) and any associated acute organ dysfunction.

1.119. Assign the code(s) for the following diagnosis: 20-day-old infant was admitted with Staphylococcus aureus sepsis.

Code(s): _____

1.120. This full-term newborn was delivered four days ago and she was discharged with no problems. After going home she was noticed to be somewhat jaundiced, and her mother brought her to the pediatrician's office. She was diagnosed with hyperbilirubinemia and will have phototherapy provided at home. What **diagnosis** codes are assigned?

Code(s): _____

> **Coding Guideline I.C.16.a.2. Principal Diagnosis for Birth Record**
> When coding the birth episode in a newborn record, assign a code from category Z38, Liveborn infants according to place of birth and type of delivery, as the principal diagnosis. A code from category Z38 is assigned only once, to a newborn at the time of birth. If a newborn is transferred to another institution, a code from category Z38 should not be used at the receiving hospital.

1.121. This full-term female infant was born in this hospital by vaginal delivery. Her mother has been an alcoholic for many years and would not stop drinking during her pregnancy. The baby was born with fetal alcohol syndrome and was placed in the NICU. What **diagnosis** codes are assigned?

Code(s): _____

> **Coding Guideline I.C.16.d. Prematurity and Fetal Growth Retardation**
> Providers utilize different criteria in determining prematurity. A code for prematurity should not be assigned unless it is documented. Assignment of codes in categories P05, Disorders of newborn related to slow fetal growth and fetal malnutrition, and P07, Disorders of newborn related to short gestation and low birth weight, not elsewhere classified, should be based on the recorded birth weight and estimated gestational age. Codes from category P05 should not be assigned with codes from category P07.
>
> When both birth weight and gestational age are available, two codes from category P07 should be assigned, with the code for birth weight sequenced before the code for gestational age.
>
> A code from P05 and codes from P07.2 and P07.3 may be used to specify weeks of gestation as documented by the provider in the record.

1.122. Assign the codes for the following diagnosis: Premature "crack" baby born in the hospital by cesarean section to a mother dependent on cocaine. The newborn did not show signs of withdrawal. Birth weight of 1,247 g, 31 completed weeks of gestation. Dehydration. What **diagnosis** codes are assigned?

Code(s): _____

Chapter 17: Congenital malformations, deformations and chromosomal abnormalities (Q00-Q99)

Many codes for congenital conditions and chromosomal abnormalities have been expanded in ICD-10-CM; for example, chromosomal anomalies are classified to category 758 in ICD-9-CM; however, in ICD-10-CM, there are nine categories for chromosomal abnormalities, not elsewhere classified.

Again, block, category, subcategory, and code title changes have been made in Chapter 17; for example, in ICD-9-CM, code 758.1 is titled "Patau's Syndrome," whereas the counterpart codes in ICD-10-CM are titled "Trisomy 13."

These codes are assigned when a malformation or deformation or chromosomal abnormality is documented, and the code may be the principal or first listed diagnosis on a record or a secondary diagnosis.

When no unique code is available, assign additional code(s) for any manifestations that may be present. When the code assignment specifically identifies the malformation, deformation, or chromosomal abnormality, manifestations that are an inherent component of the anomaly should not be coded separately. Additional codes should be assigned for manifestations that are not an inherent component.

Codes from Chapter 17 may be used throughout the life of the patient. If the congenital malformation or deformity has been corrected, a personal history code should be used to identify the history of the malformation or deformity. Although present at birth, malformation, deformation, or chromosomal abnormality may not be identified until later in life, and if diagnosed by the physician, it is appropriate to assign a code from codes Q00-Q99.

For the birth admission, the appropriate code from category Z38, Liveborn infants, according to place of birth and type of delivery, should be sequenced as the principal diagnosis, followed by any congenital anomaly codes, Q00-Q89.

Chapter 17 Coding Cases

1.123. Assign the code for the following diagnosis: Frontal encephalocele with hydroencephalocele.

Code: _____

1.124. Assign the code(s) for the following diagnosis: Cleft palate involving both the soft and hard palate, with bilateral cleft lip.

Code(s): _____

1.125. Assign the code(s) for the following diagnosis: Penoscrotal hypospadias.

Code(s): _____

1.126. This newborn was delivered by cesarean section and transferred immediately to NICU because of previous anomalies identified via sonogram and fetal echocardiogram. The newborn male has complete transposition of the great vessels with cyanosis. The baby received IV prostaglandin and underwent uneventful corrective surgery at four days, and was discharged 10 days post surgery. What **diagnosis** codes are assigned?

Code(s): _____

Chapter 18: Symptoms, signs and abnormal clinical and laboratory findings, not elsewhere classified (R00-R99)

Chapter 18 includes symptoms, signs, abnormal results of clinical or other investigative procedures, and ill-defined conditions regarding which no diagnosis classifiable elsewhere is recorded.

Signs and symptoms that point rather definitely to a given diagnosis have been assigned to a category in other chapters of the classification. In general, categories in this chapter include the less well-defined conditions and symptoms that, without the necessary study of the case to establish a final diagnosis, point perhaps equally to two or more diseases or to two or more systems of the body. Practically all categories in the chapter could be designated Not Otherwise Specified, Unknown Etiology, or Transient. The Alphabetic Index should be consulted to determine which symptoms and signs are to be allocated here and which to other chapters. The residual subcategories, numbered .8, are generally provided for other relevant symptoms that cannot be allocated elsewhere in the classification.

The conditions, signs, and symptoms included in Chapter 18 consist of: (a) cases for which no more specific diagnosis can be made even after all the facts bearing on the case have been investigated; (b) signs or symptoms existing at the time of the initial encounter that proved to be transient and whose causes could not be determined; (c) provisional diagnosis in a patient who failed to return for further investigation or care; (d) cases referred elsewhere for investigation or treatment before the diagnosis was made; (e) cases in which a more precise diagnosis was not available for any other reason; (f) certain symptoms, for which supplementary information is provided, that represent important problems in medical care in their own right.

Coma Scale

Subcategory R40.2, Coma, incorporates the Glasgow coma scale (R40.21-R40.23). The coma scale codes can be used in conjunction with traumatic brain injury or sequelae of cerebrovascular disease codes. They are primarily for use by trauma registries and research use, but they may be used in any setting where this information is collected. The coma scale codes are sequenced after the diagnosis code(s). These codes, one from each subcategory (R40.21, R40.22, R40.23), are needed to complete the scale. The seventh character indicates when the scale was recorded, and it should match for all three codes:

> 0 – unspecified time
> 1 – in the field [EMT or ambulance]
> 2 – at arrival to emergency department
> 3 – at hospital admission
> 4 – 24 hours or more after hospital admission

At a minimum, report the initial score documented on presentation at the facility. This may be a score from the emergency medicine technician (EMT) or in the emergency department. If desired, a facility may choose to capture multiple coma scale scores.

Code R40.24, Glasgow coma scale, total score, should be assigned when only the total score is documented in the medical record and not the individual score(s).

Systemic Inflammatory Response Syndrome

Systemic inflammatory response syndrome (SIRS) is classified to category R65, Symptoms and signs specifically associated with systemic inflammation and infection. Codes in this category identify SIRS of non-infectious origin with and without acute organ dysfunction and severe sepsis with and without septic shock. An instructional note indicates that the underlying condition (or underlying infection, in the case of severe sepsis) should be coded first. Sepsis is not classified to category R65. Sepsis should be coded to the infection. For example, code A41.9 should be assigned for sepsis, unspecified.

Chapter 18 Coding Cases

1.127. Assign the code(s) for the following diagnosis: Right upper quadrant rebound abdominal tenderness.

Code(s): _____

Coding Guideline I.C.18.e. Coma Scale

The coma scale codes (R40.2-) can be used in conjunction with traumatic brain injury codes, acute cerebrovascular disease, or sequelae of cerebrovascular disease codes. These codes are primarily for use by trauma registries, but they may be used in any setting where this information is collected. The coma scale codes should be sequenced after the diagnosis code(s).

These codes, one from each subcategory, are needed to complete the scale. The seventh character indicates when the scale was recorded. The seventh character should match for all three codes.

At a minimum, report the initial score documented on presentation to the facility. This may be a score from the emergency medicine technician (EMT) or in the emergency department. If desired, a facility may choose to capture multiple Glasgow coma scale scores.

Assign code R40.24, Glasgow coma scale, total score, when only the total score is documented in the medical record and not the individual score(s).

1.128. Assign the Glasgow coma scale code(s) when the patient had the following documented by the EMT: Eyes do not open, no verbal response, with no motor response. The neurologist documented the following on day 2 of the hospital admission: Eyes open to sound, verbal response produced inappropriate words, and motor response with flexion withdrawal.

Code(s): _____

1.129. Assign the code for the following diagnosis: Microcalcification found on breast mammography.

Code(s): _____

1.130. Assign the code(s) for the following diagnosis: Sinoatrial bradycardia.

Code(s): _____

Coding Guideline II.E. A. Symptom(s) Followed by Contrasting/Comparative Diagnoses
When a symptom(s) is followed by contrasting/comparative diagnoses, the symptom code is sequenced first. All the contrasting/comparative diagnoses should be coded as additional diagnoses.

1.131. The patient is admitted through the emergency room with a complaint of chest pain. The EKG and laboratory tests completed in the ER are inconclusive, but an acute myocardial infarction is ruled out. During the hospital stay, the cardiovascular workup did not reveal any coronary artery disease and the patient did not want to have a cardiac catheterization study performed at this time. The patient is known to have gastroesophageal reflux disease. Given the conflicting information, the attending physician concluded the patient had "atypical chest pain due to either angina or GERD." What **diagnosis** codes are assigned?

Code(s): _____

1.132. The patient who has experienced a fever of 101 degrees Fahrenheit with chills was brought to the emergency room. Laboratory tests, including a complete blood count and urinalysis, were performed with normal results. The ER physician wrote the final diagnosis as "fever with chills, possible viral syndrome." What **diagnosis** code is assigned?

Code(s): _____

1.133. The patient is seen complaining of right upper quadrant abdominal pain. In addition, the patient is having nausea and vomited several times. Patient also has elevated blood pressure readings but a diagnosis of hypertension is not made at this visit. The patient was given an order for an outpatient sonogram. What **diagnosis** codes are assigned?

Code(s): _____

Chapter 19: Injury, poisoning and certain other consequences of external causes (S00-T88)

In ICD-10-CM, injuries are grouped by body part rather than by categories of injury, so that all injuries of the specific site (such as head and neck) are grouped together rather than groupings of all fractures or all open wounds; for example, categories in ICD-9-CM grouped by injury such as fractures (800-829), dislocations (830-839), and sprains and strains (840-848) are grouped in ICD-10-CM by site, such as injuries to the head (S00-S09), injuries to the neck (S10-S19), and injuries to the thorax (S20-S29).

Chapter 19 encompasses two alpha characters. The **S** section provides codes for the various types of injuries related to single body regions; the **T** section covers injuries to unspecified body regions as well as poisonings and certain other consequences of external causes.

The following note refers to the entire chapter:

> Use secondary code(s) from Chapter 20, External causes of morbidity, to indicate cause of injury. Codes within the T section that include the external cause do not require an additional external cause code.

Many codes, such as fractures, include much greater specificity in ICD-10-CM. For example, some of the information that may be found in fracture codes includes the type of fracture, specific anatomical site, whether the fracture is displaced or not, laterality, routine versus delayed healing, nonunions, and malunions. Laterality and identification of type of encounter (initial, subsequent, sequela) are a significant component of the code expansion.

Seventh characters are assigned in this chapter, and are identified at the category level to indicate initial encounter, subsequent encounter, or sequela.

Fracture seventh characters are expanded to include
        A – initial encounter for closed fracture
        B – initial encounter for open fracture
        D – subsequent encounter for fracture with routine healing
        G – subsequent encounter for fracture with delayed healing
        K – subsequent encounter for fracture with nonunion
        P – subsequent encounter for fracture with malunion
        S – sequela

Some fracture categories provide for seventh characters to designate the specific type of open fracture (these designations are based on the Gustilo open fracture classification):
        B – initial encounter for open fracture type I or II (open NOS or not otherwise specified)
        C – initial encounter for open fracture type IIIA, IIIB, or IIIC
        E – subsequent encounter for open fracture type I or II with routine healing
        F – subsequent encounter for open fracture type IIIA, IIIB, or IIIC with routine healing
        H – subsequent encounter for open fracture type I or II with delayed healing
        J – subsequent encounter for open fracture type IIIA, IIIB, or IIIC with delayed healing
        M – subsequent encounter for open fracture type I or II with nonunion
        N – subsequent encounter for open fracture type IIIA, IIIB, or IIIC with nonunion

Q – subsequent encounter for open fracture type I or II with malunion
R – subsequent encounter for open fracture type IIIA, IIIB, or IIIC with malunion

In ICD-10-CM, a fracture not indicated as displaced or nondisplaced should be coded to displaced and a fracture not designated as open or closed should be coded to closed.

Seventh characters for "initial encounter" are used while the patient is receiving active treatment for the condition, for example, surgical treatment, emergency department encounter, and evaluation and treatment by a new physician.

The seventh characters for "subsequent encounter" are used for encounters after the patient has received active treatment for the condition and is receiving routine care for the condition during the healing or recovery phase, for example, cast change or removal, removal of external or internal fixation device, medication adjustment, other aftercare and follow-up visits following treatment of the injury or condition.

Seventh character S, "sequela," is for use for complications or conditions that arise as a direct result of a condition, such as scar formation after a burn. The scars are sequela of the burn. When using seventh character S, it is necessary to use both the injury code that precipitated the sequela and the code for the sequela itself. The S is added only to the injury code, not the sequela code. The seventh character S identifies the injury responsible for the sequela. The specific type of sequela (e.g., scar) is sequenced first, followed by the injury code.

The aftercare Z codes should not be used for aftercare for conditions such as injuries or poisonings, where the seventh characters are provided to identify subsequent care. For example, aftercare of an injury, assign the acute injury code with the appropriate seventh character for "subsequent encounter."

Poisoning by, adverse effects of and underdosing of drugs, medicaments and biological substances (T36-T50) includes the following note:
> *Includes:* adverse effect of correct substance properly
> administered
>> poisoning by overdose of substance
>> poisoning by wrong substance given or taken in error
>>> underdosing by (inadvertently) (deliberately) taking less
>>> substance than prescribed or instructed

Use additional code(s) for all manifestations of poisonings and assign the code for the nature of the adverse effect first followed by the code for the drug.

Use additional code for intent of underdosing:
> Failure in dosage during medical and surgical care (Y63.8-Y63.9)
> Patient's underdosing of medication regime (Z91.12-, Z91.13-)

There are combination codes for poisonings and the associated external cause (accidental, intentional self-harm, assault, undetermined), and the Table of Drugs and Chemicals groups all poisoning columns together, followed by adverse effect and underdosing. When no intent of poisoning is indicated, code to Accidental. Undetermined intent is only for use when there is specific documentation in the record that the intent of the poisoning cannot be determined.

Toxic effects of substances chiefly nonmedicinal as to source (T51-T65) provides direction to use additional code(s) for all associated manifestations of toxic effect, such as
> Respiratory conditions due to external agents (J60-J70)

When no intent is indicated, code to Accidental. Undetermined intent is only for use when there is specific documentation in the record that the intent of the toxic effect cannot be determined.

This block has an *Excludes1* note:
> *Excludes1*: Contact with and (suspected) exposure to toxic substances (Z77.-)

Chapter 19 Coding Cases

> **Note:** Lesson 19 will provide practice coding Chapter 19 codes. External cause codes are discussed and coded in Lesson 20 of this training. For Lesson 19, assign only diagnosis codes, not external cause codes.

1.134. The 6-month-old is seen for increased fussiness and vomiting. After significant study, the patient is diagnosed with shaken baby syndrome. What is the correct **diagnosis** code(s)? (Do not assign the external cause codes.)

Code(s): _____

> **Coding Guideline I.C.19.a. Application of Seventh Characters in Chapter 19**
> Most categories in Chapter 19 have a seventh character requirement for each applicable code. Most categories in this chapter have three seventh character values (with the exception of fractures): A, initial encounter; D, subsequent encounter; and S, sequela. Categories for traumatic fractures have additional seventh character values.

> **Coding Guideline I.C.19.c.1. Initial vs. Subsequent Encounter for Fractures**
> Traumatic fractures are coded using the appropriate seventh character for initial encounter (A, B, and C) while the patient is receiving active treatment for the fracture. Examples of active treatment are: surgical treatment, emergency department encounter, and evaluation and treatment by a new physician. The appropriate seventh character for initial encounter should also be assigned for a patient who delayed seeking treatment for the fracture or malunion.

1.135. This patient is seen for increased pain in her ankle. She has previous trimalleolar fracture of the left ankle. After evaluation she was found to have a nonunion of her left trimalleolar fracture. What is the correct **diagnosis** code(s)? (Do not assign external cause codes.)

Code(s): _____

> **Coding Note:** ICD-10-CM categories S52, Fracture of forearm; S72, Fracture of femur; and S82, Fracture of lower leg, including ankle, have additional seventh character extensions (B, C, E, F, H, J, M, N, Q, R) to identify open fractures with the Gustilo classification. The classification is as follows:
>
> | | |
> |---|---|
> | I | Low energy, wound less than 1 cm |
> | II | Wound greater than 1 cm with moderate soft tissue damage |
> | | High energy wound greater than 1 cm with extensive soft tissue damage |
> | IIIA | Adequate soft tissue cover |
> | IIIB | Inadequate soft tissue cover |
> | IIIC | Associated with arterial injury |

1.136. This young man is seen today with right forearm fracture. This is found to be a displaced, compound comminuted fracture of the radial shaft. It is a type II open fracture. What is the correct **diagnosis** code? (Do not assign the external cause code.)

Code(s): _____

1.137. A 40-year-old woman is seen today to establish care. She is a complete paraplegic due to a traumatic L2 vertebral fracture five years ago. At this time, she is experiencing no problems. What is the correct **diagnosis** code(s)? (Do not assign external cause codes.)

Code(s): _____

1.138. This patient is found to have delayed healing of his traumatic mandible fracture. The fracture was at the angle of the jaw. He will be referred for additional radiologic studies. What is the correct **diagnosis** code? (Do not assign the external cause codes.)

Code(s): _____

1.139. This patient is seen emergently for a frontal skull fracture with a subsequent subdural hemorrhage. There was a 45-minute loss of consciousness at the time of the accident. What is the correct **diagnosis** code(s)? (Do not assign the external cause codes.)

Code(s): _____

1.140. Code the following diagnosis: 2 cm laceration of the left heel with foreign body. This is a current injury. (Do not assign external cause codes.)

Code(s): _____

1.141. This patient is seen in follow-up to his traumatic lateral epicondyle fracture of the right elbow. This is healing normally. What is the correct **diagnosis** code? (Do not assign external cause codes.)

Code(s): _____

1.142. This toddler is seen emergently for nausea and vomiting after an accidental overdose of acetaminophen. He inadvertently ate several of these when he found an open bottle at home. What is the correct **diagnosis** code(s)? (Do not assign external cause codes.)

Code(s): _____

Coding Guideline I.C.19.e. Adverse Effects, Poisoning, Underdosing, and Toxic Effects
Codes in categories T36-T65 are combination codes that include the substance that was taken as well as the intent. No additional external cause code is required for poisonings, toxic effects, adverse effects, and underdosing codes.

Coding Guideline I.C.19.e.5.a. Adverse Effects
When coding an adverse effect of a drug that has been correctly prescribed and properly administered, assign the appropriate code for the nature of the adverse effect followed by the appropriate code for the adverse effect of the drug (T36-T50). The code for the drug should have a fifth or sixth character 5. Examples of the nature of an adverse effect are tachycardia, delirium, gastrointestinal hemorrhaging, vomiting, hypokalemia, hepatitis, kidney failure, or respiratory failure.

1.143. A patient has been taking Digoxin and is experiencing nausea and vomiting and profound fatigue. The patient indicates that he has been taking the drug appropriately. The evaluation and treatment was focused on adjustment of medication only. What is the correct **diagnosis** code(s)? (Do not assign external cause codes.)

Code(s): _____

Coding Guideline I.C.19.e.5.c. Underdosing
Underdosing refers to taking less of a medication than is prescribed by a provider or a manufacturer's instruction. For underdosing, assign the code from categories T36-T50 (fifth or sixth character 6). Codes for underdosing should never be assigned as principal or first-listed codes. If a patient has a relapse or exacerbation of the medical condition for which the drug is prescribed because of the reduction in dose, the medical condition itself should be coded.

Noncompliance (Z91.12-, Z91.13-) or complication of care (Y63.8-Y63.9) codes are to be used with an underdosing code to indicate intent, if known.

1.144. This 85-year-old patient is seen in the hospital with a diagnosis of congestive heart failure due to hypertensive heart disease. Patient also has stage 5 chronic kidney failure. The patient had been prescribed Lasix previously but admits that he forgets to take his medication every day. This is due to his advanced age. What are the correct **diagnosis** codes? (Do not assign external cause codes.)

Code(s): _____

1.145. This 50-year-old man was in the Cardiac Cath Lab for insertion of a dual chamber pacemaker to treat his sick sinus syndrome. During the procedure the pacemaker electrode broke upon insertion. The procedure was abandoned and will be rescheduled. What is the correct **diagnosis** code(s)? (Do not assign external cause codes.)

Code(s): _____

1.146. This elderly woman is seen for increased right hip pain. She has a right hip prosthesis. After extensive evaluation, she is found to have an infection of the prosthesis. She will be scheduled for surgery. What is the correct **diagnosis** code? (Do not assign external cause codes.)

Code(s): _____

Coding Guideline I.C.19.b.1. Superficial Injuries
Superficial injuries such as abrasions or contusions are not coded when associated with more severe injuries of the same site.

1.147. This young snowboarder suffered a crash at a local ski area. He suffered multiple injuries and was transported to this facility for treatment. He was found to have right-sided fracture of 3 ribs, a right chest contusion and a fractured right wrist. None of his injuries required surgical intervention. What is the correct **diagnosis** code(s)? (Do not assign external cause codes.)

Code(s): _____

1.148. The woman is admitted for an intentional overdose of marijuana and cocaine. She sustained a fall which resulted in a left cheek and scalp laceration. After she is stabilized medically, she will be transferred to a psychiatric unit. What are the correct **diagnosis** codes? (Do not assign external cause codes.)

Code(s): _____

Chapter 20: External causes of morbidity (V00-Y99)

This chapter permits the classification of environmental events and circumstances as the cause of injury, and other adverse effects. Where a code from this section is applicable, it is intended that it shall be used secondary to a code from another chapter of the classification indicating the nature of the condition. Most often, the condition will be classifiable to Chapter 19, Injury, poisoning and certain other consequences of external causes (S00-T88). Other conditions that may be stated to be due to external causes are classified in Chapters 1 through 18. For these conditions, codes from Chapter 20 should be used to provide additional information as to the cause of the condition.

An external cause code may be used with any code in the range of A00.0-T88.9, Z00-Z99, classification that is a health condition due to an external cause. Though they are most applicable to injuries, they are also valid for use with such things as infections or diseases due to an external source, and other health conditions, such as a heart attack that occurs during strenuous physical activity.

This chapter encompasses alpha characters V, W, X, and Y, and contains a massive expansion from ICD-9-CM. It is helpful to review the Tabular to gain an understanding of all of the possible codes available.

Assign the external cause code, with the appropriate seventh character (initial encounter, subsequent encounter, or sequela) for each encounter for which the injury or condition is being treated.

In ICD-9-CM, the late effect codes for external causes are located in various subsections of the External Cause chapter. In ICD-10-CM, all late effects of external causes are identified by the addition of the seventh character S, sequela, to the code for each intent (e.g., accident, suicide).

The transport accidents section (V00-V99) is structured in 12 groups. Those relating to land transport accidents (V01-V89) reflect the victim's mode of transport and are subdivided to identify the victim's "counterpart" or the type of event. The vehicle of which the injured person is an occupant is identified in the first two characters since it is seen as the most important factor to identify for prevention purposes. A transport accident is one in which the vehicle involved must be moving or running or in use for transport purposes at the time of the accident. The definitions of transport vehicles are provided in the classification and should be reviewed.

The following note is available with this section:
> Use additional code to identify:
> > Airbag injury (W22.1)
> > Type of street or road (Y92.4-)
> Use of cellular telephone and other electronic equipment at the time of the transport accident (Y93.C-)

Category Y92, Place of occurrence of the external cause is for use, when relevant, to identify the place of occurrence. It is to be used in conjunction with an activity code. Place of occurrence should be recorded only at the initial encounter for treatment. Only one code from Y92 should be recorded on a medical record. Do not use place of occurrence code Y92.9 if the place is not stated or is not applicable.

Category Y93, Activity code is provided for use to indicate the activity of the person seeking healthcare for an injury or health condition, such as a heart attack while shoveling snow, which resulted from the activity or was contributed to by the activity. These codes are appropriate for use for both acute injuries, such as those from Chapter 19, and conditions that are due to the long-term, cumulative effects of an activity, such as those from Chapter 13. They are also appropriate for use with external cause codes for cause and intent if identifying the activity provides additional information on the event. These codes should be used in conjunction with codes for external cause status (Y99) and place of occurrence (Y92). The activity code is used only once, at the initial encounter for treatment. Only one code from Y93 should be recorded on the encounter.

The activity codes are not applicable to poisonings, adverse effects, misadventures, or late effects. Do not assign Y93.9, unspecified activity, if the activity is not stated.

This section contains the following broad activity categories:
    Y93.0 Activities involving walking and running
    Y93.1 Activities involving water and water craft
    Y93.2 Activities involving ice and snow
    Y93.3 Activities involving climbing, rappelling, and jumping off
    Y93.4 Activities involving dancing and other rhythmic movement
    Y93.5 Activities involving other sports and athletics played individually
    Y93.6 Activities involving other sports and athletics played as a team or group
    Y93.7 Activities involving other specified sports and athletics
    Y93.A Activities involving other cardiorespiratory exercise
    Y93.B Activities involving other muscle strengthening exercises
    Y93.C Activities involving computer technology and electronic devices
    Y93.D Activities involving arts and handcrafts
    Y93.E Activities involving personal hygiene and interior property and
           clothing maintenance
    Y93.F Activities involving caregiving
    Y93.G Activities involving food preparation, cooking, and grilling
    Y93.H Activities involving exterior property and land maintenance, building
           and construction
    Y93.I Activities involving roller coasters and other types of external motion
    Y93.J Activities involving playing musical instrument
    Y93.K Activities involving animal care
    Y93.8 Activities, other specified
    Y93.9 Activity, unspecified

Category Y99, External cause status codes should be assigned whenever any other external cause code is assigned for an encounter, including an activity code, except for the events noted below. Assign a code from category Y99, External cause status, to indicate the work status of the person at the time the event occurred. The status code indicates whether the event occurred during military activity, whether a non-military person was at work, or whether an individual including a student or volunteer was involved in a non-work activity at the time of the causal event.

A code from Y99, External cause status, should be assigned, when applicable, with other external cause codes, such as transport accidents and falls. The external cause status codes are not applicable to poisonings, adverse effects, misadventures, or late effects.

Do not assign a code from category Y99 if no other external cause codes (cause, activity) are applicable for the encounter. Do not assign code Y99.9, Unspecified external cause status, if the status is not stated.

Chapter 20 Coding Cases

> **Coding Note:** The seventh character must always be the seventh character in the data field. If a code that requires a seventh character is not six characters, a placeholder X must be used to fill in the empty characters.

> **Coding Guideline I.C.20 External Causes of Morbidity (V00-Y99)**
> The external causes of morbidity codes should never be sequenced as the first-listed or principal diagnosis.

There is no national requirement for mandatory ICD-10-CM external cause code reporting. Unless a provider is subject to a state-based external cause code reporting mandate or these codes are required by a particular payer, reporting of ICD-10-CM codes in Chapter 20, External Causes of Morbidity, is not required. In the absence of a mandatory reporting requirement, providers are encouraged to voluntarily report external cause codes, as they provide valuable data for injury research and evaluation of injury prevention strategies.

> **Coding Guideline I.C.20.b. Place of Occurrence**
> A place of occurrence code—Y92—is used only once, at the initial encounter for treatment.

> **Coding Guideline I.C.20.c. Activity Code**
> An activity code—Y93—is used only once, at the initial encounter for treatment and should be used in conjunction with Y92, Place of occurrence.

1.149. Assign external cause codes for this case: An 18-year-old driver of a car collided with a pickup truck on the interstate highway. The driver confessed to using his cell phone to send a text message to his girlfriend.

Code(s): _____

1.150. Assign only external cause codes for this case: An Air Force officer was injured while on patrol on the military base in Afghanistan by an explosion of an IED.

Code(s): _____

1.151. Assign only external cause codes for this case: The patient was bitten by a dog while attempting to rescue it from an abandoned barn while performing his job at animal control.

Code(s): _____

1.152. Assign only external cause codes for this case: A cook in a fast food restaurant was accidently burned with hot oil while cooking French fries while on duty.

Code(s): _____

1.153. This 46-year-old male, working on his own home improvement projects, fell from a ladder outside of his single family home. After evaluation, it was determined that he had a non-displaced femoral neck fracture on the left side. At this time, no surgical intervention is planned. What **diagnosis** codes are assigned?

Code(s): _____

1.154. A patient fell from a ladder in the garage four weeks ago while working on replacing a garage door switch. The injury resulted in a fracture of L1 and L2 vertebral bodies. He is receiving physical therapy for this routine healing injury. What **diagnosis** codes are assigned?

Code(s): _____

1.155. A child has second- and third-degree burns of the left calf and second- and third-degree burns of the back. The patient was burned when he was running and fell into the lit fireplace in his parent's bedroom. What **diagnosis** codes are assigned?

Code(s): _____

1.156. This 32-year-old female was burned by hot grease in her kitchen in her condo. She is seen in the hospital's outpatient clinic for large dressing change on her left forearm. She was treated for second-degree burns to her left arm several days ago. What **diagnosis** codes are assigned?

Code(s): _____

1.157. This 35-year-old female patient was a driver involved in an automobile accident when she was rear-ended by another car on the interstate highway. She was seen in the emergency room complaining of pain in the arm and neck. She was brought into the hospital by the EMTs on a backboard and after proper splinting to the right arm. It was evident that there was a compound fracture present. After CT scan of the head and neck, the patient was removed from the backboard. She was treated for a displaced, compound fracture of the shaft of the right radius and ulna. She also received a collar for her cervical strain. What **diagnosis** codes are assigned?

Code(s): _____

> **Coding Guideline I.C.19.c.1. Initial vs. Subsequent Encounter for Fractures**
> Care of complications of fractures, such a malunion and nonunion, should be reported with the appropriate seventh character for subsequent care with nonunion (K, M, N) or subsequent care with malunion (P, Q, R).

1.158. This 10-year-old female is seen for continued pain related to her elbow fracture. Six weeks ago, this patient injured her elbow when she fell while skating at the local roller rink. After further evaluation, the attending physician found a nonunion of the previously displaced right distal humerus fracture. She will be scheduled for surgery in the next two days. What **diagnosis** codes are assigned?

Code(s): _____

> **Coding Note:** The coding note under category S61 indicates a "code also any associated wound infection" which does not provide a mandatory sequencing requirement for S61 to be sequenced ahead of the wound infection.

1.159. This 28-year-old female was seen for an infection due to a laceration on the palm of her right hand. Apparently, this laceration occurred five days ago. The patient reports that her hand was cut by broken glass at a restaurant, where she was a customer, drinking heavily. She is a chronic alcohol abuser and also a chronic abuser of meth. The wound will not be sutured due to the late presentation for treatment. She will, however, be placed on antibiotics to treat the infection. What **diagnosis** codes are assigned?

Code(s): _____

1.160. This patient is a 19-year-old college student who is brought to the emergency department by ambulance, found to be the victim of a random beating. This patient was walking in his neighborhood park when he was pulled down and then beaten during a fight. The patient was comatose when found by the paramedics but did open his eyes in response to pain; however, he has no verbal or motor response. The patient was in a coma upon admission but regained consciousness within 40 minutes of arriving in the ED, less than an hour after being found. The MRI is negative for fractures or internal bleeding. The physician describes the injury as a closed head injury with loss of consciousness of less than 1 hour. What **diagnosis** codes are assigned?

Code(s): _____

1.161. This is a 50-year-old female who fell down the icy front steps of her single-family house and sustained trauma to her head as well as a nondisplaced closed trimalleolar fracture of the medial and lateral malleolus of her left leg. The patient denies any loss of consciousness. Attention was directed to her head injury which, after CT scan, revealed a basilar skull fracture and a small subdural hematoma. The neurosurgeon felt that the hematoma currently did not require surgical intervention. Serial CT scans showed shrinking of the hematoma after several days. What **diagnosis** codes are assigned?

Code(s): _____

1.162. This patient is a 22-year-old male, admitted through the emergency department after the motorcycle he was driving (for leisure) collided with an elk on a mountain highway. The patient was wearing a helmet and suffered a minor head injury with just a short loss of consciousness reported at 15 minutes. His major injury was a displaced, cervical, C2 fracture with complete transection of the spinal cord. Upon evaluation by neurosurgery, the patient had no feeling below his shoulders, although he did admit to tingling in his arms and hands. The patient had no other apparent fractures. The patient's family was notified and arrived two days later.

Due to problems in the OR, it was necessary to transfer the patient to complete surgical stabilization. The physician's final diagnosis was stated as quadriplegia secondary to C2 vertebral fracture with spinal cord injury. What **diagnosis** codes are assigned?

Code(s): _____

Chapter 21: Factors influencing health status and contact with health services (Z00-Z99)

Certain codes have been moved from other chapters in ICD-9-CM to Chapter 21; for example, elective, legal, or therapeutic abortions have been moved from ICD-9-CM Chapter 11, Complications of Pregnancy, Childbirth, and the Puerperium, to ICD-10-CM Chapter 21.

Several codes have been expanded in ICD-10-CM; for example, personal and family history codes have been expanded.

In addition, codes have been added for concepts that currently do not exist in ICD-9-CM; for example, category Z67 identifies the patient's blood type.

By contrast, there are also concepts that existed in ICD-9-CM that no longer exist in ICD-10-CM; for example, there is no comparable category in ICD-10-CM to ICD-9-CM category V57, Care involving use of rehabilitation procedures. For encounters for rehabilitative therapy, report the underlying condition for which therapy is being provided (such as an injury) with the appropriate seventh character indicating subsequent encounter. This change greatly impacts certain settings providing aftercare.

The note at the beginning of the chapter explains the use of the codes:

> Z codes represent reasons for encounters. A corresponding procedure code must accompany a Z code if a procedure is performed. Categories Z00-Z99 are provided for occasions when circumstances other than a disease, injury or external cause classifiable to categories A00-Y89 are recorded as "diagnoses" or "problems." This can arise in two main ways:
> a) When a person who may or may not be sick encounters the health services for some specific purpose, such as to receive limited care or service for a current condition, to donate an organ or tissue, to receive prophylactic vaccination (immunization), or to discuss a problem which is in itself not a disease or injury.
> b) When some circumstance or problem is present which influences the person's health status but is not in itself a current illness or injury.

Category Z68, Body mass index (BMI) is divided into adult and pediatric codes. The BMI adult codes are for use for persons 21 years of age or older. BMI pediatric codes are for use for persons 2–20 years of age. The percentiles listed with the codes are based on the growth charts published by the Centers for Disease Control and Prevention (CDC).

Chapter 21 Coding Cases

1.163. This single newborn was born vaginally in the hospital. The baby is being treated for Rh incompatibility. The baby has type A+ blood and the mother is A-. What is the correct **diagnosis** code(s)?

Code(s): _____

1.164. Assign the code(s) for the following diagnosis: Medical examination of four-year-old child prior to admission to preschool.

Code(s): _____

1.165. Assign the code(s) for the following encounter: Patient seen for fitting of right artificial leg after patient had below-knee amputation due to medical condition.

Code(s): _____

1.166. Assign the code(s) for the following diagnosis: Postmenopausal osteoporosis in a 63-year-old female with a history of healed osteoporotic fracture of the ankle.

Code(s): _____

Coding Guideline I.C.21.c.3. Z92.82. Status Post Administration of tPA (rtPA) in a Different Facility Within the Last 24 Hours Prior to Admission to a Current Facility

Assign code Z92.82, Status post administration of tPA (rtPA) in a different facility within the last 24 hours prior to admission to current facility, as a secondary diagnosis when a patient is received by transfer into a facility and documentation indicates he or she was administered tissue plasminogen activator (tPA) within the last 24 hours prior to admission to the current facility. This guideline applies even if the patient is still receiving the tPA at the time he or she is received into the current facility.

The appropriate code for the condition for which the tPA was administered (such as cerebrovascular disease or myocardial infarction) should be assigned first.

Code Z92.82 is only applicable to the receiving facility record and not to the transferring facility record.

1.167. This 42-year-old male had lateral wall STEMI and was brought by ambulance to the emergency room. He received tPA and was transferred to a tertiary care center for continued care. The patient was received with the tPA infusion continuing, and immediately taken to the cardiac cath lab. What **diagnosis** codes are assigned at the receiving hospital?

Code(s): _____

1.168. The patient who has had his bladder removed due to carcinoma without recurrence is scheduled for a radiology procedure to evaluate the patency of his ileal conduit, including ureteropyelography using contrast media. The entire procedure is performed in the radiology suite with the radiologists' impression of "normal functioning ileal conduit." What is the correct **diagnosis** code(s)?

Code(s): _____

Coding Note: Aftercare Z codes in ICD-10-CM should not be used for aftercare of fractures. For aftercare of a fracture, assign the acute fracture code with the seventh character D (subsequent encounter).

Coding Guideline I.C.20.a.2. External Cause Code Used for Length of Treatment
Assign the external cause code, with the appropriate seventh character (initial encounter, subsequent encounter, or sequela) for each encounter for which the injury or condition is being treated.

1.169. The patient was seen in his primary care physician's office for fracture aftercare concerning the traumatic fracture of the anterior wall of the acetabulum of the right pelvis. The patient was hit by a car, knocked down, and the car ran over his pelvis. The pelvic fracture is healing appropriately. What **diagnosis** codes are assigned?

Code(s): _____

Part II: Site-Specific Cases

Long-Term Care Cases

Note: These cases are included for practice assigning ICD-10-CM codes. They are *not* intended to illustrate any payer specific guidelines or whether a diagnosis is reportable or not per the MDS. Further, sequencing in the following cases may not always be consistent with actual long-term care (LTC) practice. These cases are presented to practice coding, not to illustrate the correct sequencing in LTC for admissions/returns. The *Coding Clinic,* 4th Quarter, 1999 addresses LTC sequencing issues, but currently there are no comparable guidelines in ICD-10-CM.

Coding Guideline I.C.21.c.3 Z79. Long-Term (Current) Drug Therapy
Codes from this category indicate a patient's continuous use of a prescribed drug (including such things as aspirin therapy) for the long-term treatment of a condition or for prophylactic use.

1.170. This long-term multiple sclerosis patient was admitted for continuing long-term antibiotic therapy for a urinary tract infection due to E. coli. Assign the correct **diagnosis** code(s).

Code(s): _____

Coding Guideline I.C.21.c.7. Aftercare
The aftercare Z codes should not be used for aftercare for injuries. For aftercare of an injury, assign the acute injury code with the appropriate seventh character (for subsequent encounter).

Coding Note: Coding Guideline 1.C.19.a directs the coder to use D as the seventh character when coding aftercare of a condition. However, if the condition involves an open fracture, reference the Tabular List for other seventh character options using the Gustilo classification for open fractures:

        Type I – Low energy, wound less than 1 cm
        Type II – Wound greater than 1 cm with moderate soft tissue damage
        Type III – High energy wound greater than 1 cm with extensive soft tissue damage
        Type IIIA – Adequate soft tissue cover
        Type IIIB – Inadequate soft tissue cover
        Type IIIC – Associated with arterial injury

1.171. This 55-year-old male was admitted for occupational therapy (OT) following hospitalization for type I open traumatic fractures of the left radius and ulna. Assign the correct **diagnosis** code(s).

Code(s): _____

Coding Note: ICD-10-CM does not provide a separate diagnosis code for physical, occupational, and speech therapy.

1.172. A 75-year-old woman was admitted for occupational therapy (OT) following cardiac bypass surgery. She continues to have significant acute post-thoracotomy pain. Assign the correct **diagnosis** code(s).

Code(s): _____

1.173. This patient sustained a fractured pelvis due to a fall from his moving electric wheelchair while in the nursing facility where he resides due to multiple sclerosis. Patient is readmitted from hospital. Assign the correct **diagnosis** code(s).

Code(s): _____

Coding Guideline I.C.21.c.3. Status

A status code should not be used with a diagnosis code from one of the body system chapters, if the diagnosis code includes the information provided by the status code. For example, code Z94.1, Heart transplant status, should not be used with a code from subcategory T86.2, Complications of heart transplant. The status code does not provide additional information. The complication code indicates that the patient is a heart transplant patient.

Coding Note: Similar to the coding guideline above, when a code for adjustment or management of a device is coded, the status code does not provide additional information and should not be coded.

1.174. This patient has cardiac defibrillator in situ for ventricular fibrillation and coronary artery disease who is admitted to the nursing facility for monitoring of the defibrillator. Assign the correct **diagnosis** code(s).

Code(s): _____

1.175. This patient fell while walking down the hall of the nursing facility where she lives and dislocated her right wrist. This was reduced in the facility. Assign the correct **diagnosis** code(s).

Code(s): _____

1.176. This 48-year-old male patient was admitted for PT and OT to maintain strength for Parkinson's disease. He requires continued monitoring and is not able to live alone. He also has type 1 diabetes mellitus and COPD. Assign the correct **diagnosis** code(s).

Code(s): _____

Coding Guideline I.C.19.e.5. Adverse Effect
When coding an adverse effect of a drug that has been correctly prescribed and properly administered, assign the appropriate code for the nature of the adverse effect followed by the appropriate code for the adverse effect of the drug (T36-T50). The code for the drug should have a fifth or sixth character 5. Examples of the nature of an adverse effect are tachycardia, delirium, gastrointestinal hemorrhaging, vomiting, hypokalemia, hepatitis, renal failure, or respiratory failure.

1.177. A nursing home resident who is starting chemotherapy treatments at the local hospital outpatient center had adverse reaction to chemotherapy after receiving the first dose of Fluorouracil (5-FU) for carcinoma of the transverse colon. After initial stabilization at the outpatient center, the patient returned to the nursing home still requiring management of diarrhea and nausea. Assign the correct **diagnosis** code(s).

Code(s): _____

1.178. This patient was hospitalized for a below-the-knee amputation of the left leg. Following surgery, he developed an infection of the amputation stump which was treated during the hospitalization and the antibiotics were complete at the time of discharge. The patient is now admitted to the nursing facility for dressing changes. Assign the correct **diagnosis** code(s).

Code(s): _____

1.179. This 35-year-old woman is in a coma due to a late effect of ingestion of valium and alcohol. This was a suicide attempt that occurred prior to admission to the nursing facility. Assign the correct **diagnosis** code(s).

Code(s): _____

1.180. This patient is being treated for a pathological fracture of the right humerus due to severe senile osteoporosis. This fracture was previously diagnosed during an acute-care hospital stay. Assign the correct **diagnosis** code(s).

Code(s): _____

Coding Guideline I.C.19.a. Application of Seventh Characters in Chapter 19
Seventh character S, sequela, is used for complications or conditions that arise as a direct result of a condition such as scar formation after a burn. The scars are sequelae of the burn. When using seventh character S, it is necessary to use both the injury code that precipitated the sequela and the code for the sequela itself. The S is added only to the injury code, not the sequela code. The specific type of sequela (e.g., scar) is sequenced first, followed by the injury code.

1.181. This elderly gentleman has severe chronic ulcerative colitis and osteoporosis, which is due to long-term use of corticosteroid injections. Assign the correct **diagnosis** code(s).

Code(s): _____

1.182. Resident is admitted to the nursing home following hospitalization for acute osteomyelitis and gangrene due to a chronic nonhealing stage 3 decubitus ulcer of the right ankle. Antibiotic therapy is continued. The patient is a type 1 diabetic with peripheral vascular disease due to the diabetes. The patient also has stage 4 chronic kidney disease, hypertension, and is status post left below-the-knee amputation. PMH also includes hypercholesterolemia and chronic alcoholism which is in remission. Assign the correct **diagnosis** code(s).

Code(s): _____

1.183. This 81-year-old female is a resident of the nursing facility due to CHF and atrial fibrillation. She fell from the bed at the nursing facility, and was transferred to the hospital. She was readmitted to the nursing facility to resume care and to add physical therapy following open reduction and pinning of left comminuted subcapital femoral neck fracture. Assign the correct **diagnosis** code(s).

Code(s): _____

Coding Guideline I.C.9.d.1. Category I69, Sequelae of Cerebrovascular Disease
Category I69 is used to indicate conditions classified to categories I60-I67 as the causes of sequela (neurologic deficits), themselves classified elsewhere. These late effects include neurologic deficits that persist after initial onset of conditions classifiable to categories I60-I67. The neurologic deficits caused by the cerebrovascular disease may be present from the onset or may arise at any time after the onset of the conditions classifiable to categories I60-I67.

Coding Note: Coding of sequelae in ICD-10-CM generally requires two codes with the residual condition or nature of the late effect being sequenced first. An exception to this requirement is when the sequelae have been expanded to include the manifestation(s). Cerebrovascular sequelae codes have been expanded to include the manifestation and therefore require only one code for both the residual condition and the cause of the sequelae.

1.184. This nursing home resident is admitted following a hospital stay for an acute cerebral infarction. The resident will receive multiple therapies for the resulting left hemiplegia of the nondominant side, dysphasia, and facial droop. Other admitting diagnoses include GERD, rheumatoid arthritis, and early onset Alzheimer's disease with dementia and aggressive behavior. Assign the correct **diagnosis** code(s).

Code(s): _____

1.185. This 65-year-old female patient had been living alone and had a cerebral embolism with infarction and was admitted to the hospital. She was discharged and admitted to the nursing facility because of the residuals of altered sense of taste and left dominant hemiplegia. Assign the correct **diagnosis** code(s).

Code(s): _____

1.186. This 62-year-old female resident of the nursing facility has early onset Alzheimer's disease. The dementia causes her to wander off. She had a cerebral embolism with infarction while in the nursing facility, with the residuals of global aphasia and right dominant hemiplegia. She remained in the facility and was not admitted to the hospital. Assign the correct **diagnosis** code(s).

Code(s): _____

1.187. This 85-year-old man is admitted to the nursing facility following hospitalization for dehydration due to pneumonia. Resident is admitted for multiple therapies due to weakness because of infiltrates. He will complete the antibiotics in the nursing home for the Pseudomonas pneumonia. Resident also had progressing dementia resulting from Parkinson's disease and he realized that it was getting more difficult to remain in his own home and agreed to admission. His past medical history includes mitral valve regurgitation, kyphosis, mild asthma, and type 2 diabetes. Assign the correct **diagnosis** code(s).

Code(s): _____

1.188. This patient is admitted to the nursing facility for PT and OT following hospitalization for an infected hip prosthesis that was performed two months prior. Resident was found to have vancomycin resistant enterococcus (VRE) that will require antibiotic therapy for six weeks via PICC line. The hospital discharge summary also included the following diagnoses: BPH with urinary obstruction, situational depression with agitation, hypertension, atrial fibrillation treated with Coumadin with INRs monthly. Assign the correct **diagnosis** code(s).

Code(s): _____

> **Coding Guideline I.C.4.a.3. Diabetes Mellitus and the Use of Insulin**
> If the documentation in a medical record does not indicate the type of diabetes but does indicate that the patient uses insulin, code E11, Type 2 diabetes mellitus, should be assigned. Code Z79.4, Long-term (current) use of insulin, should also be assigned to indicate that the patient uses insulin. Code Z79.4 should not be assigned if insulin is given temporarily to bring a type 2 patient's blood sugar under control during an encounter.

1.189. A resident was admitted to the nursing facility following foot amputation due to diabetic peripheral vascular disease. PT and OT were ordered with the plan for the resident to return home. Staff is to change dressings and report any suture site breakdown to the physician. Other diagnoses include gastroparesis due to type 2 diabetes (receiving insulin), mitral valve regurgitation with aortic stenosis, inguinal hernia, generalized DJD and COPD. Assign the correct **diagnosis** code(s).

Code(s): _____

Home Healthcare Cases

Note: These cases are included for practice assigning ICD-10-CM codes. They are *not* intended to illustrate any payer specific guidelines or whether a diagnosis is reportable or not per OASIS.

Coding Note: Superficial injuries, such as abrasions or contusions are not coded when associated with more severe injuries of the same site.

1.190. This 75-year-old woman is receiving continuing care for multiple facial lacerations, abrasions, and contusions. She was previously treated in the hospital's emergency department for these injuries. Assign the correct **diagnosis** code(s).

Code(s): _____

1.191. This 88-year-old gentleman is receiving home care for his coronary artery disease and the cardiac pacemaker placed during his hospitalization last week. He continues to gain strength but requires wound checks, dressing changes, and medication management ongoing. Assign the correct **diagnosis** code(s).

Code(s): _____

Coding Guideline I.C.2.k. Malignant Neoplasm Without Specification of Site
Code C80.1, Malignant (primary) neoplasm, unspecified, equates to Cancer, unspecified. This code should only be used when no determination can be made as to the primary site of a malignancy. This code should be rarely used in the inpatient setting.

1.192. This woman is being treated for a severe allergic reaction to chemotherapy due to cancer. The specific drug is Fluorouracil. Assign the correct **diagnosis** code(s).

Code(s): _____

1.193. This patient is admitted to home care for physical therapy three times a week and for surgical dressing changes two times a week after falling from an escalator at the mall. The patient is status-post traumatic right subtrochanteric hip fracture and is receiving continued care for this fracture with routine healing. Assign the correct **diagnosis** code(s).

Code(s): _____

1.194. This patient is a 65-year-old female admitted to home care following a hip replacement for osteoarthritis of the left hip. Patient was placed on Coumadin following surgery and has a refill for the Coumadin to continue several weeks postoperatively. Nurses are to do PT/PTT to monitor Coumadin levels, to change dressings, to watch for healing and signs of infection, and to report to the physician weekly. PT is providing gait training for walking difficulties. Assign the correct **diagnosis** code(s).

Code(s): _____

1.195. Home care skilled nursing visits are ordered for a patient who is on home oxygen for chronic obstructive pulmonary disease. Assign the correct **diagnosis** code(s).

Code(s): _____

1.196. This patient is admitted to home care with cellulitis of the right arm and is receiving IV antibiotics via a PICC line with routine PICC line maintenance. Assign the correct **diagnosis** code(s).

Code(s): _____

1.197. This female patient is admitted to home care following modified radical mastectomy for adenocarcinoma of the lower-outer quadrant of the right breast. Nursing services were ordered and provided for wound healing and dressing changes. Patient will be receiving chemotherapy in the following weeks. Assign the correct **diagnosis** code(s).

Code(s): _____

1.198. Patient is a 67-year-old woman, admitted to home care for physical therapy only for gait abnormality, following a total knee replacement of her right knee for osteoarthritis of the same knee. Patient had osteoarthritis of that particular joint only. Assign the correct **diagnosis** code(s).

Code(s): _____

1.199. An 80-year-old woman is admitted to home care following a hip replacement after traumatic closed fracture of the left hip, after she slipped on the ice in front of the grocery store. Since returning home the patient has developed a superficial wound infection at the incision site which will be addressed by home care staff. The physician has ordered wound care three times per week and gait training two times per week for her gait abnormality. Assign the correct **diagnosis** code(s).

Code(s): _____

1.200. Home healthcare nurses have been ordered to do monthly Foley catheter changes on this 70-year-old patient with a long-standing neurogenic bladder. Nurses are providing only Foley catheter changes. Assign the correct **diagnosis** code(s).

Code(s): _____

1.201. Home healthcare has been ordered by the patient's physician for this 75-year-old male who has had a cholecystectomy for acute cholecystitis. He had a drain placed at surgery to drain intra-abdominal fluid. Nurses are to monitor the drain output, watch for signs of infection, and provide dressing changes and remove drain per order. Assign the correct **diagnosis** code(s).

Code(s): _____

1.202. Patient is admitted to home care following a hospitalization for congestive heart failure, peripheral vascular insufficiency, and hypothyroidism. Skilled nursing is ordered for observation, weights, and medication management. Assign the correct **diagnosis** code(s).

Code(s): _____

1.203. Patient is discharged from the hospital after a problem with type 1 diabetes in ketoacidosis. Currently the diabetes is poorly controlled. Patient has a new insulin pump and is struggling to maintain glucose control. Skilled nursing is to both monitor glucose levels and provide dietary counseling and insulin pump training. Assign the correct **diagnosis** code(s).

Code(s): _____

1.204. Patient is admitted to home care following CABG for coronary artery disease. Nursing is following to provide skilled observation of cardiac status and wound care. Assign the correct **diagnosis** code(s).

Code(s): _____

1.205. An 80-year-old female is discharged from the hospital following surgical treatment for a malignant neoplasm of the sigmoid colon. The physician indicates that the patient will be undergoing chemotherapy for sigmoid cancer. Skilled nursing services are ordered for this patient three times a week for six weeks to teach colostomy care and assess the patient's compliance with medications. Assign the correct **diagnosis** code(s).

Code(s): _____

Coding Guideline I.C.19.a. Application of Seventh Characters in Chapter 19
The aftercare Z codes should not be used for aftercare of conditions such as injuries or poisonings, where seventh characters are provided to identify subsequent care. For example, for aftercare of an injury, assign the acute injury code with the seventh character D (subsequent encounter).

Coding Guideline I.C.19.c. Coding of Traumatic Fractures
A fracture not indicated as open or closed should be coded to closed. A fracture not indicated whether displaced or not displaced should be coded to displaced.

1.206. An 85-year-old independent female fell in her home, sustaining a left hip fracture. An open reduction with internal fixation was performed seven days ago. The patient was discharged home where her sister now cares for her. The patient is non-weight bearing on left lower extremity but can perform supervised pivot transfers with contact guard assist in and out of bed. The physician orders the agency to provide physical therapy for gait training because of gait abnormality, and exercise three times per week for four weeks. Assign the correct **diagnosis** code(s).

Code(s): _____

1.207. An 83-year-old female is admitted by the HHA following discharge from the hospital. The patient is seven days status post left total hip replacement due to generalized osteoarthritis. She developed a mildly exudated postop wound infection (MRSA), with partial separation of her surgical incision with external wound dehiscence. She was discharged from the hospital with IV antibiotics. This is the patient's initial episode of home healthcare.

Skilled Nursing Need: The patient's physician ordered daily skilled nursing visits for three weeks to treat her infected left hip surgical wound. The specific skilled nursing services ordered by the physician include the following:
- Monitor the wound for increasing signs and symptoms of infection;
- Administer IV antibiotics daily for 21 days; and
- Teach the patient's daughter to perform IV administration and wound care.

Therapy Need: The patient's physician ordered physical therapy services for gait training and strengthening exercises two times a week for four weeks. Ambulation is limited due to non-weight bearing status of her left lower extremity. The patient can perform supervised pivot transfers with contact guard assistance in and out of bed. Her daughter will be staying with her until her mobility improves. Assign the correct **diagnosis** code(s).

Code(s): _____

1.208. A 66-year-old left-handed woman who lives alone is discharged from the hospital three days after a right, modified radical mastectomy for breast cancer. She has residual weakness of her left arm, due to H/O stroke and is unable to care for her breast wound. Her medications include Tamoxifen for breast cancer chemotherapy and pain medications. Her physician reports that the patient's breast cancer is not resolved and the surgical drain is scheduled to be removed in several days.

Skilled Nursing Need: The patient's physician ordered skilled nursing visits daily for 10 days until the surgical drain is removed, then three times a week for four weeks to provide surgical wound care and supervision of the exercises ordered to improve her right shoulder range of motion and to monitor for any signs of infection.

Skilled Therapy Need: Skilled therapy services are not required or ordered by the patient's physician. The nurse will supervise the patient's performance of the exercises ordered to improve her shoulder range of motion on the affected side. Assign the correct **diagnosis** code(s).

Code(s): _____

1.209. A 70-year-old male is admitted to home health following discharge from an acute rehab facility. The patient received two weeks of physical therapy following his hospitalization for an acute CVA with infarct. Although his functional ability is improved, he is unable to ambulate due to monoparesis of his right lower leg, which is affecting his dominant right side. He has the ability to wheel independently in his wheel-chair. The patient requires physical therapy to regain his normal gait. His physician orders seven weeks of home health skilled therapy due to Monoplegia of lower limb affecting his dominant side.

Skilled Nursing: The HHA did not receive an order from the patient's physician to provide skilled nursing services. The patient's initial comprehensive assessment visit by the HHA did *not* identify a skilled nursing need.

Therapy Need: The patient's physician ordered physical therapy for gait evaluation/ training and strengthening exercises three times per week for four weeks, then two times per week for three weeks. The patient is currently wheelchair dependent (chairfast). He is unable to ambulate but he is able to wheel independently in his wheel-chair. This is his first episode of home healthcare. Twenty therapy visits are ordered by his physician for this episode of care. Assign the correct **diagnosis** code(s).

Code(s): _____

Hospital Inpatient Cases

> **Coding Guideline I.C.1.d.1.a. Sepsis**
>
> For a diagnosis of sepsis, assign the appropriate code for the underlying systemic infection. If the type of infection or causal organism is not further specified, assign code A41.9, Sepsis, unspecified organism.
>
> A code from subcategory R65.2, Severe sepsis, should not be assigned unless severe sepsis or an associated acute organ dysfunction is documented.

1.210. The following documentation is from the health record of a 71-year-old male patient.

Discharge Summary

History and Physical Findings: This 71-year-old male is a nursing home resident as a result of a cerebrovascular accident two years ago. He has had numerous hospital admissions for pneumonia and other infectious complications. On the day of admission, the patient was noted to be clammy, with tachypnea, to have decreased level of responsiveness, and to show increased fever. He was seen in the ER, where evaluation revealed the presence of probable urinary tract infection and sepsis. The patient was also found to have renal insufficiency with BUN and creatinine elevated. His WBC count was 23,000 with decreased hemoglobin and hematocrit. He was admitted for treatment of E. coli sepsis. Physical examination revealed an elderly male who was aphasic and had right-sided hemiplegia (he is right-handed), both from a previous CVA. The heart had a regular rhythm. The lungs were clear. The abdomen was soft.

Significant Lab, X-ray, and Consult Findings: Follow-up chemistry showed progressive decline in the BUN and creatinine to near normal levels. Initial white blood cell count was 23,700. Final blood count was 9,000. The urinalysis showed too numerous to count white cells. The urine culture had greater than 100,000 colonies of E. coli and Group B strep, which revealed the cause of the UTI. Repeated blood cultures grew E. coli with the same sensitivities as that of the urine. There were no acute abnormalities noted. EKG showed sinus tachycardia and low lead voltage, otherwise was normal and unchanged.

Course in Hospital: The patient was initially started empirically on Primaxin. He underwent fluid rehydration and his electrolytes were followed closely. Electrolytes improved through his hospital stay. He was continued on IV Primaxin until the date of discharge, when he was changed to Cipro by tube. All of the bacteria grown in the urine and in the blood were sensitive to the Cipro. The chest x-ray showed no change from previous admissions, and he was followed closely with additional oxygen as needed. The patient does have a history of chronic obstructive lung disease and has required intermittent oxygen therapy at the nursing home. At this time, the patient had reached maximal hospital benefit. He was switched to oral antibiotics. He was to continue on tube feedings, which he was tolerating quite well. The patient was discharged back to the nursing home on 5/4. Assign the correct **diagnosis** code(s).

Discharge Diagnoses:
1. E. coli sepsis
2. UTI, due to E. coli, and Group B strep
3. Renal insufficiency
4. Chronic obstructive lung disease
5. CVA with right hemiplegia

Code(s): _____

Coding Guideline I.C.2.c.2. Anemia Associated with Chemotherapy, Immunotherapy and Radiation Therapy

When the admission/encounter is for management of an anemia associated with an adverse effect of the administration of chemotherapy or immunotherapy and the only treatment is for the anemia, the anemia code is sequenced first, followed by the appropriate codes for the neoplasm and the adverse effect (T45.1x5), Adverse effect of antineoplastic and immunosuppressive drugs).

When the admission/encounter is for management of an anemia associated with an adverse effect of radiotherapy, the anemia code should be sequenced first, followed by the appropriate neoplasm code and code Y84.2, Radiological procedure and radiotherapy as the cause of abnormal reaction of the patient, or of later complication, without mention of misadventure at the time of the procedure.

1.211. A patient with known carcinoma of the pancreatic head is admitted with an Hgb of 9.1. She has been receiving Docetaxel chemotherapy and the physician diagnoses this new anemia as an adverse effect of the chemotherapy. The patient is treated with darbepoetin alpha and IV iron. The patient is discharged with an improvement in the Hgb to 11.3. Assign the correct **diagnosis** code(s).

Code(s): _____

1.212. The following documentation is from the health record of an 85-year-old female patient.

Discharge Summary: This 85-year-old female patient was noted to have three to four falls in the past two months at ABC Nursing Home. Patient fell yesterday from her parked wheelchair and hit the left frontal temporal area of her head causing a contusion. For this reason, the patient was brought to the hospital for observation and further workup. The patient's exam was remarkable for moderate ataxia. Past medical history includes senile dementia – Alzheimer's, late onset type, depression and emphysema. Current medications include Zoloft and Theophylline. CT scan of the brain noted that the patient had multiple masses in the brain due to metastatic disease. It was felt that the patient's ataxia was most likely due to the metastatic disease of the brain. These results were discussed with the patient's family. After much discussion regarding the treatment options, the family decided that they did not want the patient to undergo further tests and/or evaluation. It was the family's decision that the patient be transferred back to the nursing home and put under hospice care. Assign the correct **diagnosis** code(s).

Code(s): _____

1.213. The following documentation is from the health record of a 58-year-old male patient.

Discharge Diagnoses:
1. Carcinoma of the lung, right upper lobe, currently undergoing chemotherapy
2. Type 2 diabetes, with neuropathy and nephropathy
3. Hyperlipidemia
4. Hepatomegaly

History: This patient is a 58-year-old male who presented for outpatient chemotherapy. He had surgery for lung cancer three months ago and is now undergoing chemotherapy with Taxol and carboplatin, including dexamethasone as part of his chemotherapy and prophylaxis for nausea. He has done very well with the outpatient chemotherapy. When he presented for treatment on the day of admission, he was found to be hypoglycemic. He is a known type 2 diabetic which is also complicated by neuropathy and nephropathy. Due to his blood glucose levels, it was decided to postpone this chemotherapy session and he was admitted for control of his diabetes. Dr. Johnson consulted with the patient to manage his diabetes regimen. He has been on 70/30 insulin, 25 units in the morning and 15 units in the evening for several years. An IV insulin drip was started and he also had q 1 hour Accu-Checks. His hepatomegaly has enlarged from the last time that I saw him. Question whether this is fatty infiltration due to poor diabetes control, or whether there is now some involvement with metastatic carcinoma.

Lab Data: Sodium 128, potassium 5.5, chloride 89, BUN 13, creatinine 0.8, glucose range 30-460, with final glucose of 210. Calcium 9.4, WBC 9.8, hemoglobin 11.6, hematocrit 34.3, platelets 277,000.

Plan: One difficulty here is the cyclic nature of his chemotherapy treatment regimen, likely to produce major shifts in his glucose, which is already difficult to control. The patient will need to monitor his glucose levels closely. He is discharged on 70/30 insulin, 35 units in the morning and 20 units in the evening. He is to follow up with me for further chemotherapy in the oncology clinic next week. Assign the correct **diagnosis** code(s).

Code(s): _____

1.214. The following documentation is from the health record of an 87-year-old female patient.

Discharge Summary

History of Present Illness: The patient is an 87-year-old female who was admitted from a nursing home with congestive heart failure, dehydration as well as urinary tract infection and thrombocytopenia with petechial hemorrhage. On admission she was found to have a platelet count of 77,000 and a Hematology consult was done. The patient denied any bleeding diathesis in the past. She stated that she had recent bruising of the hands related to needle sticks, but otherwise has not had any past history of any bleeding disorder. No specific history of hematuria, hematemesis, gross rectal bleeding, or black stools.

Past Medical History: Significant for congestive heart failure, diabetes

Medications: Coreg, isosorbide, Actos, digoxin, glyburide, hydralazine, furosemide, Ditropan, and potassium

Family History: No family history of any bleeding disorder

Physical Examination: She is an elderly-appearing white female, somewhat short of breath, using supplemental oxygen. Examination of the head and neck revealed no scleral icterus. Throat was clear. Tongue was papillated. There was no thyromegaly or JVD. There was no cervical supraclavicular, axillary, or inguinal adenopathy. Chest examination revealed rales, bilaterally. There were decreased breath sounds at the right base. There were coarse rales heard in the right midlung field. Heart exam showed rhythm was irregular. Abdomen exam was difficult to perform. I was unable to palpate the liver or spleen. Bowel sounds were active. Extremities revealed no clubbing, cyanosis, or edema. There were diffuse ecchymoses, especially in the dorsum of the right hand.

Laboratory Studies: Hematocrit was 43, white count 9,000 with 82% neutrophils, and the platelet count 77,000. The MCCV was 102. Creatinine was 1.7. Bilirubin was 1.7. The alkaline phosphatase was 122. AST 498, ALT 493, and albumin 3.6. The prothrombin time was 18 seconds, the PTT was 25 seconds. The chest x-ray showed a right pleural effusion.

Course in Hospital: The patient was admitted and started on IV fluids. Her diuretics were increased, and she showed a good response and better control of her congestive heart failure. Hematology consult recommended holding platelet transfusion unless there was evidence of active bleeding. No platelets were given during this admission.

The patient was discharged back to the nursing home on day six in improved condition to continue with the same medication regimen as previous to hospitalization. Assign the correct **diagnosis** code(s).

Final Diagnoses:
1. Congestive heart failure
2. Dehydration
3. Primary thrombocytopenia with petechial hemorrhage and hematoma of the eyelids and bilateral arms and hands
4. Urinary tract infection
5. Type 2 diabetes mellitus

Code(s): _____

> **Coding Guideline I.C.9.a.1. Hypertension with Heart Disease**
> Heart conditions classified to I50.- or I51.4-I51.9 are assigned to a code from category I11, Hypertensive heart disease, when a causal relationship is stated (due to hypertension) or implied (hypertensive). Use an additional code from category I50, Heart failure, to identify the type of heart failure in those patients with heart failure.

1.215. The following documentation is from the health record of an 85-year-old female patient.

Discharge Summary
Admit Date: 12/10/XX
Discharge Date: 12/22/XX

Discharge Diagnoses:
1. Hypertensive left heart failure with acute pulmonary edema
2. Myocardial infarction ruled out
3. Chronic obstructive pulmonary disease
4. Pseudomonas pneumonia

History of Present Illness: This 85-year-old female was admitted via the Emergency Room from the nursing home with shortness of breath, confusion, and congestion. There was no history of fever or cough noted. Patient also has a history of COPD. Prior to admission, the patient was on the following medications: Prednisone, Lasix, Benicar, and Colace. Patient had a long history of tobacco dependence prior to admission to the nursing home.

Physical Examination: Blood pressure 140/70, heart rate of 125 per minute, respirations were 30, temperature of 101.4. The eyes showed postsurgical eyes, nonreactive to light. The lungs showed bilaterally bibasilar crackles. The heart showed S1 and S2, with no S3. The abdomen was soft and nontender. The extremities showed leg edema. The neurological exam revealed no deficits and she was alert ×3.

Hospital Course: Basically, this patient was admitted to the coronary care unit with acute pulmonary edema, rule out myocardial infarction. Serial cardiac enzymes were done, which were within normal limits, therefore ruling out myocardial infarction. A chest x-ray performed on the day before admission confirmed left heart failure and pneumonia.

The patient was started on Unasyn and Tobramycin for the pneumonia, which improved. The left heart failure, however, was not improving with administration of Lasix. The patient was not taking foods and liquids well, and, at the family's request, she was made DNR. On hospital day 12, she was found without respirations, with no heart sounds, and pupils were fixed. She was declared dead by the physician, and the family was notified. Assign the correct **diagnosis** code(s).

Code(s): _____

1.216. The following documentation is from the health record of a 69-year-old female.

History of Present Illness: The patient is a 69-year-old female with previous MI, known hypertensive, who started complaining of cough, chills, and fever about 4 days prior to admission. One day prior to admission, she started to complain of progressive dyspnea. She went to the ER and was noted to be extremely dyspneic and wheezing. She was given an aerosol treatment with good response. However, chest x-ray showed evidence of bilateral lower pneumonia with a PO2 of 66 and white blood cell count of 12,400. The patient was subsequently admitted. The patient has been taking Methyldopa 500 mg. bid, Ascriptin 1 tablet daily, Transderm Nitro 5 once daily, Capoten 30 mg. bid, and Lanoxin 0.725 mg. daily. The patient had an inferior wall myocardial infarction three years ago and chronic, mild congestive heart failure. She is known to have chronic anxiety problems and has been under the care of the Mental Hygiene Clinic.

Physical Examination: Revealed a well-developed, well-nourished female whose respirations had improved since the aerosol therapy was given. Blood pressure is somewhat elevated. Respirations 24. Pulse 110/minute. HEENT: Unremarkable. No carotid bruits. No distended neck veins. Chest: No deformity. Equal expansion. Lungs: Crepitant rales over the lower half of hemithorax. No wheezing. No pericardial or pleural rub noted. Heart: Regular rhythm. No murmurs. Abdomen: Soft. Liver, spleen and kidneys not enlarged. No tenderness. Extremities: No clubbing. No cyanosis. Peripheral pulses strong and equal.

Impression: Lobar pneumonia. Previous inferior wall myocardial infarction. Hypertension. Chronic anxiety.

Hospital Course: Sputum smear showed moderate white blood cells, many epithelial cells and many mixed respiratory microflora. Sputum culture showed normal growth. Blood cultures after 10 days showed no growth. Chest x-ray report revealed acute congestive cardiac failure. Significant improvements in congestive heart failure noted on second x-ray, but not complete resolution, although the pneumonia has resolved. EKG showed right bundle branch block with old inferior myocardial infarction. This patient's previous medications were continued during hospitalization.

After cultures were obtained, she was empirically started on IV Kefzol and aerosolized bronchodilator therapy consisting of Alupent. She remained afebrile during her stay in the hospital. She had no further wheezing after 24 hours, but continued to have mild crepitant rales in both bases. She had one episode of mild angina pains relieved by nitroglycerin during her stay. With improvement in her respirations and x-ray findings, she was discharged. Her BP was 154/110 on discharge, but this is not considered unusual since her BP is quite unstable as an outpatient, with variable high and low readings. This will, however, be followed up in the office. Assign the correct **diagnosis** code(s).

Final Diagnoses:
1. Bilateral pneumonia
2. Old myocardial infarction with angina
3. Hypertension
4. Chronic anxiety
5. Acute on chronic diastolic congestive heart failure

Code(s): _____

1.217. The following documentation is from the health record of a 33-year-old female patient.

OB Record
Admit Note 2/27
This is a 33-year-old G2 P0, with an estimated delivery date of 2/28, and estimated gestational age of 40 weeks. She presents for induction secondary to gestational diabetes mellitus. The diabetes has been managed by diet throughout the pregnancy. The patient also has diastasis recti that occurred three weeks ago, which has kept her at bedrest since that time. PNL: O positive, rubella immune. PE: AVSS, Abdomen FH 40 cm, EFW 3800-4000 grams. Cervix is closed/50%/-3/post/ceph. Plan is for Pitocin induction with epidural at the beginning of active labor.

Progress Note 2/28 09:15
Patient is having uterine contractions every 3-8 minutes. Cervix is 1 cm/100%/floating. Patient desires not to start Pitocin yet. Feels that she is in labor. FHR reactive, baseline 120's with accelerations.

Progress Note 2/28 19:25
Patient's uterine contractions have resolved. Cervix unchanged. Discussed options, would like to go home to sleep and return in a.m. for Pitocin induction. Discharged home for tonight to sleep. Admit in a.m., start IV Pitocin as per protocol and clear liquid diet. Assign the correct **diagnosis** code(s).

Code(s): _____

1.218. The following documentation is from the health record of an 18-day-old baby boy.

Discharge Summary
This is an 18-day-old male infant, who was admitted after he was noticed to be developing omphalitis. He was immediately placed on intravenous Cefotaxime and Ampicillin, later changed to Cefotaxime and Clindamycin. A culture taken from the umbilical stump grew Staphylococcus aureus (MRSA) and Group H Streptococcus.

After the first day, there was great improvement and the patient continued to improve completely. Now there is no redness or swelling whatsoever. The child has remained afebrile, has continued to eat very well. He shows no sign of abdominal tenderness or peritonitis. I feel that we have treated this well. He has had five days of intravenous antibiotics. I will finish the treatment with Keflex by mouth seeing that both Streptococcus pyogenes and Staphylococcus aureus are sensitive. The mother will watch the child closely and let me know if any problems occur. I have instructed her to watch for any more redevelopment of the redness, swelling, or discharge. We will recheck this in two weeks for one-month checkup. Assign the correct **diagnosis** code(s).

Code(s): _____

> **Coding Guideline I.C.19.e. Adverse Effects, Poisoning, Underdosing, and Toxic Effects**
> Codes in categories T36-T65 are combination codes that include the substance that was taken as well as the intent. No additional external cause code is required for poisonings, toxic effects, adverse effects, and underdosing codes.
>
> When coding a poisoning or reaction to the improper use of a medication (e.g., overdose, wrong substance given or taken in error, wrong route of administration), first assign the appropriate code from categories T36-T50. The poisoning codes have an associated intent as their fifth or sixth character (accidental, intentional self-harm, assault, and undetermined). Use additional code(s) for all manifestations of poisonings.

1.219. The following documentation is from the health record of a 17-year-old male patient.

History of Present Illness: The patient is a 17-year-old white male who was brought to the ED after being found in the town park. The patient was in restraints and accompanied by two police officers. The patient was combative and aggressive, threatening physical harm to himself as well as the physician and hospital staff. The patient has a long history of alcohol and drug abuse, was in the local treatment center, and walked off campus two days ago.

Allergies: NKDA

PMH: Attention deficit hyperactivity disorder (ADHD), amphetamine drug and alcohol dependence, unsocialized aggressive behavior

Family History: Noncontributory

ROS: As above

Physical Examination: Vital signs: temp. 100.1 degrees, BP 144/88 mmHg; General: alternating between lethargy and combativeness; HEENT: pupils pinpoint, 1 mm bilaterally; Skin: cool, clammy to touch, feet and hands cold, slightly diaphoretic; Heart: rate tachy, no murmurs; Lungs: clear, respiratory rate 28 and shallow; Abdomen: benign; Neurological: mental status as above; follows commands inconsistently, responds to voice; cranial nerves: pupils as noted, gag intact; motor: moving all four extremities with equal power; sensory: responds to touch in all four extremities; deep tendon reflexes +3 throughout, but plantar reflexes down going bilaterally.

Laboratory: U/A shows 2+ blood, done after Foley catheter was placed; drug screen + for amphetamines; ETOH 45 mg/100 ml; ABG within normal limits; EKG sinus tachycardia.

Hospital Course: Family was contacted, IV fluids were initiated for dehydration and tachycardia, and the patient was admitted to ICU with suicide protocol, Ativan 1–2 mg IV q 2 hours prn. He was maintained on soft restraints with checks every 15 minutes and monitored with telemetry and neuro checks through the night. By the morning he was no longer tachycardic. By hospital day three he was medically stable, but still saying he wants to "kill himself." Psychiatric consult requested.

Disposition: Discharge to psych. Psychiatric liaison service agreed to accept him in transfer to the inpatient adolescent psychiatric unit at children's hospital. Assign the correct **diagnosis** code(s).

Discharge Diagnoses:
1. Drug overdose with amphetamines and alcohol
2. Suicide attempt
3. Alcohol intoxication

Code(s): _____

1.220. The patient is being seen due to right knee pain and decreased mobility. Previously the patient had a right total knee replacement for osteoarthritis. The patient also has extensive medical problems which were all monitored and treated while he was in the hospital: Parkinson's disease, hypertensive heart disease, congestive heart failure, bilateral capsular glaucoma, old MI six months ago, and recent abnormal cardiac stress test. Evaluation of the right knee indicated that patient had aseptic loosening of the tibial component of the knee. The orthopedic consultant indicated that the patient would need to be scheduled for a revision arthroplasty once he was cleared by cardiology for surgery. The cardiac clearance will be done as an outpatient and the procedure will then be scheduled. Assign the correct **diagnosis** code(s).

Code(s): _____

1.221. The patient is a 47-year-old-female admitted to the hospital for a scheduled total abdominal hysterectomy and bilateral salpingo-oophorectomy due to submucous leiomyoma of the uterus. The patient also has extensive endometriosis of the uterus, ovaries, and pelvic peritoneum. On the day of admission the patient was taken to surgery and in addition to the scheduled procedure lysis of extensive pelvic peritoneal adhesions was also carried out. In the process of removing the adhesions, the physician accidentally punctured the small bowel. This small puncture was quickly repaired. The patient was diagnosed with acute blood-loss anemia with a documented loss of 1,500 ml of blood during surgery. The remainder of the postoperative course was uneventful and the patient was discharged on day 4. Assign the **diagnosis** codes only.

Code(s): _____

> **Coding Guideline I.C.16.a.2. Principal Diagnosis for Birth Record**
> When coding the birth episode in a newborn record, assign a code from category, Z38, Liveborn infants according to the place of birth and type of delivery, as the principal diagnosis. A code from category Z38 is assigned only once, to a newborn at the time of birth. If a newborn is transferred to another institution, a code from category Z38 should not be used at the receiving hospital. A code from category Z38 is used only on the newborn record, not on the mother's record.

1.222. Hospital Summary: A male newborn, born at this hospital with pre-axial polydactyly of the thumbs and cleft deformities of both hands and feet, had a harsh murmur heard posteriorly and faint femoral pulses on initial newborn exam. The newborn was 39 weeks gestation and was born vaginally. Cardiology was consulted and an echocardiogram diagnosed coarctation of the aorta and a very small conoventricular ventricular septal defect. The newborn had surgical repair of the coarctation but the VSD could not be repaired at this young age due to closeness to the aortic valve. Cardiology will follow to manage the VSD. Orthopedics was consulted for the hand and feet deformities and will schedule serial repairs after the age of about 1 year. The family will be seen by Medical Genetics as an outpatient for possible determination of a syndrome that encompasses this combination of defects. Assign the correct **diagnosis** code(s).

Code(s): _____

Physician-Related Cases

Coding Guideline IV.N. Ambulatory Surgery

For ambulatory surgery, code the diagnosis for which the surgery was performed. If the postoperative diagnosis is known to be different from the preoperative diagnosis at the time the diagnosis is confirmed, select the postoperative diagnosis for coding, since it is the most definitive.

1.223. The patient was seen with amenorrhea, characteristics of masculinization, and high levels of serum testosterone. Pelvic ultrasound revealed a left discrete ovarian mass. The GYN performed a laparoscopic unilateral salpingo-oophorectomy as an outpatient. Pathologic diagnosis returned as ovarian Sertoli-Leydig cell tumor. Upon receipt of the pathology report, what **diagnosis** does the GYN report?

Code(s): _____

1.224. The physician sees this 16-year-old patient with myasthenia gravis and adolescent idiopathic thoracic scoliosis. Surgery for spinal fusion was cancelled after the patient had a positive TB skin test during the preop physical workup, suggesting latent TB. On today's visit, the patient is started on Isoniazid 300 mg daily and instructed on possible side effects. She will reschedule surgery after two months of INH treatment. Assign the correct **diagnosis** code(s).

Code(s): _____

Coding Guideline IV.E. Encounters for Circumstances Other than a Disease or Injury

ICD-10-CM provides codes to deal with encounters for circumstances other than a disease or injury. The Factors Influencing Health Status and Contact with the Health Services codes (Z00-99) is provided to deal with occasions when circumstances other than a disease or injury are recorded as diagnosis or problems.

Coding Guideline I.C.21.c.2. Inoculations and Vaccinations

Code Z23 is for encounters for inoculations and vaccinations. It indicates that a patient is being seen to receive a prophylactic inoculation against a disease. Procedure codes are required to identify the actual administration of the injection and the type(s) of immunizations given. Code Z23 may be used as a secondary code if the inoculation is given as a routine part of preventive health care, such as a well-baby visit.

1.225. A 62-year-old female visits her family practice physician for an annual physical and follow-up on her chronic gout with tophi. She has her annual Pap smear and flu shot for the season. What **diagnoses** codes would the physician report?

Code(s): _____

1.226. The surgeon performed surgery on an 8-year-old boy who presented with progressive ataxia over a period of the past month. Surgical removal and frozen section identified the lesion as malignant ependymoma of the midbrain of the brain stem. During the surgical procedure, an accidental infratenorial intraoperative laceration left the patient with postsurgical left-sided muscle weakness and he will be sent for an outpatient rehabilitation evaluation next week. What **diagnosis** code(s) would the surgeon submit for the case?

Code(s): _____

1.227. The following documentation is from the record of a 36-year-old male patient during a visit to his primary care physician.

History of Present Illness: The patient is here for follow-up of lab work from earlier in the week. He was bitten by a tick last month and has had body aches, some swelling to the right upper arm, pain and stiffness in the right elbow, as well as feeling fatigued. He had a Lyme test that came back positive and the patient is to have a repeat blood test today, the Western Blot test, as a secondary follow-up.

Physical Examination: He is alert and in no acute distress. Temp 98.4. Pulse 108. Respirations 20. Blood pressure is 118/70. Weight is 296 on a 5' 9" frame. Weight up 3 pounds from last week and 22 pounds up since the beginning of the year. Arm continues to display a circular erythematous lesion with 2+ pitting edema. The lesion has not grown outside the perimeter markings from his first visit.

Impression:
1. Localized arthritis, right elbow in Lyme disease due to tick bite
2. Morbid obesity, BMI of 43.7

The patient has blood drawn and was put on Doxycycline 100 mg b.i.d. × 4 weeks. Additional educational material on Lyme disease was given. He should follow-up immediately if the affected area grows larger than the current, marked area or if any new symptoms develop. We discussed again the need for an exercise program, when able, and portion control due to his over-nourishment status. Assign the correct **diagnosis** code(s).

Code(s): _____

1.228. The following documentation is from the office note of a podiatrist:

S: The patient presents for initial consult of tender lumps in the arches of both feet, left greater than right. Patient relates they have been present for several years and can change in size. Patient is also a diabetic and relates that his sugars are hard to control, running in the low 200s. Does get numbness in his feet.

O: Palpable pedal pulses bilaterally. Skin is warm with hair growth present. On plantar aspect of medial band of plantar fascia on the left, there is an approximately 1 × 1 cm elevated, solid lesion consistent with plantar fibroma. Pain with palpation. With palpation, medial band of plantar fascia on the right arch, there are two small, solid lesions noted, approximately 0.5 × 0.5 cm in diameter. These do not protrude through the skin as lesion on left foot does. Lesions on the right foot are nontender with palpation.

A: Plantar fibroma, bilateral, with left greater than right
   Diabetes mellitus, type 2 with diabetic neuropathy

P: Discussed findings with patient. I advised that patient apply Triamcinolone cream to his feet to help decrease the size of the lesions. To help break down the lesion on the left arch, I injected 0.2 cc of 0.25% Marcaine plain and 0.2 cc of Kenalog into the lesion. The patient was instructed to work more diligently at controlling his sugars to prevent further neuropathy. I suggested Vitamin B_6 200 mg and Vitamin B_{12} 1,000 mcg, one tab of each daily to aid in nerve function. These are over the counter and can be purchased at the drug store. Patient is to follow-up with me in 4 to 6 weeks. Assign the correct **diagnosis** code(s).

Code(s): _____

1.229. The patient is a 42-year-old female with multiparity who presented for tubal ligation. She also had a large vulvar skin tag that the physician removed while the patient was under anesthesia. The physician listed diagnoses of multiparity, desiring sterilization by tubal ligation and vulvar skin tag, removed. What ICD-10-CM **diagnosis** codes would the surgeon report?

Code(s): _____

1.230. The patient is a 49-year-old female with a chief complaint of painful mouth ulcers over the last month. She was treated with acyclovir for 10 days and penicillin on two occasions, including tapering doses of steroids on the second occasion. The patient states that she feels somewhat better but continues to have these ulcers with pain. Denies fever, chills, dysphagia, or lymphadenopathy. No high risk behavior.

Physical Exam: Reveals whitish patches measuring 1 mm × 1 mm on the buccal musoca and the hard palate. They are erythematous and inflamed.

Assessment: Aphthous ulcers and herpangina

Plan: Will start patient on clindamycin orally for buccal cellulitis and Amlexanox 5% as oral paste along with the Xylocaine mouth wash. Patient should follow up with me in 2 weeks. Assign the correct **diagnosis** code(s).

Code(s): _____

1.231. The patient was seen for menstrual irregularities, as well as new symptoms of vaginal itching and skin rash. The physician diagnoses vaginal candidiasis and tinea corporis on this visit, provides treatment as well as continuing treatment for the patient's polycystic ovarian syndrome. Assign the correct **diagnosis** code(s).

Code(s): _____

1.232. The patient presents for results of an MRI of the right knee, done to diagnose a new problem of severe pain and inability to safely descend stairs. She reports falling while running in the park. The MRI revealed a complex medial meniscal tear and a Baker's cyst, along with mild chondromalacia of the patella, which the physician discussed with the patient. Options for treatment were discussed and the patient will determine what she'd like to do, after discussing the situation with her husband and family. Assign the correct **diagnosis** code(s).

Code(s): _____

1.233. From a discharge summary written by an internal medicine physician:

The patient was admitted for dizziness and a vague feeling of epigastric discomfort. She has a history of duodenal carcinoma which was resected two years ago. The patient underwent chemo and has been in relatively good health over the last year until recently when she took a rapid decline. She no longer has evidence of an existing primary duodenal malignancy.

During her hospitalization, she underwent a GI workup to evaluate her current issues. An abdominal ultrasound showed a large liver mass. Oncology was consulted. The mass was further evaluated by needle biopsy and found to be metastatic carcinoma.

After lengthy consultation with me and the oncologist, the patient and family wish the patient to be a "Do Not Resuscitate" with no further workup and comfort care only. The patient was transferred from my service on the telemetry unit to the hospice program for ongoing palliative care.

What **diagnosis** codes would the attending physician submit?

Code(s): _____

1.234. The following is taken from the records of a psychiatrist:

Follow-up Visit: The patient is a 10-year-old girl who is seen today to check progress after her Adderall XR was increased from 10 to 15 mg about six weeks ago. Since that time, the mother reports a very noticeable improvement in attention and task persistence, and a decrease in her hyperactivity and distractibility. This has also been commented on by her teacher and observed at home. She is now able to complete homework at one sitting, prior to dinner and without prompting. The teacher also reports less negativity than the patient had sometimes shown in the past.

Status of Medication: Adderall XR 15 mg with the above noted benefits. Appetite has been fine. Weight is stable.

Vitals Signs: Height 52½ inches, Weight 56.8 lbs, Blood pressure 96/54, Heart rate 91.

Impression: Medication showing clear benefits according to both teacher and parent.

Diagnoses:
Coordination disorder, developmental
Attention deficit disorder with hyperactivity, combined type

Plan: Continue current dosing. Three months of refills provided. Follow-up in three months. Assign the correct **diagnosis** code(s).

Code(s): _____

1.235. Reason for evaluation: Follow-up and medical management

History: The patient is a 5-year-old who has been in fairly good health. Her last skeletal dysplasia visit was 3 years ago. Since then, there has been some concern regarding signs of sleep apnea with a diagnosis of obstructive sleep apnea confirmed on sleep study. She has not had any imaging studies since her last visit.

The patient has a family history of achondroplasia in the father and the paternal grandmother. No other chromosomal abnormalities are noted. Her initial newborn bone survey showed bilateral foreshortening and splaying of the epiphyses of the distal and proximal ends of the femurs, irregular appearance of the developing acetabulum, thickening, with slight bowing of the femurs and lordosis. She has not reported any neurological issues and has never had a brain MRI. Her physical exam today is relatively unchanged and is remarkable for a large appearing head with frontal bossing, protuberant abdomen, lumbar hyperlordosis, extremity shortening with inability to extend elbow, trident-like hands and lax joints.

Impression:
1. Osteosclerosis congenita
2. Obstructive sleep apnea
3. Congenital lumbar lordosis
4. Family history of Osteosclerosis congenita

Recommendations: Weight management with dietitian to help prevent additional stress on bones and joints. Follow-up with me in one year. Assign the correct **diagnosis** code(s).

Code(s): _____

Coding Guideline IV.H. Uncertain Diagnosis

Do not code diagnoses documented as "probable," "suspected," "questionable," "rule out," or "working diagnosis" or other similar terms indicating uncertainty. Rather, code the condition(s) to the highest degree of certainty for that encounter/visit, such as symptoms, signs, abnormal test results, or other reasons for the visit.

1.236. From the record of a primary care physician:

Chief complaint: Vertigo

HPI: The patient is a 55-year-old Caucasian female who presents with vertigo over the last month. She has had vertigo symptoms mostly when lying down on her back. She gets a dizzy feeling which she describes as spinning and reports some decreased hearing and buzzing in the left ear. Symptoms last about 30 minutes, relieved when she does not move. She denies nausea, vomiting, or any other neurologic symptoms associated with this dizziness. She also describes left-sided temporal pain which she states feels like she is going to develop a headache but never quite develops into a headache. It comes and goes many times throughout the day.

Past Medical History: None

Review of Systems: As above

Physical Exam: She is afebrile. Vital signs are stable. Neurologic exam is unremarkable. Cerebellar exam is normal. PERRLA. EOM intact. No nystagmus with lateral gaze. Vision is WNL on screening with no diplopia. Tympanic membranes are normal ×2. Posterior pharynx is normal. Neck is supple. No lymphadenopathy. No rigidity. Lungs are clear to auscultation bilaterally. Heart is regular rate and rhythm without murmur. Normal S1, S2. Abdomen: Soft and nontender. Extremities: No edema. Skin: without rash or significant lesions. No tenderness over the temporal artery. Neuro: Cranial nerves II-XII are intact.

Assessment and Plan:
1. Labyrinthine vertigo. Patient agrees to PT evaluation. Will try Antivert for spinning.
2. Headache with normal neurologic exam. ESR ordered to rule out temporal arteritis due to the location.

Patient to return in two weeks for follow-up. Assign the correct **diagnosis** code(s).

Code(s): _____

1.237. From the clinic record of a family practice physician:

Problem: Hospital Follow-up

S: The patient is here for follow-up of new diagnosis of Bell's palsy, made during hospitalization over the weekend. He thought he was having a stroke but complete evaluation ruled out stroke and diagnosed Bell's palsy. He was started on medication for this. His main concern today is a lot of ear pain and jaw pain on the left that have been increasing since his discharge on Monday. He describes the jaw pain as burning and stinging in nature.

O: Patient is in no acute distress but is obviously in some pain. Vital signs are stable. Left TM is erythematous. Right TM is gray. He does have a notable Bell's palsy with the droop of his face on the left as well as persistent inability to close the left eyelid. Palpation of the jaw area elicits a hot, shooting pain. Lungs are clear. Cardiovascular reveals regular rate and rhythm.

A: Bell's palsy. New facial pain, rule out superimposed trigeminal neuralgia. Nonsuppurative otitis media.

P: I did start him on Bactrim double strength dose twice a day for 10 days. I have recommended Tylenol for pain. He should continue to use the eyedrops prescribed by the neurologist and I gave him an eye patch to use at nighttime to rest the eye. I have arranged another appointment for later today with the neurologist to further evaluate the increasing jaw pain and recommend treatment. Follow-up with me as necessary.

Assign the correct **diagnosis** code(s).

Code(s): _____

1.238. The patient is a 54-year-old female who presents today with an infected cuticle on her left thumbnail. The patient states this started about one week ago. She denies any discharge from the nail but throbbing pain at night. She does work as a bartender where she is frequently having her hands immersed in water. She denies any trauma to her hand. No possibility of a fracture. No nausea, vomiting or diarrhea, fever or chills. The patient does have a cough. She is a smoker for the past 20+ years. She smokes a pack of cigarettes a day. The cough is typical and sometimes productive of whitish clear sputum.

Allergies: Penicillin and iodine both which produce hives.

Social History: Admits to drinking two beers a day. No illicit drug use.

Review of Systems: The patient has never had a chest x-ray done. She is up to date on her Pap smears and mammogram.

Physical Exam: Blood pressure is 118/66. Pulse 70. Respiration 12. Temp is 98.5. Lungs are clear to auscultation. No rales, rhonchi, or wheezing. Heart is RRR. Abdomen is soft, nontender, and nondistended. To the lateral aspect of the left thumbnail bed there is increased swelling and erythema with no discharge noted. There is exquisite tenderness on palpation.

Impression:
1. Paronychia left thumbnail - levaquin 750 mg once a day for five days
2. Smokers' cough - chest x-ray ordered, CMP, lipids, TSH and CBC ordered.
3. Tobacco abuse

Assign the correct **diagnosis** code(s).

Code(s): _____

> **Coding Guideline I.C.15.a.1. Codes from Chapter 15 and Sequencing Priority**
> Obstetrics cases require codes from Chapter 15, codes in the range of O00-O9A, Pregnancy, childbirth and the puerperium. Chapter 15 codes have sequencing priority over codes from other chapters. Additional codes from other chapters may be used in conjunction with Chapter 15 codes to further specify conditions. Should the provider document that the pregnancy is incidental to the encounter, then code Z33.1, Pregnant state, incidental, should be used in place of any Chapter 15 codes. It is the provider's responsibility to state that the condition being treated is not affecting the pregnancy.

1.239. The patient is a 32-year-old female with Hashimoto thyroiditis and gestational diabetes, currently 34 weeks gestation. She is seen for ongoing monitoring of the conditions. Blood sugars and thyroid lab results are reviewed. Synthroid is increased to 0.125 mg p.o. daily. The endocrinologist will see her back six weeks postpartum to re-evaluate her conditions. The endocrinologist documents the following diagnoses: Hashimoto thyroiditis complicating pregnancy and gestational diabetes, well controlled utilizing dietary measures. Assign the correct **diagnosis** code(s).

Code(s): _____

1.240. The following documentation is from the health record of a 25-year-old female patient.

History of Present Illness: The patient is a Caucasian female without significant medical history and is 18 weeks pregnant. She presents with a 6-month history of right hand pain and paresthesias, happening prior to her pregnancy. This seems to be worse over the last 1 month. She states that she bought a hand splint for nighttime but typing and writing during the day makes it hurt significantly. She says she's always had cold hands/fingertips. When she runs them under warm water, this improves them. She denies any color changes in the fingertips. The paresthesias seem to involve most of the fingers. The pain seems to be mostly in the palm of the hand. The only relieving factors are heating her hand.

Past Surgical History: None.
Medications: Prenatal vitamins.
Allergies: No known drug allergies.
Family History: No neurological issues.

Physical Examination: On exam, her blood pressure is 122/68. Pulse is 82. Both her hands are warm. Right fingertips are considerably cooler. There are no color changes. She has good distal pulses. Hands are neurovascularly intact. There is no thenar atrophy. Strength is 5/5 in the fingers and wrists. Phalen and Tinel sign are negative. Skin has no rashes.

Assessment and Plan: Right hand pain and paresthesias. Incidental pregnancy. She should wear her right wrist splint at night and in the day as tolerated. She will get an ergonomic keyboard. She will take Tylenol for pain and avoid all other analgesics due to pregnancy. She will have a TSH to rule out hypothyroidism and will have right upper extremity EMG/nerve conduction. If this is normal, we could consider the possibility of Raynaud phenomenon. She will follow up with me after her testing is complete. Assign the correct **diagnosis** code(s).

Code(s): _____

1.241. The following is an admission H&P dictated by the patient's primary care provider:

Reason for Admission: Malaise, low-grade fever, and diarrhea

HPI: This is a 60-year-old male with severe peripheral vascular disease who had recently been hospitalized for C. difficile diarrhea, which seemed to resolve well with treatment. His diarrhea was basically resolved after his 5-day admission. He went home and was doing fine but over the last week he started developing more malaise, low-grade fever and the watery and frequent diarrhea returned. He presented to the ED today and was admitted.

Past Medical History: He has peripheral vascular disease of both lower legs. He also has had a peptic ulcer in the remote past.

Social History: He lives at home with his wife and does have a supportive family. He does not smoke or drink.

Physical Exam: His blood pressure is low at 90/60. His temperature is 97.2. HEENT: Pupils are equal and reactive to light and accommodation. There is some weakness of an ocular muscle. Neck: Supple. Lungs: Clear. Heart: S1 and S2. No murmur. No gallop. Abdomen: There is some minimal diffuse tenderness to his abdomen on palpation. Extremities: No edema or cyanosis in the thighs. The lower legs are both looking better than on past admission.

Impression: Recurrence of Clostridium difficile colitis.

Plan: Started on flagyl and vancomycin. C. diff cultures will be obtained. We will also check blood cultures and urine cultures. The patient is dehydrated and IV fluids started in the ED will be continued. Will ask Vascular to consult about the need for DVT prophylaxis due to decreased mobility while hospitalized.

What **diagnosis** codes should the physician report?

Code(s): _____

1.242. Primary care provider note from the record of a 44-year-old female patient:

CC: Mourning

History: The patient is here because of fatigue. Does not want to get out of bed, is still crying and wants to give up on her life. The patient did see a counselor for one visit a couple of months ago but she says it didn't really help. She has not been feeling any better and is depressed. She is eating appropriately and is well groomed today. She denies any serious suicidal ideation.

Physical Exam: She is 44 and weighs 151 pounds. She is 5 feet tall. Blood pressure is 112/60. HEENT is WNL. Lungs are clear. Heart is regular rate and rhythm. Abdomen: Benign.

Assessment and Plan: Major depression with bereavement of husband. She was given fluoxetine 10 mg daily for a week, then 20 mg daily for a week. She is to return to the office to see me in 2 weeks. Assign the correct **diagnosis** code(s).

Code(s): _____

1.243. This 30-year-old male patient has exhausted all types of conservative treatment for his morbid obesity. Despite regular consultation with a registered dietitian, he continues to eat in excess of 7,000 calories per day. This may be attributed to his very low-literacy level. He has been treated in this clinic for the last three years. He has also been treated for hypertension and hypercholesterolemia. With these risk factors and with careful review of his condition and symptoms and with consultation regarding the risks and benefits of surgery, it has been decided to perform a vertical-banded gastroplasty two weeks from this office visit. Assign the correct **diagnosis** code(s).

Code(s): _____

> **Coding Note:** When coding otitis media, ICD-10-CM provides laterality specificity at the sixth character level.

1.244. From the clinic record of a family practice physician:

Subjective: The patient is a 12-month-old female patient who presents to the clinic today with a possible ear infection. She has been waking up at night and is irritable. She has had some cold-like symptoms as well as some purulent drainage from her eyes over the past four days. She has had a fever since last night. This morning the temperature is back to near normal. No cough and appetite has been slightly decreased.

Objective: In no acute distress; alert and interactive. Temperature is 100.7.

HEENT: Lids and sclera are normal. No erythema noted. She does have some purulent drainage mostly on the left lower lid. She also has a purulent nasal discharge that is yellow to green. TMs are erythematous bilaterally, bulging and with purulent effusions. Oropharynx is nonerythematous without lesions. Tonsils are unremarkable. Two teeth on the bottom.

Neck: Neck is supple with good ROM. Positive cervical adenopathy.

Lungs: Clear.

Heart: Regular rate and rhythm without murmur.

Assessment:
1. Acute bilateral suppurative otitis media
2. Upper respiratory infection

Plan: The patient will be placed on Augmentin 40 mg/kg. divided t.i.d. for 10 days. Also recommended lots of fluids and rest, decongestants and elevating the head of the bed for symptomatic control. I believe the eyes are due to backup from her nose and not due to conjunctivitis at this point. The parents will need to contact the clinic if she develops any erythema or persistent drainage. The parents are comfortable with this plan and will contact the clinic with any further questions and/or concerns. Assign the correct **diagnosis** code(s).

Code(s): _____

> **Coding Note:** ICD-10-CM provides combination codes that include the type of diabetes mellitus and the manifestation/complication.

> **Coding Note:** The Tabular instructs the coding professional to use an additional code with type 2 diabetes to identify any insulin use.

1.245. Assign the **diagnosis** code(s) for a patient with type 2 diabetic gastroparesis who is presently on insulin.

Code(s): _____

1.246. A 20-year-old patient with end-stage renal disease is seen for monitoring of his condition. The patient is currently receiving dialysis three times a week. He has an A-V fistula in his left arm for vascular access. Assign the correct **diagnosis** code(s).

Code(s): _____

> **Coding Guideline I.C.21.c.8. Follow-up**
> The follow-up codes are used to explain continuing surveillance following complete treatment of a disease, condition, or injury. A follow-up code may be used to explain multiple visits. Should a condition be found to have recurred on the follow-up visit, then the diagnosis code for the condition should be assigned in place of the follow-up code.

1.247. From the health records of a patient receiving endoscopy services:

The patient presents to the hospital outpatient department for follow-up cystoscopy for a history of high-grade bladder cancer. This was resected five years ago and was found to be Grade III with superficial muscle invasion. A cycle of chemotherapy was provided, but no radiation. No recurrence has been noted since then. CT scan of the pelvis six months ago was negative for masses. Sometimes the patient experiences painful ejaculation, but no hematospermia has been found. Cytology to date has been negative.

Cystoscopy examination today shows a new primary site of transitional cell carcinoma of the anterior wall of the bladder. There is some lateral lobe prostatic hypertrophy, just barely touching in the midline. The bladder is nontrabeculated. There is clear efflux from each orifice. The area of resection was around the right ureteral orifice, which appears a little atrophic, but patent. Patient is scheduled for surgery as soon as convenient.

Impression: Stable transitional cell carcinoma of the bladder with mild benign prostatic hypertrophy. Assign the correct **diagnosis** code(s).

Code(s): _____

1.248. This 70-year-old patient is seen for his follow-up care for his arthritis. He has primary generalized degenerative arthritis mostly of the knees, hip, and of the lumbosacral spine. It is getting progressively worse. He refuses surgery and is not a prime candidate because of his arteriosclerotic heart disease and hypertension. A prescription was written to renew his Celebrex and other medications for his ASHD and hypertension. Assign the correct **diagnosis** code(s).

Code(s): _____

1.249. A 13-year-old male patient is being evaluated in the Children's Clinic for growth problems. He is 4'11" and does not exhibit any signs of puberty or secondary sexual characteristics. His parents wonder if the necrotizing enterocolitis that he had at birth is the cause of his short stature. Other than his short stature, the patient seems perfectly normal. His short stature does create problems at school, however, as he is experiencing definite problems with social rejection and exclusion because of his height. Blood tests were drawn. Diagnosis: Short stature with delayed puberty.

The patient came back to the clinic for follow-up of test results, which indicated a deficiency of growth hormone. The patient was started on growth hormone treatments. Diagnosis on the second visit is HGH deficiency. Provide the ICD-10-CM codes for both the first and second visit. Assign the correct **diagnosis** code(s).

Code(s) for first visit: _____

Code(s) for second visit: _____

Coding Note: In ICD-10-CM, when coding an infection due to an indwelling urinary catheter, the coding professional is instructed to use an additional code to identify the infection. Additionally, if the infectious agent is also known, this should be assigned as an additional diagnosis.

1.250. A nursing home patient with an indwelling Foley catheter is diagnosed at the physician office, with a serious urinary tract infection due to E. coli caused by the catheter. The catheter is removed and a urine culture and sensitivity is sent. The catheter is replaced through the urethra, and aggressive antibiotic therapy is begun. The patient is returned to the nursing home for continued follow-up. Assign the correct **diagnosis** code(s).

Code(s): _____

Coding Guideline I.C.9.a.3. Hypertensive Heart and Chronic Kidney Disease
Assign codes from combination category I13, Hypertensive heart and chronic kidney disease, when both hypertensive kidney disease and hypertensive heart disease are stated in the diagnosis. Assume a relationship between the hypertension and the chronic kidney disease, whether or not the condition is so designated. If heart failure is present, assign an additional code from category I50 to identify the type of heart failure. The appropriate code from category N18, Chronic kidney disease, should be used as a secondary code with a code from category I13 to identify the stage of the chronic kidney disease.

1.251. A patient is seen in the hospital with a diagnosis of congestive heart failure due to hypertensive heart disease. The patient responds positively to Lasix therapy. The patient also has chronic kidney disease stage 5. Assign the correct **diagnosis** codes.

Code(s): _____

Hospital Outpatient Cases

Coding Guideline I.C.1.a.2.d. Asymptomatic Immunodeficiency Virus
Z21, Asymptomatic human immunodeficiency virus [HIV] infection status, is to be applied when the patient without any documentation of symptoms is listed as being "HIV positive," "known HIV," "HIV test positive," or similar terminology. Do not use this code if the term "AIDS" is used or if the patient is treated for any HIV-related illness or is described as having any condition(s) resulting from his/her HIV positive status; use B20 in these cases.

Coding Guideline IV.H. Uncertain Diagnosis for Outpatient Services
Do not code diagnoses documented as "probable," "suspected," "questionable," "rule out," or "working diagnosis" or other similar terms indicating uncertainty. Rather, code the condition(s) to the highest degree of certainty for that encounter/visit, such as symptoms, signs, abnormal test results, or other reason for the visit.

1.252. The following documentation is from the health record of a male patient who received emergency department services.

Emergency Department Report
A patient, who is a known heroin addict, is brought into the emergency room in significant distress. His genitalia are covered with many lesions. Due to his IV drug habit and sexual practices, he is at risk for HIV exposure and hepatitis. He is unable to provide a medical history, but the physician is able to get some information from his girlfriend. Although severely ill, he is not comatose.

Physical examination reveals multiple excoriations covering the penis and scrotum with fluid-filled blisters and the patient is in significant distress. The patient is heavily intoxicated and the last "fix" was one hour ago per the girlfriend. The patient has been using heroin daily for the past two months. A number of laboratory tests were run, and it was determined that the patient should be transferred to a tertiary care center for definitive treatment with an infectious disease consultation and substance abuse rehabilitation when stable.

The physician's dictated report that details the test results shows the following diagnostic assessment:
1. HSV-2 infection, culture confirmed, severe outbreak
2. Hepatitis suspected, pending laboratory results for type, abnormal liver function studies confirmed
3. HIV seropositive
4. High-risk lifestyle; sexual habits and drug addict
5. Heroin intoxication

Assign the correct **diagnosis** code(s).

Code(s): _____

1.253. The encounter is to receive chemotherapy following the recent diagnosis of carcinoma of the pancreas neck. The cancer was diagnosed two months ago and the patient has been receiving chemotherapy. After the chemotherapy administration, the patient developed severe nausea and vomiting due to the chemotherapy, which led to dehydration. Medications were given for the nausea and vomiting. IV fluids were given to rehydrate the patient. What **diagnosis** codes are assigned?

Code(s): _____

Coding Guideline I.C.18.b. Use of a Symptom Code with a Definitive Diagnosis Code
Signs or symptoms that are associated routinely with a disease process should not be assigned as additional codes, unless otherwise instructed by the classification.

1.254. The following documentation is from the health record of a 39-year-old male patient.

Emergency Department Services
History of Present Illness: The patient is a 39-year-old African-American gentleman who has a known history of sickle-cell Hb-C disease who presented to the Emergency Department with diffuse extremity pains with a little more complaints of pain along the right inguinal area. They started on Friday, became a little bit better on Saturday, then improved; and again started in the past 24 hours. He denies any problems with cough or sputum or production. He denies any problems with fever.

Past Medical History: See recent medical records in charts. He does have a new onset of diabetes, probably related to his hemochromatosis. He does have evidence of iron overload with high ferritins.

Review of Systems: Otherwise unremarkable except for those related to his pain. He denies any problems with any fever or night sweats. No cough or sputum production. Denies any changes in gastrointestinal or genitourinary habits. No blood per rectum or urine.

Physical Examination: This is a 39-year-old African-American gentleman who is conscious and cooperative. He is oriented ×3 and appears in no acute distress. Vital signs are stable. HEENT is remarkable for icterus present in oral mucosa and conjunctivae, which is a chronic event for him. The neck is supple. No evidence of any gross lymphadenopathy of the cervical, supraclavicular, or axillary areas. The heart is irregular in rate without any murmurs heard. Lungs are clear to auscultation and percussion. The abdomen is soft and benign without any gross organomegaly. Extremities reveal no edema. No palpable cords. He does have some tenderness along the inner aspects of his right lower extremity near the inguinal area; however, no masses were palpable and no point tenderness is noted.

IV fluids and pain medications were administered in the ED. He had a problem with his right inguinal area. He had evidence of pain. There was some pain on abduction of his right lower extremity. The wrist really was unremarkable. There was no evidence of any Holman, no palpable cords, no masses were palpable.

Because of his sickle-cell anemia, rule out the possibility of avascular necrosis of the femur. Complete x-rays of his femur and hip were carried out. However, these were both negative.

Patient is being transferred to a larger facility for treatment of his sickle-cell crisis. Unfortunately, he has very little family support with his medical issues. Doppler studies should also be carried out to rule out any venous thrombosis.

Diagnoses:
1. Painful sickle-cell crisis
2. Type 2 diabetes mellitus
3. Limited family support

Condition on Discharge: Stable on pain meds.

Assign the correct **diagnosis** code(s).

Code(s): _____

1.255. The following documentation is from the health record of a 66-year-old male patient.

Outpatient Hospital Department Services
History: This is a 66-year-old gentleman who had coronary artery bypass graft two months ago and continues to do well. Sometime after he was discharged home, he had two days of black stools. He has not had any other evidence of hematemesis, melena, or hematochezia but was feeling rather weak and fatigued. He had blood work done which showed a hemoglobin of 9.7, hematocrit of 20.9, MCV of 80 and serum iron of 8.2% saturation. No indigestion, heartburn, or abdominal pain of any kind. There is no past history of anemia or GI bleed.

Past Medical History: General health has been good.
Allergies: None known
Previous Surgeries: Coronary artery bypass graft
Medications: At the time of admission include Glucotrol, Lasix, and potassium

Review of Systems: Endocrine: He does have diabetes, controlled with oral medication. Cardiovascular: Coronary artery disease with coronary artery bypass graft. No recent symptoms of chest pain or shortness of breath. Respiratory: No chronic cough or sputum production. GU: No dysuria, hematuria, history of stones, or infections. Musculoskeletal: No arthritic complaints or muscle weakness. Neuropsychiatric: No syncope, seizures, weakness, paralysis, depression.

Family History: Is positive for cardiovascular disease and diabetes in his mother. No history of cancer.

Social History: The patient is married. Has never smoked and does not drink. Works in a factory where he is exposed to high levels of industrial toxic agents.

Physical examination reveals a well-developed, well-nourished, alert male in no acute distress. Blood pressure: 146/82. Respirations: 18. Heart rate: 78. Skin: Good turgor and texture. Eyes: No scleral icterus. Pupils are round, regular, equal, and react to light. Neck: No jugular venous distention. No carotid bruits. Thyroid is not enlarged. Trachea is in the midline. Lungs are clear. Heart: No murmur noted. Abdomen is soft. Bowel sounds present. No masses, no tenderness. Liver and spleen are not palpably enlarged. Extremities: Good pulses. Trace edema of the feet.

Laboratory values show severe anemia with a hemoglobin of 9.7. His iron studies showed low iron and low ferritin, consistent with chronic blood loss anemia. His B_{12} and folate levels were normal. His SMA-12 was essentially unremarkable.

Recommendations: Patient should have an esophagogastroduodenoscopy and colonoscopy, possible biopsy or polypectomy, as well as a blood transfusion, which has been explained to the patient along with potential risks and complications. These will be scheduled as soon as possible.

Final Diagnoses:
1. Severe blood loss anemia; weakness
2. Type 2 diabetes mellitus
3. Coronary artery disease status post coronary artery bypass graft
4. Unhealthy work environment

The patient was scheduled for EGD and colonoscopy as well as a blood transfusion. The patient will be discharged home and he will have clear liquid diet. He is to call for any problems. He will continue with his home medications, and he was placed on ferrous sulfate 1 tablet twice a day. Assign the correct **diagnosis** code(s).

Code(s): _____

1.256. The following documentation is from the health record of a 2-week-old baby.

Emergency Department Services
A 2-week-old baby is rushed to the hospital after the parents checked and found her cyanotic. While in the ER, she suffered respiratory arrest followed by cardiac arrest and was given cardiopulmonary resuscitation. The baby was born with a birth weight of 2,400 g. Her current weight is 2,700 g. The baby was emergently transferred to the neonatal intensive care unit at the university hospital across town for monitoring and further workup. Final diagnosis for the ER service is "Hypoxia with respiratory failure in a low birth weight infant—etiology unknown." Assign the correct **diagnosis** code(s).

Code(s): _____

1.257. The following documentation is from the health record of a 51-year-old female patient:

Emergency Department Services
The patient has a history of serious illnesses, including type 1 diabetic complications, that include severe peripheral vascular disease of the extremities. She presented to the ER via ambulance with chest pain and shortness of breath.

She has been hypertensive for many years and is currently well controlled on medication. Her BP in the ER was stable but was monitored frequently. The patient's blood sugar was also monitored.

Impression:
Chest pain and shortness of breath
Rule out CHF vs. pulmonary embolus
Diabetes mellitus, type 1, out of control, with significant peripheral vascular disease

Plan: Transfer to University Hospital.

Assign the correct **diagnosis** code(s).

Code(s): _____

Coding Guideline I.C.20.k. External Cause Status

A code from category Y99, External cause status, should be assigned whenever any other external cause code is assigned for an encounter, including an activity code, except for the events noted below. Assign a code from category Y99, External cause status, to indicate the work status of the person at the time the event occurred. The status code indicates whether the event occurred during military activity, whether a non-military person was at work, whether an individual including a student or volunteer was involved in a non-work activity at the time of the causal event.

A code from Y99, External cause status, should be assigned, when applicable, with other external cause codes, such as transport accidents and falls. The external cause status codes are not applicable to poisonings, adverse effects, misadventures, or late effects.

Do not assign a code from category Y99 if no other external cause codes (cause, activity) are applicable for the encounter.

An external cause status code is used only once, at the initial encounter for treatment. Only one code from Y99 should be recorded on a medical record.

Do not assign code Y99.9, Unspecified external cause status, if the status is not stated.

1.258. The patient is seen in the ER today for a burn of the right ankle. The patient was cooking dinner in the kitchen of her single family home and carrying a pot of boiling hot liquid that splashed on her ankle. The physician documents the diagnosis as: Second degree burn, right ankle. Assign the correct **diagnosis** code(s).

Code(s): _____

1.259. The following documentation is from the health record of a male patient who received emergency department services.

Emergency Department Report: This is a 48-year-old male patient who presents to the ED with a history of left lower quadrant abdominal pain for two days. The patient has localized tenderness with some guarding on the left lower quadrant.

Past Medical History: Hypertension
Past Surgical History: Right rotator cuff surgery
Allergies: Ibuprofen
Medications: Diovan HCT
Social History: Patient smokes cigarettes, alcohol socially
Family History: Father had diverticulitis and cancer of the colon

Review of Systems: Negative nausea, vomiting, or diarrhea. Had a relatively normal bowel movement earlier today. No rectal bleeding. All other systems reviewed and are negative.

Physical Examination: No acute distress but in pain. Vital signs: Temp is 98.6, pulse 88, respirations 20, blood pressure 116/78. HEENT: Within normal limits. Neck: Supple, no masses, no bruit. Heart: Regular S1, S2 present. No chest pain. Lungs: Clear. No shortness of breath, no cough. Abdomen: Soft. Tenderness with guarding of the left lower quadrant. Bowel sounds are present. Extremities: No calf tenderness. Pulses are palpable. Sensory motor system is intact. Neurological: Patient is alert and oriented.

A stat CBC was done which showed white cell count of 20,000.

Impression:
1. Acute diverticulitis
2. Family history of colon cancer
3. Hypertension

The patient is started on Levaquin and Flagyl and will continue his at-home hypertension med. A surgical consult is requested and the surgeon recommended admission to 23-hour observation. Assign the correct **diagnosis** code(s).

Code(s): _____

1.260. The patient presented to the hospital urgent-care center, complaining of a swollen left upper eyelid for the past 2 days. She stated that the swelling was increasing and putting more and more pressure on her eye. The eyelashes were affecting her vision as the angle of the lashes had changed due to the swelling. She reported a history of surgery to her sinus on the left side about 2 months ago. On physical exam the physician noted that the left eyelid and surrounding tissue was severely swollen and had a focal area consistent with an internal hordeolum.

The assessment was internal hordeolum of left eyelid with secondary orbital cellulitis and the physician prescribed Keflex 500 mg 4 times a day for 7 days and cortisporin ophthalmic ointment twice daily to the eye. The physician advised washing the eyelid with Johnson's No More Tears baby shampoo twice daily, using good handwashing technique and not touching either eye during the healing process, except for treatments as above. The patient was told to follow up with her PMD in 3 days for a recheck or sooner if the area increases in size. Assign the correct **diagnosis** code(s).

Code(s): _____

1.261. The following documentation is from the health record of a female patient who received emergency department services.

Emergency Department Report
Chief Complaint: Multiple Sclerosis

S: The patient presents today with numbness and pain in her left arm and leg and in her back. She says it feels the way it felt when she was first diagnosed with MS several years ago. She came in today because of a rather sharp pain over her lungs and in her chest area while she was driving to work. She came here rather than continuing on to work. She describes the pain as fairly sharp and stabbing. It was exacerbated when she took a deeper breath, which really scared her. She denies any coughing with this and she denies any diaphoresis with it.

O: Patient is in mild distress and is breathing rather shallowly to avoid pain. Her BP is 126/78, pulse 88, respirations 24. Temp is 99.3 degrees. Lungs: Essentially clear. CV: Regular rate and rhythm and no murmurs. Extremities: without edema. EKG is unchanged from previous and chest x-ray shows blunting in the costophrenic angle but no infiltrates or pneumothorax seen.

A: Exacerbation of multiple sclerosis with viral pleurisy.

P: The patient will start Prednisone 60 mg a day with the tapering schedule to be determined by the neurologist at her outpatient evaluation the day after tomorrow. She will begin Indomethacin 25 mg twice a day and will take Tylenol if additional pain relief is needed. The patient is placed off of work and will avoid any strenuous activity. She should return if her symptoms get worse or for additional pain management if a cough develops. Assign the correct **diagnosis** code(s).

Code(s): _____

> **Coding Guideline I.C.13.a. Site and Laterality**
> Most of the codes within Chapter 13 have site and laterality designations. The site represents either the bone, joint, or the muscle involved. For some conditions where more than one bone, joint, or muscle is usually involved, such as osteoarthritis, there is a "multiple sites" code available. For categories where no multiple site code is provided and more than one bone, joint, or muscle is involved, multiple codes should be used to indicate the different sites involved.

1.262. The following documentation is from the health record of a female patient who is receiving care from the Rheumatology Clinic.

Follow-up Clinic Note

HPI: The patient returns now for a follow-up visit. She has been on Plaquenil for about 6 weeks. Overall she feels somewhat better. She does report a new issue with incontinence and wonders if this is related to either of her medications. She describes this as an urgency and as leakage if she sneezes or coughs. She seems to otherwise be tolerating her medications without difficulty.

Physical Exam: Examination today shows her vital signs to be stable. She is afebrile. Joints show inflammation in the right ankle and left wrist. The remainder of the upper and lower extremity joints are quiet.

Impression: Palindromic rheumatism on methotrexate and Plaquenil. Urge and stress incontinence.

Plan: UA done in the office today is normal. Review of medication literature does not give any evidence that either medication is associated with urinary incontinence. I recommended that she make an appointment with the Urology clinic to discuss this new issue. The patient and I again talked about the need to avoid methotrexate in situations where she could become dehydratd because of potential renal clearance problems. She was instructed not to take methotrexate if she has been vomiting for more than 12 hours without consultation here. The patient will have a hemogram, liver function panel, and creatinine today and then will follow up with this clinic in 8 weeks. If she has other illnesses, she will call us, hold her methotrexate and arrange to be seen either here or in the emergency department for evaluation. Assign the correct **diagnosis** code(s).

Code(s): _____

1.263. The following documentation is the discharge note of a female patient who received emergency department and observation services.

HPI: The patient presents today with blurred vision which resolved after a duration of 20 minutes, left temporal headache, and left lower extremity weakness and numbness. The lower extremity complaints resolved within the first hour in the ED. She states that the headache has been an 8 or 9 out of 10 but her vision has improved. She recalls headaches like this in the past but not this painful and without the associated symptoms.

Vitals Signs: In the ED, her blood pressure was 143/88, pulse 80, respirations 20, temperature 97.4. HEENT: all within normal limits. Chest: Clear to auscultation bilaterally. Cardiac: Normal S1, S2. Slight bradycardia. No heaves, murmurs, or rubs. Abdomen: Soft. Nontender. No HSM. Extremities. No clubbing, cyanosis, or edema. Sensation has completely returned. Gait is now normal. Neurological: Cranial nerves II-XII are intact. Alert and oriented ×3. The patient was admitted to 23 hour observation for intractable headache.

Observation Course: The patient was seen by neurology and an MRI, 2D echo, ESR, and RPR were all checked. Her results were essentially negative. CT scan showed no bleed, no mass effect or shift. Her carotid dopplers were within normal limits. MRI showed no acute infarct but some small vessel ischemic changes. The patient was also seen by cardiology and was cleared by them. Her EKG showed signs of bradycardia and her 2D echo was normal.

Pain was managed with morphine 2.5–4mg IV q 6–8hrs with resolution at approximately observation hour number 14. The patient was discharged on no medication and will follow up with neurology as an outpatient.

Impression: Cluster headache, intractable. Secondary cause ruled out. Assign the correct **diagnosis** code.

Code(s): _____

Coding Guideline IV.A.2. Observation Stay

When a patient is admitted for observation for a medical condition, assign a code for the medical condition as the first-listed diagnosis.

When a patient presents for outpatient surgery and develops complications requiring admission to observation, code the reason for the surgery as the first reported diagnosis (reason for the encounter), followed by codes for the complications as secondary diagnoses.

Coding Guideline I.C.21.c.9. Donor

Codes in category Z52, Donors of organs or tissues, are used for living individuals who are donating blood or other body tissue. These codes are only for individuals donating for others, not for self-donations. They are not used to identify cadaveric donations.

1.264. This 24-year-old male bone marrow donor was taken to the Same Day Surgery suite and, under general anesthesia, 200 cc of bone marrow was aspirated from the posterior iliac crests. During postop recovery, the patient developed a postop fever, nausea, and vomiting and was subsequently admitted to observation. The nausea and vomiting subsided following medication. The patient became afebrile and was discharged home. Assign the correct **diagnosis** code(s).

Code(s): _____

1.265. The patient is taken to the outpatient surgical suite for an ERCP to remove a stone from the common bile duct. The patient has a history of tachycardia which recurred after the procedure. The patient was admitted to observation until the heart rate could be stabilized.

Preoperative Diagnosis: Jaundice due to calculus obstruction of the common bile duct

Postoperative Diagnosis: Jaundice due to calculus obstruction of the common bile duct, tachycardia. Assign the correct **diagnosis** code(s).

Code(s): _____

Coding Guideline IV.H. Uncertain Diagnosis

Do not code diagnoses documented as "probable," "suspected," "questionable," "rule out," or "working diagnosis" or other similar terms indicating uncertainty. Rather, code the condition(s) to the highest degree of certainty for that encounter/visit, such as symptoms, signs, abnormal test results, or other reasons for the visit.

1.266. The patient is a 1Y, 11M old female who presents to the emergency department with a 2-day history of pain in the left groin area. Four months ago, the patient had a similar problem on the right side and was diagnosed with an inguinal fold abscess. She has no fever today, is on no medication, and does have an allergy to Bactrim, which was tried last time.

On examination, the patient has a 2 cm × 1 cm abscess of the left labia majora toward the inguinal fold. Yellow pus was expressed and there is no surrounding erythema. The remainder of the exam was normal.

Findings are a nearly 2-year-old female with labial abscess from what appears to be staph. The patient is given Keflex 250 mg/5 ml, 4 ml PO TID × 10 days and Bactroban BID × 5 days. The mother is to clean the area with Hibaclens at every diaper change. Follow-up with the PMD in 1 week or sooner if fever, increased erythema, or rash. Assign the correct **diagnosis** code(s).

Code(s): _____

1.267. The following documentation is from the health record of a female patient who received emergency department services.

Emergency Department Report

The patient presents to the emergency department today complaining of chest pain, cough, and joint pain. She has a history of pulmonary sarcoidosis. She states that she has been missing a lot of work because she has been so sick with a variety of complaints.

On physical exam, she weighs 174 pounds. Temp is 98.2. Pulse is 60. Respiratory rate is 24. Blood pressure is 132/90. Lungs: She has coarse breath sounds. Pharynx is slightly erythematous without exudates. Nasal mucosa is pink and moist. Neck is supple with some shotty anterior cervical lymphadenopathy. Heart has a regular rate and rhythm. S1 and S2 without murmur, gallop, or rub. Joints are non-tender, non-erythematous, and have full range of motion with no effusion.

Studies: CMP and UA came back normal. Chest x-ray PA and lateral reveals bronchitis and known granulomas of the left lower lobe. EKG was normal.

Assessment:

Acute bronchitis

Sarcoidosis

Arthralgias

Elevated blood pressure, not on hypertensive medication

Plan: Clarithyromycin 500 mg once a day for 10 days along with Robitussin AC cough syrup 1 teaspoon every 4 hours prn for cough. She will follow-up with her primary care physician next week for her blood pressure which is elevated today. This may be a transient finding due to her breathing issues. Assign the correct **diagnosis** code(s).

Code(s): _____

1.268. The following documentation is the discharge progress note from an observation case.

Nephrology Attending

Patient is doing somewhat better. Slight cough. Afebrile. Pulmonology has been here to consult. Ordered PEP valve training for airway clearance.

Temp 37, P 115, R22, BP 100/68
No acute distress. Cushingoid facies. RRR with no murmur. Lungs clear bilaterally. Abdomen soft, non-tender, not distended. No edema and no rash.

Blood culture was negative × 24 hours. CXR – mild peribronchial thickening. Urine not sent for culture.

Assessment/Plan: Viral URI and neutropenia in a six year old male with Wegener's granulomatosis.

Urine for culture. Respiratory therapy training today. Discharge home after training and ceftriaxone dose this evening. CBC with diff on Monday in my office. Assign the correct **diagnosis** code(s).

Code(s): _____

1.269. The patient is a 22-year-old male who had bilateral nasolacrimal duct serial probing with silicone stent placement, completed in the outpatient surgery suite. Assign the correct **diagnosis** code(s).

Pre- and Postoperative Diagnosis:
1. Lacrimal duct stenosis, left greater than right
2. Microcephaly
3. Angelman microcephaly syndrome

Code(s): _____

Coding Guideline IV.K. Patients Receiving Diagnostic Services Only

For patients receiving diagnostic services only during an encounter/visit, sequence first the diagnosis, condition, problem, or other reason for encounter/visit shown in the medical record to be chiefly responsible for the outpatient services provided during the encounter/visit. Codes for other diagnoses (e.g., chronic conditions) may be sequenced as additional diagnoses.

For outpatient encounters for diagnostic tests that have been interpreted by a physician, and the final report is available at the time of coding, code any confirmed or definitive diagnosis(es) documented in the interpretation. Do not code related signs and symptoms as additional diagnoses.

1.270. The following information is documented on the electrocardiogram report interpreted by the physician:

Clinical History: Irregular heart beat

Findings: Normal sinus rhythm, bigeminy with frequent PVCs.

Assign the correct **diagnosis** code.

Code(s): _____

1.271. The following documentation is from the health record of a male patient who received emergency department services at the community hospital.

Emergency Department Report
Chief Complaint: Vomiting and stomach ache

HPI: 21 month old male with emesis ×4 days. Hard to console today, crying constantly. Vomited at least 3 times for the last four days. Non-bloody, non-bilious vomiting. Today, 1 loose stool. Positive hard stomach with audible bowel sounds last night. Three wet diapers today and positive tears today. Decreased appetite. No fever. No sick contacts. No allergies. No current meds. Immunizations up to date.

Exam: General: Screaming during exam. Emesis during exam and not consolable. Head: Fontanel closed. Eyes: Positive tears. ENT: Ears clear, patent tubes bilaterally. Positive rhinorrhea. Moist mucous membranes but lips are dry. Neck: Supple. Chest: Clear to auscultation bilaterally. Tachycardia without murmur. Abdomen: Hard, no audible bowel sounds appreciated. Screaming inconsolably during abdomen exam. GU: Testes high but descended. Lymph nodes: No adenopathy. Skin: Dry with petechiae lower back.

KUB highly suggestive for intussusception. Will bolus fluids and arrange immediate transfer to Children's Hospital for surgical consult and treatment.

Diagnosis: Intussusception, acute gastroenteritis, excessive crying, abdominal pain. Assign the correct **diagnosis** code(s).

Code(s): _____

1.272. The patient had dental extractions and restoration procedures under general anesthesia as an outpatient. The patient is a child with a history of liver transplant, developmental delay, and dental caries in four deciduous teeth that required extraction and two deciduous teeth that required crowns until permanent teeth develop. Assign the correct **diagnosis** code(s).

Pre- and Postoperative Diagnosis:
1. Dental caries, deciduous teeth
2. Global developmental delay
3. Status post liver transplant

Code(s): _____

ICD-10-CM Coder Training Manual Answer Key

Introduction to ICD-10-CM Overview

Activity – New Features in ICD-10-CM

1. False

2. True

3. By trimester

4. 7

5. 21

Section 1 Review Questions

1.   c. Musculoskeletal system and connective tissue

2.   a. True

3.   c. Diseases and conditions of the eyes and ears are classified in the same chapter as diseases of the nervous system

4.   b. False

5.   d. All of the above

6.   a. All codes in ICD-10-CM include full code titles

7.   d. N

8.   b. The first character is always an alpha.

9.   b. L03.313

10.   b. False

Section 2 Review Questions

1.   b. To preserve the meaning of the sixth character

2.   c. NEC

3.   a. True

4.   b. Bracket

5.   b. False

6.   a. True

7.   c. Code first underlying disease

8.   b. The abbreviation NEC

9.   b. False

10.   a. True

Sections 3 and 4 Review Questions

1.   a. True

2.   b. H10.33

3.   b. False

4.   c. E28.310

5.   b. False

6.   b. False

7.   a. Intractable or not intractable

8.   a. True

9.   a. Dominant

10. b. The pain code

Sections 5 and 6 Review Questions

1.   a. True

2.   a. Chapter 13

3.   b. False

4.   b. False

5.   d. Cardiac arrest includes cardiogenic shock

6.   b. False

7.   c. K50.011, K50.014

8.   a. True

9.   a. Septic myocarditis

10. b. Depth of the ulcer

Sections 7 and 8 Review Questions

1.   a. True

2.   b. False

3.   c. Eclampsia in the first trimester

4.   b. R10.0

5.   a. A placeholder

6.   a. True

7.   d. P35-P39, Infections specific to the perinatal period

8.   b. False

9.   c. Assigned with the condition discovered coded secondary

10. a. True

Final Review Questions

1.   c. October 1, 2014

2.   d. Codes for intraoperative complications and postprocedural disorders have been combined

3.   b. False

4.   b. Note placement

5.   c. As filler so a seventh character may be assigned

6.   b. A diagnosis with an associated sign or symptom

7.   d. Poisoning by medicaments and biological substances

8.   c. N30.11, B96.20

9.   b. Asthmatic bronchitis

10. d. H65.191

11. b. M48.46XG

12. b. False

13. a. Dominant side

14. d. All of the above

15. a. Bilateral cleft palate

16. a. True

17. a. Gender

18. a. First two characters

19. a. True

20. c. I21, I22

ICD-10-CM Coding Conventions and Coding Guidelines Review

ICD-10-CM Coding Conventions

1. c. T75.4XXA

    Rationale: ICD-10-CM Coding Guideline I.A.5 states that the seventh character must always be the seventh character in the data field. If a code that requires a seventh character is not six characters long, a placeholder X must be used to fill in the empty characters. Additionally, Guideline A.4 indicates that ICD-10-CM utilizes a placeholder character X and where a placeholder exists, the X must be used in order for the code to be considered a valid code. All alpha characters in ICD-10-CM are *not case* sensitive, which means that if the placeholder X is entered in either the upper- or lowercase format, the meaning would not change.

2. c. parentheses

    Rationale: Parentheses are used in ICD-10-CM in both the Alphabetic Index and Tabular to enclose supplementary words that may be present or absent in the statement of a disease without affecting the code number to which it is assigned. The terms within the parentheses are referred to as *nonessential modifiers*. Boxes are not a defined convention of ICD-10-CM. Square brackets in ICD-10-CM in the Tabular List are used to enclose synonyms, alternative wordings, abbreviations, and explanatory phrases. Brackets are used in the Index to identify manifestation codes. Colons are used in the Tabular List after an incomplete term that needs one or more of the modifiers following the colon to make it assignable to a given category.

3. a. True

    Rationale: An *Excludes2* note indicates that the condition excluded is not part of the condition represented, but a patient may have both conditions at the same time. When an *Excludes2* note appears under a code, it is acceptable to use both the code and the excluded code together if the documentation indicates that the patient has both conditions (ICD-10-CM Coding Guideline I.A.12.b).

4. b. Always a letter

    Rationale: This is an ICD-10-CM convention, with all codes beginning with a letter of the alphabet except the letter U.

5. c. *Excludes1*

    Rationale: ICD-10-CM has two types of "excludes" notes. An *Excludes1* note indicates that the code excluded should never be used at the same time as the code above the *Excludes1* note (ICD-10-CM Coding Guideline I.A.12.a). An *Excludes2* note represents "not included here" and it is acceptable to use both the code and the excluded code together when both are documented (ICD-10-CM Coding Guideline I.A.12.b).

6. b. When the information in the medical record provides detail for which a specific code does not exist

    Rationale: Codes titled "other" or "other specified" are for use when the information in the medical record provides detail for which a specific code does not exist (Coding Guideline I.A.9.a). This can be contrasted with "unspecified" codes when the information in the medical record is insufficient to assign a more specific code (Coding Guideline I.A.9.b).

7.   a. True

       Rationale: All categories in ICD-10-CM are three characters. A three-character category that has no further subdivision is equivalent to a code. Subcategories are either four or five characters. Codes may be three, four, five, six, or seven characters.

8.   b. False

       Rationale: The word "and" should be interpreted to mean and/or when it is used in a narrative statement (Coding Guideline I.A.8).

9.   b. False

       Rationale: Inclusion notes contain terms that are the condition for which that code number is to be used. The terms may be synonyms of the code title, or in the case of "other specified" codes, the terms are a list of various conditions assigned to that code. The inclusion terms are not necessarily exhaustive (Coding Guideline I.A.11).

10.   b. False

       Rationale: ICD-10-CM Coding Guideline I.A.17 states a "code also" note instructs that two codes may be required to fully describe a condition, but this note does not provide sequencing direction. In contrast, the "code first/use additional code" notes provide sequencing order of the codes.

ICD-10-CM Coding Guidelines

11.   b. The appropriate Z51 code

       Rationale: If a patient admission or encounter is solely for the administration of chemotherapy, immunotherapy, or radiation therapy, assign code Z51.0, Encounter for antineoplastic radiation therapy; or Z51.11, Encounter for antineoplastic chemotherapy; or Z51.12, Encounter for antineoplastic immunotherapy as the first-listed or principal diagnosis. If a patient receives more than one of these therapies during the same admission, more than one of these codes may be assigned, in any sequence (Coding Guideline I.C.2.e.2). An encounter for chemotherapy and immunotherapy for a non-neoplastic condition should be coded to the condition.

12.   b. False

       Rationale: When a patient is admitted with an HIV-related condition, the principal diagnosis should be B20, Human immunodeficiency virus [HIV] disease, followed by additional diagnosis codes for all reported HIV-related conditions (Coding Guideline I.C.1.a.2.a). When a patient with HIV disease is admitted for an unrelated condition (for example, trauma), the code for the unrelated condition should be the principal diagnosis with B20 listed as an additional code (Coding Guideline I.C.1.a.2.b).

13.   a. Liver metastasis

       Rationale: When an admission or encounter is for the management of anemia associated with the malignancy, and the treatment is only for anemia, the appropriate code for the malignancy is sequenced as the principal or first listed diagnosis, followed by the appropriate code for the anemia (such as D63.0, Anemia in neoplastic disease) (Coding Guideline I.C.2.c.1). In addition, in the Tabular, the note under D63.0 states to code first neoplasm (C00-D49).

14.   a. True

Rationale: Code P95, Stillbirth, is only for use in institutions that maintain separate records for stillbirths. No other code should be used with P95. Code P95 should not be used on the mother's record (Coding Guideline I.C.16.g).

15.   b. False

Rationale: A fracture not indicated whether displaced or not displaced should be coded to displaced (Coding Guideline I.C.19.c). This information is also available in notes in the Tabular (see category S52). A fracture not described as open or closed is coded to the default of closed.

16.   b. I21.29, STEMI of other sites; I25.2, Old Myocardial Infarction

Rationale: ICD-10-CM has two categories for acute myocardial infarction: I21, Acute myocardial infarction and I22, Subsequent acute myocardial infarction. I21 is for all cases of initial myocardial infarction and is to be used from onset of the AMI until four weeks following onset. A code from I22 is to be used if a patient who has suffered an AMI has a new AMI within the four-week time frame of the initial AMI. A code from category I22 must be used in conjunction with a code from category I21 (Coding Guideline I.C.9.e.4).

17.   c. Highest-degree burn

Rationale: ICD-10-CM Coding Guideline I.C.19.d.1 states to first sequence the code that reflects the highest degree of burn when more than one burn is present.

18.   a. True

Rationale: Codes from category Y92, Place of occurrence of the external cause, are secondary codes for use after other external cause codes to identify the location of the patient at the time of injury. A place of occurrence code is used only once, at the initial encounter for treatment and only one code from Y92 should be recorded. A place of occurrence code should be used in conjunction with an activity code, Y93. Only one code from Y93 should be recorded on a medical record (Coding Guidelines I.C.20.b and c).

19.   d. All of the above

Rationale: The diabetes mellitus codes are combination codes that include the type of diabetes mellitus, the body system affected, and the complications affecting that body system (Coding Guideline I.C.4.a).

20.   a. True

Rationale: ICD-10-CM has combination codes for atherosclerotic heart disease with angina pectoris. The subcategories for these codes are I25.11, Atherosclerotic heart disease of native coronary artery with angina pectoris and I25.7, Atherosclerosis of coronary artery bypass graft(s) and coronary artery of transplanted heart with angina pectoris. When using one of these combination codes, it is not necessary to use an additional code for the angina pectoris. A causal relationship can be assumed in a patient with both atherosclerosis and angina pectoris unless the documentation indicates the angina is due to something other than the atherosclerosis (Coding Guideline I.C.9.b).

21. a. True

Rationale: Patients with any known prior diagnosis of an HIV-related illness should be coded to B20. Once a patient has developed an HIV-related illness, the patient should always be assigned code B20 on every subsequent admission or encounter. Patients previously diagnosed with any HIV illness (B20) should never be assigned to R75 or Z21, Asymptomatic human immunodeficiency virus [HIV] infection status (Coding Guideline I.C.1.a.2.f).

22. c. Congestive heart failure due to hypertension

Rationale: Heart conditions classified to I50.- or I51.4 through I51.9 are assigned to a code from category I11, Hypertensive heart disease, when a causal relationship is documented (due to hypertension) or implied (hypertensive). The same heart conditions with hypertension but without a stated causal relationship are coded separately (Coding Guideline I.C.9.a.1).

23. a. For the trimester in which the complication developed

Rationale: ICD-10-CM Coding Guideline I.C.15.a.4 states in the instances when a patient is admitted to a hospital for complications of pregnancy during one trimester and remains in the hospital into a subsequent trimester, the trimester character for the antepartum complication code should be assigned on the basis of the trimester when the complication developed, not the trimester of the discharge. If the condition developed prior to the current admission or encounter or represents a pre-existing condition, the trimester character for the trimester at the time of the admission or encounter should be assigned.

24. b. False

Rationale: If a newborn has a condition that may be either due to the birth process or community-acquired and the documentation does not indicate which it is, the default is due to the birth process and the code from Chapter 16 should be assigned (Coding Guideline I.C.16.a.5). By definition, the perinatal period is defined as before birth through the 28th day following birth.

25. a. True

Rationale: ICD-10-CM Coding Guideline I.C.20.b states that a place of occurrence code is used only once, at the initial encounter for treatment with only one code from Y92, Place of occurrence of the external cause, being recorded on a medical record. Coding Guideline I.C.20.c states that an activity code, Y93, is used only once, at the initial encounter for treatment with only one code from Y93 being recorded on a medical record.

26.   a. True

Rationale: Underdosing refers to taking less of a medication than is prescribed by a provider or a manufacturer's instruction. Noncompliance (Z91.12-, Z91.13-) or complication of care (Y63.8-Y63.9) codes are to be used with an underdosing code to indicate intent, if known (Coding Guideline I.C.19.e.5.c). Codes for underdosing should never be assigned as principal or first-listed codes.

27.   b. Z21, Asymptomatic HIV infection status

Rationale: Z21, Asymptomatic HIV infection status is to be used when the patient without any documentation of symptoms is listed as being "HIV positive," "known HIV," "HIV test positive," or similar terminology. Do not use this code if the term "AIDS" is used or if the patient is treated for any HIV-related illness or is described as having any condition(s) resulting from HIV positive status; use B20 in these cases (Coding Guideline I.C.1.a.2.d).

28.   a. Confer with the physician and ask if the condition should be listed as a final diagnosis

Rationale: Abnormal findings (laboratory, x-ray, pathologic, and other diagnostic results) are not coded and reported unless the provider indicates their clinical significance. If the findings are outside the normal range and the attending provider has ordered other tests to evaluate the condition or prescribed treatment, it is appropriate to ask the provider whether the abnormal findings should be added (Coding Guidelines III.B).

29.   b. False

Rationale: The coding of severe sepsis requires a minimum of two codes: first a code for the underlying systemic infection, followed by a code from subcategory R65.2, Severe sepsis. If the causal organism is not documented, assign code A41.9, Sepsis, unspecified organism, for the infection (Coding Guideline I.C.1.d.1.b). Additional codes for the other acute organ dysfunctions should also be assigned. This condition usually will result in a total of three codes, except in the case of combination codes, such as severe sepsis with septic shock.

30.   a. A, Initial encounter

Rationale: Seventh character A, initial encounter, is used while the patient is receiving active treatment for the condition, Seventh character D, subsequent encounter, is used for encounters after the patient has received active treatment for the condition and is receiving routine care for the condition during the healing or recovery phase. Seventh character S, sequela, is used for complications or conditions that arise as a direct result of a condition (Coding Guideline I.C.19.a).

Part I: ICD-10-CM Diagnostic Coding

Chapter 1 Coding Cases

1.1. N39.0   Infection, infected, infective (opportunistic), urinary (tract)

B96.20   Infection, infected, infective (opportunistic), bacterial NOS, as cause of disease classified elsewhere, Escherichia coli [E. coli] (*see also* Escherichia coli)

Rationale: The symptoms associated with the UTI should not be coded. The "use additional code" note under N39.0 instructs the coder to an additional code (B95-B97) to identify the infectious agent.

1.2. A04.7   Colitis (acute) (catarrhal) (chronic) (noninfective) (hemorrhagic), Clostridium difficile

Z16.39   Resistance, resistant (to), organism(s), to, drug, antimicrobial (single), specified NEC

Rationale: ICD-10-CM provides a code to identify resistance to antimicrobial drugs (Z16.-). The "use additional code" note is found at the beginning of Chapter 1.

1.3. M62.561   Atrophy, atrophic (of), muscle, muscular (diffuse) (general) Idiopathic) (primary), lower leg

B91   Late effect(s) – *see* Sequelae, Sequelae (of), poliomyelitis (acute)

Rationale: In ICD-10-CM, late effect conditions are classified to "sequelae." In Chapter 1, Sequelae of Infectious and Parasitic Diseases are classified to categories B90-B94. The condition resulting from the sequela is sequenced first.

1.4. A02.9   Poisoning (acute), food (acute) (diseased) (infected) (noxious), bacterial – *see* Intoxication, foodborne, by agent, Intoxication, foodborne, due to Salmonella

Rationale: Food poisoning is classified to Chapter 1, Certain infectious and parasitic diseases (A00-B99). If gastroenteritis was documented, the code would be A02.0.

1.5. A56.11   Disease, diseased, sexually transmitted, chlamydial infection – *see* Chlamydia, female, pelvic inflammatory disease

Rationale: With documentation of a sexually transmitted condition, the correct diagnosis code is found beginning with Disease, sexually transmitted.

1.6. B20   AIDS (related complex)

B59   Pneumonia, Pneumocystis (carinii) (jiroveci)

Rationale: Per the Official Coding Guidelines, if a patient is admitted for an HIV-related condition, the principal diagnosis should be B20, Human immunodeficiency virus [HIV] disease, followed by additional diagnosis codes for all reported HIV-related conditions.

1.7. A41.51   Sepsis (generalized), Escherichia coli (E. Coli). Review Tabular for complete code assignment.

Rationale: Without documentation of severe sepsis or an associated organ dysfunction, only one code from category A41 is necessary for correct code assignment.

1.8. A41.50   Sepsis (generalized), gram-negative (organism). Review Tabular for complete code assignment.

R65.20   Sepsis, with, organ dysfunction (acute) (multiple)

J96.00   Failure, failed, respiration, respiratory, acute

Rationale: Under the R65.2 subcategory, there is a "code first underlying infection" note; therefore, A41.50 should be listed as the principal diagnosis followed by R65.20 as a secondary diagnosis. Coding Guideline C.1.d.1.b provides sequencing guidance for severe sepsis: "the coding of severe sepsis requires a minimum of two codes: first a code for the underlying systemic infection, followed by a code from subcategory R65.2, Severe sepsis." Code J96.00 is used to identify the acute respiratory failure.

1.9. A39.2   Sepsis (generalized), meningococcal, acute

R65.21   Shock, septic (due to severe sepsis)

Rationale: The combination code of severe sepsis with septic shock is assigned as a secondary diagnosis although severe sepsis is not documented. The underlying infection, meningococcal sepsis is sequenced first.

1.10. N20.0   Nephrolithiasis (congenital) (pelvis) (recurrent) - *see also* Calculus, kidney, Calculus, calculi, calculous, kidney (impacted) (multiple) (pelvis) (recurrent) (staghorn)

J15.1   Pneumonia, Pseudomonas, NEC

Y95   Index to External Causes, Nosocomial condition

Rationale: The renal colic is a symptom of the patient's nephrolithiasis and would not be coded. The nosocomial infection external cause diagnosis should be added to identify the patient's hospital-acquired pneumonia.

1.11. B18.1   Hepatitis, viral, virus, chronic, type B

Rationale: In ICD-10-CM chronic (viral) hepatitis B without delta-agent is coded B18.1. Delta agent is a type of virus called hepatitis D that causes symptoms only in people who have hepatitis B infection. Because of this, there are no other hepatitis D codes (in the Index or Tabular List). It is a combination code available for use with hepatitis B codes. The delta-agent can be shown with or without hepatic coma by individual codes.

Chapter 2 Coding Cases

1.12. C34.31   Carcinoma, *see also* Neoplasm, by site, malignant. Refer to Neoplasm Table, by site (lung), malignant, primary site, lower lobe.

C77.1   Refer to Neoplasm Table, by site, lymph gland, malignant, intrathoracic, secondary site.

C79.31   Refer to Neoplasm Table, by site, brain, malignant, secondary site.

C79.51   Refer to Neoplasm Table, by site, bone, malignant, rib, secondary site.

Rationale: The primary site is the small cell carcinoma of the right lower lobe of the lung. The intrathoracic lymph nodes, brain, and rib are secondary sites. Index the term Carcinoma because the histological term is documented. This refers you to the Neoplasm Table, by site, malignant. It is correct to list each metastatic site.

1.13. D3A.021   Carcinoid, *see* Tumor, carcinoid, benign, cecum

Rationale: When indexing Carcinoid, the note directs to Tumor. It is not necessary to use the Neoplasm Table to code this tumor. Under Carcinoid, there is a differentiation between benign or malignant, with specific sites listed. Benign carcinoid tumors fall into category D3A, Benign neuroendocrine tumors. The following notes are present: Code also any associated multiple endocrine neoplasia [MEN] syndromes; and Use additional code to identify any associate endocrine syndrome, such as Carcinoid syndrome (E34.0).

1.14. C93.91   Leukemia, leukemic, monocytic (subacute)

Rationale: Leukemia is not coded from the Neoplasm Table, but rather indexed under the term Leukemia. Subacute monocytic is classified to subcategory C93.9-.

1.15. C43.52   Melanoma (malignant), skin, breast (female) (male)
         C43.62   Melanoma (malignant), skin, arm. Review the Tabular for complete code assignment.

Rationale: To code Melanoma, the code is found directly in the Index rather than the Neoplasm Table. It is incorrect to assign primary site of skin (C44.52, C44.62) when melanoma is documented. Melanoma in situ is classified in category D03.1-.

1.16. E86.0   Dehydration
         G89.3   Pain(s) (*see also* Painful), chronic, neoplasm related
         C50.111   Carcinoma, *see also* Neoplasm, by site, malignant. Refer to Neoplasm Table, by site (breast), malignant, primary site, central portion.
         C79.31   Refer to Neoplasm Table, by site, brain, malignant, secondary site.
         C78.7   Refer to Neoplasm Table, by site, liver, malignant, secondary site.

Rationale: ICD-10-CM chapter-specific guidelines for neoplasms state that when the encounter is for management of dehydration due to the malignancy or the therapy, or a combination of both, and only the dehydration is being treated, the dehydration is sequenced first, followed by the code(s) for the malignancy. An additional ICD-10-CM Coding Guideline states that when the reason for the encounter is for neoplasm-related pain control or pain management, the pain code may be assigned as the first-listed diagnosis. Because the focus of this encounter was both the dehydration and the intractable pain, either may be sequenced first.

1.17. C79.31   Refer to Neoplasm Table, by site, brain, malignant, secondary site
         Z85.3   History, personal (of), malignant neoplasm (of), breast
         Z90.12   Absence (of) (organ or part) (complete or partial), breast(s) (and nipple(s)) (acquired)
         Z92.21   History, personal (of), chemotherapy for neoplastic condition

Rationale: The reason for this encounter is the metastatic brain cancer. The breast cancer was previously excised with no further treatment directed at that site; therefore, it is coded as history of breast cancer. Because the patient had a previous mastectomy, a code for the acquired absence of the breast is also coded. Laterality can be specified in the Z90.1 subcategory. It was documented that the brain metastasis was causing the symptoms, so they are not assigned additionally. If it is not clear by the documentation, a query might be in order. There is also a code available for history of chemotherapy if the facility takes coding to that level of detail.

1.18. Z51.11   Chemotherapy (session) (for), cancer

C17.8   Carcinoma, *see also* Neoplasm, by site, malignant. Refer to Neoplasm Table, by site, intestine, small, overlapping lesion, malignant, primary site.

Z90.49   Absence (of) (organ or part) (complete or partial), intestine (acquired) (small)

Rationale: The reason for the encounter (chemotherapy) is the first-listed diagnosis. The neoplasm is coded as current (even though it was excised) because the patient is still receiving chemotherapy. The overlapping sites code is used because the cancer is part in the duodenum and part in the jejunum. The acquired absence of the small intestine may be coded because the category includes the organ or part, complete or partial.

Chapter 3 Coding Cases

1.19. C50.912   Carcinoma, *see also* Neoplasm, by site, malignant. Neoplasm, breast (connective tissue) (glandular tissue) (soft parts)

D63.0   Anemia (essential) (general) (hemoglobin deficiency) (infantile) (primary) (profound), in (due to) (with), neoplastic disease (*see also* Neoplasm)

Rationale: When the patient is treated for anemia due to a malignancy, Coding Guideline I.C.2.c.1 directs the coding professional to sequence the malignancy as principal or first-listed diagnosis followed by a code for the anemia. There is a "code first neoplasm" note under code D63.0

1.20. D61.01   Anemia (essential) (general) (hemoglobin deficiency) (infantile) (primary) (profound), aplastic, red cell (pure), congenital

Rationale: ICD-10-CM has provided greater specificity in aplastic anemia. In the Index, it is important to find Red cell and then Congenital under the term Aplastic. The first term, Congenital (D61.09) is not specific to red cell.

1.21. D70.4   Neutropenia, neutropenic (chronic) (genetic) (idiopathic) (immune) (infantile) (malignant) (pernicious) (splenic), periodic

Rationale: ICD-10-CM has provided greater specificity in neutropenia. A note provided at category D70 states that an additional code should be assigned for any associated fever or mucositis.

1.22. D56.3   Thalassemia (anemia) (disease), minor

Rationale: ICD-10-CM has provided greater specificity in the coding of Thalassemia.

1.23. D57.01   Anemia, sickle-cell – *see* Disease, sickle-cell, with crisis (vasoocclusive pain), with, acute chest syndrome

Rationale: In some cases, combination codes are used for sickle-cell crisis with manifestation.

1.24. D81.1   Immunodeficiency, combined, severe (SCID), with, low T- and B-cell numbers

Rationale: ICD-10-CM has added specificity to the severe combined immunodeficiency subcategory. SCID is a genetic disorder in which B and T cells are crippled due to a defect in genes. It is also known as "bubble boy" disease, and the patients are extremely vulnerable to infectious diseases.

Chapter 4 Coding Cases

1.25. E11.321   Diabetes, diabetic (mellitus) (sugar), type 2, with, retinopathy, nonproliferative, mild, with macular edema

      E11.36   Diabetes, diabetic (mellitus) (sugar), type 2, with, cataract

      Z79.4   Long-term (current) (prophylactic) drug therapy (use of), insulin

Rationale: There is a combination code for the type 2 diabetes with nonproliferative diabetic retinopathy with macular edema. The diabetic cataract was documented and should be coded, but it requires a separate code. Since the patient has type 2 DM, and is on insulin, code Z79.4 should be assigned to indicate that as indicated by the note at category E11: "Use additional code to identify any insulin use (Z79.4)."

1.26. E10.22   Diabetes, diabetic (mellitus) (sugar) type 1, with, chronic kidney disease

      N18.3   Disease, diseased, kidney (functional) (pelvis), chronic, stage 3 (moderate)

      K04.7   Abscess, tooth, teeth (root)

Rationale: The Tabular instructs the coder to use an additional code to identify the stage of the chronic kidney disease, N18.3. In this case the hyperglycemia would not be coded because it was not documented by the physician as out of control in this limited documentation. A physician query might be warranted.

1.27. K85.0   Pancreatitis (annular) (apoplectic) (calcareous) (edematous) (hemorrhagic) (malignant) (recurrent) (subacute) (suppurative), acute, idiopathic

      E08.65   Diabetes, diabetic (mellitus) (sugar), due to underlying condition, with, hyperglycemia

      Z79.4   Long-term (current) (prophylactic) drug therapy (use of), insulin

Rationale: The notes in the Tabular show the sequencing in this case. Code first the underlying condition, and Use additional code to identify any insulin use (Z79.4). Coding Guideline I.C.4.a.6.b also gives direction for this case. For acute pancreatitis, assign code E85.0 for idiopathic pancreatitis, or that whose cause cannot be determined. Assign a code from category E08 and a code for long-term use of insulin.

1.28. E66.01   Obesity, morbid

      Z68.41   Body, bodies, mass index (BMI), adult, 40.0–44.9

Rationale: The Index indicates that morbid obesity is assigned code E66.01. When consulting the Tabular, the subcategory is Obesity due to excess calories. This is the correct code even though it is not documented that excess calories caused the obesity. This is the default code per the classification. The note at category E66 indicates that an additional code should be assigned for BMI when known (Z68.-).

1.29. F50.2   Bulimia (nervosa)

      E44.0   Malnutrition, protein, calorie, moderate

Rationale: Protein–calorie malnutrition codes differentiate between mild and moderate levels.

1.30. E86.0   Dehydration

      A02.0   Gastroenteritis (acute) (chronic) (noninfectious), Salmonella or Infection, Salmonella, with (gastro)enteritis

Rationale: Dehydration would be the first listed code because it is the reason for the encounter and is the diagnosis that was treated. The Gastroenteritis due to salmonella would be coded as an additional code. The symptoms (abdominal cramping, nausea, vomiting, diarrhea) are integral to the gastroenteritis and are not separately coded.

1.31. E10.10   Diabetes, diabetic (mellitus) (sugar), type 1, with, ketoacidosis
        E86.0   Dehydration

Rationale: The reason for the encounter is the diabetic ketoacidosis which would be sequenced first. The symptoms of nausea and vomiting, frequency of urination, and polydipsia would not be coded.

1.32. E09.9   Diabetes, diabetic, (mellitus) (sugar) due to drug or chemical
        T38.0X5S   Refer to Table of Drugs and Chemicals, Corticosteroid, adverse effect
        Z79.4   Long-term (current) (prophylactic) drug therapy (use of), insulin

Rationale: The reason for this encounter is the steroid-induced diabetes mellitus. E09.9 is sequenced first due to Coding Guideline I.C.19.e.5.a, which states that the nature of the adverse effect is assigned first followed by the appropriate code for the adverse effect (T36-T50). There is also a "use additional code" note under category E09 regarding the sequencing of adverse effect codes. The seventh character of S is assigned to code T38.0X5 as this is a sequela of the corticosteroid use. The seventh character D is used for encounters after the patient received active treatment and is receiving routine care. Additionally, under category E09 there is another instructional note to "Use additional code to identify any insulin use (Z79.4)."

1.33. E05.20   Hyperthyroidism (latent) (pre-adult) (recurrent) with, goiter (diffuse),
                 nodular (multinodular)
        R00.2   Palpitations (heart)

Rationale: Although palpitations are integral to hyperthyroidism, the palpitations are coded as an additional (other) diagnosis in this case due to the fact that they were more pronounced requiring additional clinical evaluation to be carried out. The UHDDS defines "other diagnoses" as those conditions that affect patient care in terms of requiring clinical evaluation, therapeutic treatment, diagnostic procedures, extended length of hospital stay, or increased nursing care and/or monitoring.

1.34. E10.621   Diabetes, diabetic (mellitus) (sugar), type 1, with foot ulcer
        L97.521   Ulcer, foot, *see* Ulcer, lower limb, lower limb, foot, left, with skin
                 breakdown only
        E10.51   Diabetes, diabetic (mellitus) (sugar), type 1, with peripheral angiopathy
        E10.22   Diabetes, diabetic (mellitus) (sugar), type 1, with chronic kidney disease
        N18.2   Disease, diseased, kidney (functional) (pelvis), chronic, stage 2 (mild)

Rationale: The diabetic ulcer is listed first since this appears to be the reason for treatment. The note under code E10.621 states to "Use additional code to identify site of ulcer (L97.4-, L97.5-)." It is correct to list as many diabetic conditions as are present, and the stage 2 chronic kidney disease and the peripheral angiopathy are coded. An additional code, N18.2, is added to identify the stage 2 chronic kidney disease. It is not correct to assign Z79.4 because type 1 diabetics must use insulin to sustain life, and this is inherent in the category E10 codes.

Chapter 5 Coding Cases

1.35. F10.129   Abuse, alcohol (non-dependent), with, intoxication

Rationale: ICD-10-CM does not specify the severity of alcohol use as previously seen in ICD-9-CM. If alcohol dependence was documented, the coding would go to F10.2.

1.36. F15.20   Dependence (on) (syndrome), amphetamine(s) (type), *see* Dependence, drug, stimulant, NEC

Rationale: ICD-10-CM classifies each drug by its type. If intoxication with the dependence is documented, an additional digit would be added.

1.37. Z71.6   Counseling (for), tobacco use
F17.220   Dependence, (on) (syndrome), nicotine, *see* Dependence, drug, nicotine. Dependence, drug, nicotine, chewing tobacco

Rationale: In ICD-10-CM, nicotine dependence is further specified by the type of product used. There is a note at code Z71.6 to "Use additional code for nicotine dependence (F17.-)."

1.38. F10.20   Dependence, (on) (syndrome), alcohol (ethyl) (methyl) (without remission)
K29.20   Gastritis (simple), alcoholic
F14.21   History, personal (of), drug dependence – *see* Dependence, drug, by type, in remission. Dependence, (on) (syndrome), drug, cocaine, in remission

Rationale: The cocaine dependence is coded as "in remission" because there is not a history code for drug dependence.

1.39. F60.3   Disorder, personality, borderline
F10.21   Alcohol, alcoholic, alcohol-induced, addiction, with remission
Z79.899   Long-term (current) (prophylactic) drug therapy (use of), drug, specified NEC

Rationale: The additional information of "cluster B personality disorder" does not affect code assignment. Cluster B personality disorders include dramatic, erratic behaviors and include Histrionic, Narcissistic, Antisocial and Borderline Personality Disorders.

1.40. F10.229   Intoxication, alcoholic (acute) (without dependence) –*see* Alcohol, intoxication. Alcohol, alcoholic, alcohol-induced, intoxication (acute) (without dependence), with, dependence
Y90.1   Index to External Causes, Blood alcohol level, 20–39mg/100ml

Rationale: A note under category F10, Alcohol-related disorders, instructs the coder to "Use additional code for blood alcohol level, if applicable (Y90.-)." Continuous use of alcohol does not affect code assignment. The code F10.229 is assigned because there is no documentation that this is uncomplicated (F10.220). This might be an opportunity for a physician query for a more specific code.

Chapter 6 Coding Cases

1.41. G30.0   Alzheimer's disease or sclerosis, *see* Disease, Alzheimer's, early onset, with behavioral disturbance

F02.81   Dementia, in Alzheimer's disease, *see* Disease, Alzheimer's

Z91.83   Wandering, in diseases classified elsewhere

Rationale: There is mandatory sequencing for these codes. The etiology (Alzheimer's disease) is sequenced first and the manifestation (dementia) is sequenced second. The Index provides the following documentation: Alzheimer's, early onset, with behavioral disturbance G30.0 [F02.81]. The use of the brackets in the Index indicates manifestation codes. Further, the note in the Tabular at the G30 category states to use an additional code to identify dementia with behavioral disturbance (F02.81). At the F02 category, the note states to "Code first the underlying physiological condition." The dementia is coded with behavioral disturbance because of the documentation of wandering off. At code F02.81, the note states to "Use additional code, if applicable, to identify wandering in dementia in conditions classified elsewhere" (Z91.83). This code further specifies the behavioral disturbance as wandering off. Early onset Alzheimer's usually begins in middle age, before the age of 65.

1.42. G40.B19   Epilepsy, epileptic, epilepsia (attack) (cerebral) (convulsion) (fit) (seizure), juvenile myoclonic, intractable

Rationale: The documentation indicates that the disorder is juvenile myoclonic epilepsy that is intractable. People with juvenile myoclonic epilepsy (JME) have myoclonic seizures which are identified as quick little jerks of the arms, shoulders, or occasionally the legs. The myoclonic jerks sometimes are followed by a tonic-clonic seizure. JME is one of the most common epilepsy syndromes, and makes up about seven percent of all cases of epilepsy. JME may begin between late childhood and early adulthood, usually around the time of puberty.

1.43. G81.94   Hemiplegia. Review Tabular for complete code assignment.

Rationale: Under the term Hemiplegia in the Index, the only code option for this diagnosis is G81.9-. Review of the Tabular under G81.9-, which offers five code choices. Coding Guideline I.C.6.a states: "Should the affected side be documented, but not specified as dominant or nondominant and the classification system does not indicate a default, code selection is as follows: If the left side is affected, the default is nondominant."

1.44. G00.1   Meningitis, pneumococcal

J13   Pneumonia, pneumococcal, (broncho) (lobar)

Rationale: The patient had both meningitis and pneumonia, so both conditions should be coded. Both conditions were present at the time of admission; therefore, either the meningitis or pneumonia could be listed as the principal diagnosis. ICD-10-CM Guidelines indicate that when there are two or more diagnoses equally meeting the criteria for principal diagnosis as determined by the circumstances of admission, any one of the diagnoses may be sequenced first.

1.45. G21.11   Parkinsonism (idiopathic) (primary), secondary, due to drugs, neuroleptic
        T43.4X5A   Refer to Table of Drugs and Chemicals, Haloperidol, adverse effect
        F20.0   Schizophrenia, paranoid (type)

Rationale: The documentation implies that this is the initial encounter, so the seventh character A is assigned. There is no evidence that the drug was taken incorrectly, so adverse effect is selected. If there is any doubt, a query could be in order. The note at G21.11, Neuroleptic induced parkinsonism, states to "Use additional code for adverse effect, if applicable, to identify drug" (T43.3X5, T43.4X5, T43.505, T43.595).

1.46. G89.3   Pain(s) (*see also* Painful), acute, neoplasm related
        C50.911   Refer to Neoplasm Table, by site, breast, malignant, primary site.
        C78.7   Refer to Neoplasm Table, by site, liver, malignant, secondary site.

Rationale: ICD-10-CM Coding Guideline I.C.6.b.5 states that code G89.3 is assigned to pain documented as being related, associated or due to cancer, primary or secondary malignancy or tumor. This code may be assigned as the principal or first-listed code when the stated reason for the encounter is pain control or pain management. The underlying neoplasm should be reported as an additional diagnosis.

1.47. G45.9   Attack, attacks, transient ischemic (TIA)
        E11.40   Diabetes, diabetic, (mellitus) (sugar) type 2, with, neuropathy
        G43.119   Migraine, classical – *see* Migraine, with aura
                     Migraine, with aura, intractable

Rationale: The TIA is the first listed diagnosis, as it was the reason for the encounter. The migraine is documented as classical. In ICD-10-CM, classical migraine is classified to with aura. An aura is a visual, motor, or cognitive phenomenon that prefaces the headache. An intractable migraine indicates that it is sustained and severe and not effectively terminated by standard outpatient interventions. ICD-10-CM also provides codes for with, without, or unspecified status migrainosus. Status migrainosus normally indicates a migraine attack lasting for more than 72 hours.

Chapter 7 Coding Cases

1.48. H01.001   Blepharitis (angularis) (ciliaris) (eyelid) (marginal) (nonulcerative), right, upper
        H01.004   Blepharitis (angularis) (ciliaris) (eyelid) (marginal) (nonulcerative), left, upper

Rationale: Blepharitis is an inflammation of the eyelash follicles along the edge of the eyelid. In ICD-10-CM, blepharitis is subdivided between right and left eyes and also upper and lower eyelids.

1.49. H11.063   Pterygium (eye), recurrent. See Tabular for correct code assignment.

Rationale: Pterygium is a non-cancerous growth of the clear, thin tissue that lies over the conjunctiva. No treatment is required unless the pterygium begins to block vision. ICD-10-CM provides codes to identify pterygium of the left, right, or bilateral eyes.

1.50. H25.12   Cataract (cortical) (immature) (incipient), age-related – *see* Cataract, senile, nuclear (sclerosis)

Rationale: With a diagnosis of age-related cataract, ICD-10-CM Index directs the coder to Senile Cataract, which is further specified by right, left, or bilateral.

1.51. H40.11X2   Glaucoma, open angle, primary. See Tabular for complete code assignment.

Rationale: Review of the Tabular at code H40.11 indicates the need for a seventh character to designate the stage of the glaucoma. Primary open-angle glaucoma is characterized by visual field abnormalities and intraocular pressure that is too high for the continued health of the eye. In this case, ICD-10-CM does not have separate codes to identify specific eyes.

1.52. H59.012   Keratopathy, bullous (aphakic), following cataract surgery

Rationale: Bullous keratopathy, or corneal edema, is often sequelae of cataract extraction. In ICD-10-CM, codes for both keratopathy and keratopathy due to cataract surgery are provided. These codes are further subdivided by laterality.

1.53. H25.011   Cataract (cortical) (immature) (incipient), age-related, *see* Cataract, senile, cortical

H59.311   Hemorrhage, postoperative, *see* Complications, postprocedural, hemorrhage, by site

Complication(s) (from) (of), postprocedural, hemorrhage (hematoma) (of), eye and adnexa, following ophthalmic procedure

Y92.530   Index to External Causes, Place of occurrence, outpatient surgery center

Rationale: Complication codes in ICD-10-CM are differentiated between intraoperative and postoperative. In this case, the primary diagnosis is the cataract and the postoperative complication is listed as a secondary diagnosis. A place of occurrence code can be added to indicate that this occurred in a day-surgery center. This code includes an outpatient surgery center connected with a hospital. Per Coding Guideline I.C.19.g.4, an external cause of injury code is not required as the complication code has the external cause included in the code.

Chapter 8 Coding Cases

1.54. H65.02   Otitis (acute), media (hemorrhagic) (staphylococcal) (streptococcal) acute, subacute, serous – *see* Otitis, media, nonsuppurative, acute, serous. Otitis media, nonsuppurative, acute or subacute, serous

H66.91   Otitis (acute), media (hemorrhagic) (staphylococcal) (streptococcal), chronic

H72.821   Perforation, perforated (nontraumatic) (of), tympanum, tympanic (membrane) (persistent post-traumatic) (postinflammatory), total

Rationale: Otitis media has an expansion of codes in ICD-10-CM to classify these conditions. Laterality is also part of the classification in ICD-10-CM. In category H65, distinction is made between recurrent infections. A note is present stating that an additional code for any associated perforated tympanic membrane should be coded separately. It is then possible to show which tympanic membrane is perforated by assigning the correct code for right side associated with the chronic otitis media. Otitis media refers to inflammation of the middle ear (area between ear drum and inner ear including the eustachian tube). Serous otitis involves a collection of fluid that occurs in the middle ear space caused by altered eustachian tube function. This is also referred to as secretory or with effusion.

1.55. H81.02   Vertigo, Ménière's – *see* subcategory H81.0

Rationale: The Index provides the category and the Tabular provides the specific laterality. Ménière's disease involves the inner ear and symptoms are vertigo, tinnitus, and a feeling of fullness or pressure in the ear.

1.56. H80.03   Otosclerosis (general) involving oval window, nonobliterative
H90.0   Loss (of), hearing – *see* also Deafness. Deafness, conductive, bilateral
H95.31   Complication(s), ear procedure, laceration – *see* Complications, intraoperative, puncture or laceration, ear. Complication(s) intraoperative, puncture or laceration (accidental) (unintentional) (of) ear, during procedure on ear and mastoid process
Y92.234   Index to External Causes, Place of occurrence, hospital, operating room

Rationale: The otosclerosis is listed first since it is the underlying condition causing the hearing loss, and absent any sequencing instruction in the classification system. Note that there are intraoperative and postprocedural complications available. Subcategory H95.3 provides codes for accidental puncture and laceration of the ear and mastoid process when a procedure on the ear and mastoid process was being performed (H95.31) and for accidental puncture and laceration of ear and mastoid process during other procedures. The cause of the complication is included in the complication code H95.31; therefore, an additional external cause code is not required. A place of occurrence code, however, can be assigned.

Chapter 9 Coding Cases

1.57. I10   Hypertension, hypertensive, (accelerated) (benign) (essential) (idiopathic) (malignant) (systemic)

Rationale: ICD-10-CM does not differentiate between benign and malignant hypertension.

1.58. I13.0   Hypertension, hypertensive, (accelerated) (benign) (essential) (idiopathic) (malignant) (systemic), cardiorenal (disease), with heart failure, with stage 1 through stage 4 chronic kidney disease
I50.9   Failure, failed, heart (acute) (senile) (sudden), congestive (compensated) (decompensated)
N18.3   Disease, diseased, kidney (functional) (pelvis), chronic, stage 3 (moderate)

Rationale: In ICD-10-CM, a combination code is used to identify those diagnoses that include hypertensive heart and kidney disease. Under I13.0 there is a "use additional code" note to identify both the type of heart failure and the stage of chronic kidney disease. The cross-reference under Disease, diseased – see also syndrome did not reveal any additional information. The term "kidney" is represented under Disease, diseased.

1.59. I21.4   Infarct, Infarction, myocardium, myocardial (acute) (with stated duration of 4 weeks or less), non-ST elevation (NSTEMI)

I48.91   Fibrillation, atrial or auricular (established)

Rationale: Per the Official Coding Guidelines, "If an AMI is documented as nontransmural or subendocardial, but the site is provided, it is still coded as a subendocardial AMI." The STEMI and NSTEMI are treated differently. Generally, the STEMI is caused by complete obstruction of the coronary artery, and causes damage that involved the full thickness of the heart muscle, while the NSTEMI is caused by a partial obstruction and the damage does not involve the full thickness of the heart wall.

1.60. I22.1   Infarct, Infarction, myocardium, myocardial (acute) (with stated duration of 4 weeks or less), subsequent (recurrent) (reinfarction), inferior (diaphragmatic) (inferolateral) (inferoposterior) (wall)

I21.4   Infarct, Infarction, myocardium, myocardial (acute) (with stated duration of 4 weeks or less), non-ST elevation (NSTEMI)

I48.91   Fibrillation, atrial or auricular (established)

Rationale: The Official Coding Guidelines specifically address the sequencing of I22 and I21 and this is stated as: "The sequencing of the I22 and I21 codes depends on the circumstances of the encounter."

1.61. I23.7   Angina (attack) (cardiac) (chest) (heart) (pectoris) (syndrome) (vasomotor), post-infarctional

I21.09   Infarct, infarction, myocardium, myocardial (acute) (with stated duration of 4 weeks or less), ST elevation (STEMI), anterior (anteroapical) (anterolateral) (anteroseptal) (Q wave) (wall)

Rationale: ICD-10-CM provides a category (I23) to identify current complications following STEMI and NSTEMI. A note appears in the Tabular under category I23 regarding the use of this code category. A code from category I23 must be used in conjunction with a code from category I21 or category I22. The I23 code should be sequenced first if it is the reason for encounter.

1.62. I25.119   Disease, diseased, coronary (artery) – *see* Disease, heart, ischemic, atherosclerotic (of), with angina pectoris – *see* Arteriosclerosis, coronary (artery), native vessel, with angina pectoris

Rationale: ICD-10-CM has combination codes for atherosclerotic heart disease with angina pectoris. There are subcategories for disease of the native artery, coronary artery bypass graft(s), and coronary artery of transplanted heart. It is not necessary to use an additional code for angina pectoris when using these combination codes.

1.63. I25.110   Angina (attack) (cardiac) (chest) (heart) (pectoris) (syndrome) (vasomotor), with atherosclerotic heart disease – *see* Arteriosclerosis, coronary (artery), native vessel with angina pectoris, unstable

I69.351   Hemiparesis – *see* Hemiplegia, following, cerebrovascular disease, cerebral infarction

Z95.1   Status (post), aortocoronary bypass

Rationale: The coronary artery disease of the native vessel is coded because the previous cardiac catheterization showed that the bypass grafts are patent. Also, per the Official Coding Guidelines, "ICD-10-CM has combination codes for atherosclerotic heart disease with angina pectoris. When using one of these combination codes it is not necessary to use an additional code for angina pectoris. A causal relationship can be assumed in a patient with both atherosclerosis and angina pectoris, unless the documentation indicates the angina is due to something other than atherosclerosis."

1.64. I50.33 Failure, failed, heart (acute) (senile) (sudden), diastolic (congestive), acute (congestive), and (on) chronic (congestive)

Rationale: An additional code for congestive heart failure is not required, as "congestive" is already identified in the preceding code.

1.65. I63.322 Infarct, infarction, cerebral – (*see also* Occlusion, artery, cerebral or precerebral, with infarction). Occlusion, artery, cerebral, anterior, with infarction, due to, thrombosis. or Infarct, infarction, cerebral, due to thrombosis, cerebral artery. Review the Tabular for correct code assignment.
G81.91 Hemiplegia. Review the Tabular for correct code assignment.

Rationale: It is necessary to review the Tabular for complete code assignment for both the cerebral infarction and the hemiplegia. If the record and the classification system do not indicate a default, the default should be dominant for hemiplegia. Coding Guideline I.C.6.a. states: "Should this information not be available in the record, and the classification system does not indicate a default, the default should be dominant."

1.66. I69.354 Hemiparesis – *see* Hemiplegia, following, cerebrovascular disease, stroke
I69.320 Aphasia, following cerebrovascular disease, cerebral infarction

Rationale: Category I69 is used to indicate neurological deficits that persist after initial onset of conditions classifiable to categories I60-I67. The left is specified as the side of the hemiparesis. After seeing the Index, it is necessary to select the correct code for subcategory I69.35 from the Tabular.

1.67. I25.110 Angina (attack) (cardiac) (chest) (heart) (pectoris) (syndrome) (vasomotor), with atherosclerotic heart disease – *see* Arteriosclerosis, coronary (artery), native vessel with angina pectoris, unstable
I25.2 Infarct, infarction, myocardium, myocardial, healed or old

Rationale: Crescendo angina is included in unstable angina, *see* the Index, Angina, crescendo – *see* Angina, unstable.

1.68. I25.720 Atherosclerosis – *see also* Arteriosclerosis, coronary artery, with angina pectoris, – *see* Arteriosclerosis, coronary (artery), bypass graft, autologous artery, with, angina pectoris, unstable
I11.0 Failure, failed, heart (acute) (senile) (sudden), hypertensive – *see* Hypertension, heart (disease) (conditions in I51.4-I51.9 due to hypertension), with, heart failure (congestive)
I50.9 Failure, failed, heart (acute) (senile) (sudden), congestive (compensated)

Rationale: ICD-10-CM differentiates between the different types of bypassed coronary arteries, including native arteries, autologous vein, autologous artery, and nonautologous graft material. Hypertensive congestive heart failure requires two diagnosis codes to correctly identify the condition. The note at code I11.0 states "Use additional code to identify type of heart failure (I50.-)."

1.69. I21.19   Infarct, infarction, myocardium, myocardial (acute) (with stated duration of 4 weeks or less), ST elevation (STEMI), inferior (diaphragmatic) (inferolateral) (inferoposterior) (wall), NEC

I23.0   Hemopericardium, following acute myocardial infarction (current complication)

Rationale: The ICD-10-CM codes for acute myocardial infarction identify the site. Subcategory I21.1 is used for ST elevation myocardial infarction of the inferior wall. A code from category I23 must be used in conjunction with a code from category I21 or category I22. The I23 code should be sequenced after the I21 or I22 code if the complication of the MI occurs during the encounter for the MI.

1.70. I63.442   Infarct, infarction, cerebellar – *see* Infarct, cerebral. (*See also* Occlusion, artery, cerebral or precerebral, with infarction.) Occlusion, occluded artery, cerebellar (anterior inferior) (posterior inferior) (superior) with infarction, due to, embolism. Review the Tabular for complete and correct code assignment.

R13.10   Dysphagia

G81.91   Hemiplegia. Review the Tabular for complete code assignment.

Rationale: ICD-10-CM provides specific codes to identify the involved artery in a cerebrovascular infarction. Right dominant side (G81.91) was selected based on Coding Guideline I.C.6.a, which states "should the affected side be documented, but not specified as dominant or nondominant, and the classification system does not indicate a default, code selection is as follows: if the right side is affected the default is dominant." Codes from category I69 are not used in this scenario as the dysphagia and hemipeglia are acute deficits from the current CVA.

Chapter 10 Coding Cases

1.71. J14   Pneumonia (acute) (double) (migratory) (purulent) (septic) (unresolved), Hemophilus influenza (broncho) (lobar)

Rationale: The H. influenza pneumonia is coded to J14. The symptoms are not coded because they are inherent in the pneumonia code.

1.72. J44.1   Disease, diseased, pulmonary, chronic obstructive, with exacerbation (acute)

F17.200   Dependence (on) (syndrome), tobacco – *see* Dependence, drug, nicotine

Z71.6   Counseling (for), substance abuse, tobacco

Rationale: Acute respiratory insufficiency is a symptom that is an integral part of the COPD and is not coded.

1.73.　J45.51　　　Asthma, asthmatic (bronchial) (catarrh) (spasmodic), persistent, severe, with exacerbation (acute)

Rationale: There are categories of the three degrees of persistent asthma, with the ability to identify with or without exacerbation and status asthmaticus.

1.74.　J96.00　　　Failure, respiration, respiratory, acute
　　　　　J44.0　　　Bronchitis (diffuse) (fibrinous) (hypostatic) (infective) (membranous), acute or subacute, with chronic obstructive pulmonary disease
　　　　　J20.9　　　Bronchitis (diffuse) (fibrinous) (hypostatic) (infective) (membranous), acute or subacute
　　　　　J44.1　　　Disease, diseased, pulmonary, chronic obstructive, with exacerbation (acute)

Rationale: Review Coding Guidelines I.C.10.b.1-3 regarding sequencing of respiratory failure. Code J96.00 may be assigned as the principal diagnosis when it is the condition established after study to be chiefly responsible for occasioning the admission to the hospital, and the selection is supported by the Index and Tabular. In this case, no other guidelines conflict, such as obstetrics, poisoning, HIV, and such. The patient was started on mechanical ventilation in the ER. The documentation is limited in this brief scenario however, so if there was any doubt about the correct sequencing, the physician should be queried. Code J20.9 is added to identify the infection (acute bronchitis). Under J44.0 there is a note: "Use additional code to identify the infection." There is an *Excludes2* note under section Other Acute Lower Respiratory Infections (J20-J22) – *Excludes2*: COPD with acute lower respiratory infection (J44.0). Both codes J44.0 and J20.9 are necessary to correctly code the acute bronchitis with COPD. Code J44.1 is added as an additional code to identify the COPD exacerbation. There is an *Excludes2* note under J44.1, but both codes can be assigned when both acute bronchitis and an acute exacerbation are documented. The Index entries also show COPD with acute bronchitis and acute exacerbation at the same indentation level, meaning that one doesn't include the other.

1.75.　J69.0　　　Pneumonia, aspiration, due to food (regurgitated)
　　　　　K21.9　　　Reflux, gastroesophageal

Rationale: The chest rales, dyspnea, cyanosis, and hypotension are all symptoms of aspiration pneumonia and are not assigned codes. The gastroesophageal reflux contributed to the condition and should be coded.

1.76.　J09.X2　　　Influenza (bronchial) (epidemic) (respiratory) (upper) (unidentified influenza virus), due to identified novel influenza A virus, with, respiratory manifestations, NEC

Rationale: Coding Guideline I.C.10.c states that only confirmed cases of influenza due to certain identified viruses (category J09) are coded. This is an exception to the hospital inpatient guideline Section II, H. In this context, "confirmation" does not require documentation of positive laboratory testing specific for avian or other novel influenza A. However, coding should be based on the provider's diagnostic statement. In this case, there is no documentation that a laboratory test confirmed the novel influenza A virus, but the statement was documented as a confirmed diagnosis, not "possible," "probable," or other such terms. ICD-10-CM provides some combination codes for associated manifestations (such as respiratory, gastroenteritis, other).

1.77. J43.9 Emphysema (atrophic) (bullous) (chronic) (interlobular) (lung) (obstructive) (pulmonary) (senile) (vesicular)

I50.9 Failure, failed, heart (acute) (senile) (sudden), congestive (compensated) (decompensated)

I10 Hypertension, hypertensive (accelerated) (benign) (essential) (idiopathic) (malignant) (systemic)

I48.91 Fibrillation, atrial or auricular (established)

Rationale: Code J43.9 includes the COPD as indicated by the nonessential modifiers. Additionally, there is an *Excludes1* note under J44 (COPD) for emphysema (J43.-). Follow Index and Tabular carefully. When indexing COPD via Disease, lung, obstructive (chronic) there is a subterm with emphysema (J44.9). When verifying J44.9 in the Tabular there is an *Excludes1* note: J44 *Excludes1*: emphysema without chronic bronchitis (J43.X). The emphysema in category J44 would be emphysema **with** chronic bronchitis. When verifying J43.9 in the Tabular, there is an *Excludes1* note: Emphysema with chronic (obstructive) bronchitis (J44.X). To differentiate these two categories with emphysema, chronic bronchitis is key and must be documented. In this case, follow the Tabular, not the Index.

1.78. J45.42 Asthma, asthmatic, moderate persistent, with, status asthmaticus

J44.1 Disease, lung, obstructive (chronic), with, acute, exacerbation NEC

Rationale: An instructional note under category J44 provides instructions to "code also type of asthma, if applicable (J45.42)." An *Excludes2* note appears under J45 for "asthma with chronic obstructive pulmonary disease." A type 2 "excludes" note represents "Not included here." An *Excludes2* note indicates that the condition excluded is not part of the condition represented by the code, but a patient may have both conditions at the same time. When an *Excludes2* note appears under a code, it is acceptable to use both the code and the excluded code together, when appropriate. The "code also" note does not provide sequencing direction.

1.79. E86.0 Dehydration

J43.9 Emphysema (atrophic) (bullous) (chronic) (interlobular) (lung) (obstructive) (pulmonary) (senile) (vesicular)

Z99.11 Dependence, on, ventilator

Rationale: The dehydration is the reason for admission, and therefore should be listed as the principal diagnosis.

1.80. J69.0 Pneumonia, aspiration, due to food (regurgitated)

I69.391 Dysphagia, following, cerebrovascular disease, cerebral infarction

R13.19 Dysphagia, neurogenic

L89.211 Ulcer, decubitus – *see* Ulcer, pressure by site
Ulcer, pressure, stage 1 (healing) (pre-ulcer skin changes limited to persistent focal edema), hip, right

L89.221 Ulcer, pressure, Ulcer, pressure, stage 1 (healing) (pre-ulcer skin changes limited to persistent focal edema), hip, left

Rationale: The documentation substantiates the assignment of aspiration pneumonia as the first-listed diagnosis. The neurogenic dysphagia is due to an old cerebral infarction and should be coded. R13.19 is coded in addition to I69.391 due to an instructional note under I69.391 stating "Use additional code to identify the type of dysphagia, if known (R13.1-)." Two decubitus ulcer codes are required since the patient has ulcers of both the right and left hip. L89.211 is pressure ulcer of the right hip, stage 1 and L89.221 is pressure ulcer of the left hip, stage 1.

Chapter 11 Coding Cases

1.81. K40.41   Hernia, hernial, (acquired) (recurrent), inguinal (direct) (external) (funicular) (indirect) (internal) (oblique) (scrotal) (sliding), unilateral, with, gangrene (and obstruction), recurrent

Rationale: When coding hernias, ICD-10-CM provides specificity by type, laterality, with or without obstruction and recurrence.

1.82. K25.0   Ulcer, ulcerated, ulcerating, ulceration, ulcerative, gastric – *see* Ulcer, stomach (eroded) (peptic) (round), acute, with, hemorrhage

Rationale: Gastric ulcers are subdivided by severity and then further subdivided by hemorrhage and/or perforation.

1.83. K80.33   Choledocholithiasis (common duct) (hepatic duct) – *see* Calculus, bile duct (common) (hepatic), with, cholangitis, acute, with, obstruction

Rationale: ICD-10-CM has provided a combination code for bile duct calculus with cholangitis.

1.84. K50.012   Crohn's disease – *see* Enteritis, regional, Enteritis (acute) (diarrheal) (hemorrhagic) (noninfective) (septic), regional (of), small intestine, with complication, intestinal obstruction

Rationale: An additional code for the small bowel obstruction is not required, as the combination code in ICD-10-CM identifies both the Crohn's disease and the small bowel obstruction. Exacerbation is not a qualifier for Crohn's disease.

1.85. K25.4   Ulcer, ulcerated, ulcerating, ulceration, ulcerative, gastric – *see* ulcer, stomach (eroded) (peptic) (round), chronic, with hemorrhage

         I50.9   Failure, failed, heart (acute) (senile) (sudden), congestive (compensated) (decompensated)

         I48.91   Fibrillation, atrial or auricular (established)

Rationale: Even though a complete diagnostic workup was not completed because of the patient's wishes, the hemorrhage should be included in the coding as it was documented by the physician.

1.86. K40.20   Hernia, hernial (acquired) (recurrent), inguinal (direct) (external) (funicular) (indirect) (internal) (oblique) (scrotal) (sliding), bilateral

         R07.2   Pain(s) (*see also* Painful), chest (central), precordial

         J44.9   Disease, diseased, pulmonary, chronic obstructive

         M54.5   Pain(s) (*see also* Painful), low back

         I10   Hypertension, hypertensive (accelerated) (benign) (essential) (idiopathic) (malignant) (systemic)

         Z53.09   Canceled procedure (surgical), because of contraindication

Rationale: The inguinal hernia should be the first-listed diagnosis, as it was the reason for admission, even though the surgery was canceled.

1.87. K94.22   Complication(s) (from) (of), gastrostomy (stoma), infection

         L03.311   Cellulitis (diffuse) (phlegmonous) (septic) (suppurative), abdominal wall

         C15.4   Neoplasm Table, by site (esophagus), malignant, primary

         B95.62   Infection, infected, infective (opportunistic), staphylococcal, as cause of disease classified elsewhere, aureus, methicillin resistant

Rationale: The infection of the gastrostomy is sequenced first. The note under K94.22 states to use an additional code to specify type of infection, such as cellulitis of abdominal wall. The organism (methicillin resistant *Staph.* aureus) is also coded per instructional note which appears directly under the section "Infections of the Skin and Subcutaneous Tissue (L00-L08)." The note states, "Use additional code (B95-B97) to identify infectious agent."

Chapter 12 Coding Cases

1.88. L27.0   Dermatitis (eczematous), due to, drugs and medicaments (generalized) (internal use)

T36.0X5A   Table of Drugs and Chemicals, Penicillin (any), Adverse Effect, initial encounter

Rationale: The reason for this encounter is the extensive dermatitis which is an adverse effect to the penicillin. An instructional note in the Tabular under code L27.0 states "Use additional code for adverse effect, if applicable, to identify drug." Following this instructional note, T36.0X5A is sequenced as the secondary diagnosis code. The seventh character of T36.0X5A indicates this is the initial encounter (A) for this condition.

1.89. I96   Ulcer, gangrenous – *see* Gangrene. Gangrene, gangrenous (connective tissue) (dropsical) (dry) (moist) (skin) (ulcer) (*see also* necrosis). Necrosis, skin or subcutaneous tissue NEC

L89.213   Ulcer, ulcerated, ulcerating, ulceration, ulcerative, pressure (pressure area) stage 3, (healing) (full thickness skin loss involving damage or necrosis of subcutaneous tissue), hip. Review the Tabular for complete code assignment.

L89.152   Ulcer, ulcerated, ulcerating, ulceration, ulcerative, pressure (pressure area) stage 2, (healing) (abrasion, blister, partial thickness skin loss involving epidermis and/or dermis) sacral region (tailbone). Review the Tabular for complete code assignment.

Rationale: Decubitus ulcers are classified to pressure ulcers. The note at the beginning of category L89 indicates the sequencing. Any associated gangrene is listed first. Subcategory L89.2 classifies pressure ulcers of the hip. It is necessary to review the Tabular to select the correct stage and laterality to identify code L89.213 for stage 3 of the right hip. The pressure ulcer of the sacral region is documented as stage 2, and code L89.152 is assigned. The sacral region includes the tailbone and the coccyx. Coding Guideline I.B.14 states that the stage of the pressure ulcer may be documented by another healthcare clinician and coded as long as the pressure ulcer is documented by the provider.

1.90. I70.233   Atherosclerosis, *see also* arteriosclerosis. Arteriosclerosis, arteriosclerotic (diffuse) (obliterans) (of) (senile) (with calcification), extremities (native arteries) leg, right, with ulceration (and intermittent claudication and rest pain), ankle

L97.311   Ulcer, ulcerated, ulcerating, ulceration, ulcerative, lower limb (atrophic) (chronic) (neurogenic) (perforating) (pyogenic) (trophic) (tropical) ankle, right, with skin breakdown only

Rationale: In the Index under arteriosclerosis, the bypass graft codes of the extremities are listed first. It is important to scan until one comes to the Leg, and then locate left, right, and such. At subcategory I70.23, the following note appears: "Use additional code to identify severity of ulcer (L97.- with fifth character 1)." A note at category L97 further dictates sequencing of these codes: Code first any associated underlying condition. A code from L97 may be used as a principal or first-listed code if no underlying condition is documented as the cause of the ulcer. If one of the underlying conditions listed here is documented with a lower extremity ulcer, a causal condition should be assumed—atherosclerosis of the lower extremities, chronic venous hypertension, diabetic ulcers, postphlebitic syndrome, varicose ulcer. The codes must be listed in this order.

1.91. L02.612   Abscess (connective tissue) (embolic) (fistulous) (infective) (metastatic) (multiple) (pernicious) (pyogenic) (septic), toe (any) *see also* Abscess, foot. Abscess, foot

   I96   Gangrene, gangrenous (connective tissue) (dropsical) (dry) (moist) (skin) (ulcer) (*see also* necrosis). Necrosis, skin or subcutaneous tissue NEC

Rationale: In ICD-10-CM, there are individual categories for abscess (L02) and cellulitis (L03). In ICD-9-CM, these were combined. Note in the Index that abscess of the toe classifies to abscess of the foot, while abscess of the toe nail classifies to cellulitis, toe. There are no "includes" or "excludes" notes that preclude the use of the abscess and gangrene code together, nor is there any sequencing guideline available.

1.92. L03.115   Cellulitis, leg – *see* Cellulitis, lower limb. Lower limb
   B95.1   Infection, bacterial NOS, as cause of disease classified elsewhere, Streptococcus group B
   L89.312   Ulcer, ulcerated, ulcerating, ulceration, ulcerative, decubitus – *see* Ulcer, pressure, by site. Pressure (pressure area) stage 2, (healing) (abrasion, blister, partial thickness skin loss involving epidermis and/or dermis), buttock
   L89.321   Ulcer, ulcerated, ulcerating, ulceration, ulcerative, decubitus – *see* Ulcer, pressure, by site. Pressure (pressure area) stage 1, (healing) (pre-ulcer skin changes limited to persistent focal edema), buttock

Rationale: Documentation supports that cellulitis is the first-listed diagnosis. Review of the Tabular shows that ICD-10-CM classifies the laterality of cellulitis of the lower extremity, with L03.115 being the right lower extremity. A note appears in the Tabular under the section Infections of the Skin and Subcutaneous Tissue (L00-L08) instructing to "Use an additional code (B95-B97) to identify infectious agent." ICD-10-CM also classifies decubitus ulcers of the buttocks both by stage and laterality. Gluteus is not listed in the classification, but it refers to the buttock region.

1.93. L27.1   Dermatitis, (eczematous) due to drugs and medicaments, (generalized) (internal use) localized skin eruption
   T46.4X5A   Table of Drugs and Chemicals, Ramipril, Adverse Effect, initial encounter
   I10   Hypertension, hypertensive (accelerated) (benign) (essential) (idiopathic) (malignant) (systemic)

Rationale: The reason, after study, for this encounter is the dermatitis which is an adverse effect to the Ramipril. An instructional note in the Tabular under code L27.1 states "Use additional code for adverse effect, if applicable, to identify drug (T36-T50 with fifth or sixth character 5)." Following this instruction note, the T46.4X5A is sequenced as a secondary diagnosis code. The seventh character of A indicates this is the initial encounter for this condition. Documentation states localized dermatitis, and there is a specific code for that. This documentation does not indicate long-term use of the drug since it was recently started.

1.94. L24.3 Dermatitis (eczematous), contact, irritant, due to, cosmetics
H01.114 Dermatitis (eczematous), eyelid, contact – *see* Dermatitis, eyelid, allergic, left, upper
H01.111 Dermatitis (eczematous), eyelid, contact – *see* Dermatitis, eyelid, allergic, right, upper
T49.8X5A Table of Drugs and Chemicals, Cosmetics, adverse effect
L70.0 Acne, cystic

Rationale: The reason for this encounter was the contact dermatitis due to the adverse reaction with the use of new eye cosmetics. The seventh character A indicates this is the initial encounter for the condition. There are several different Index terms for the dermatitis. This was documented as irritant contact dermatitis, but not allergic, so Index Contact, irritant, due to cosmetics, L24.3. Under Contact, allergic, due to cosmetics there is a different code L23.2, if documentation supported that code. Contact dermatitis (not documented as irritant) due to cosmetics is coded L25.0. Careful review of the record and Index is indicated. In addition, there is reference to a specific site (upper eyelids) having a separate classification. Under L24, there is an *Excludes2* note for dermatitis of eyelid (H01.1-). This means that if both conditions are present, both codes may be assigned. The cystic acne is assigned as a secondary condition since it was also treated during the encounter.

1.95. L03.221 Cellulitis (diffuse) (phlegmonous) (septic) (suppurative), neck (region)
F11.10 Abuse, drug, morphine type (opioids) – *see* Abuse, drug, opioid. Opioid
Z72.89 Behavior, drug seeking

Rationale: ICD-10-CM provides a code for drug seeking behavior.

Chapter 13 Coding Cases

1.96. M00.861 Arthritis, arthritic (acute) (chronic) (nonpyogenic) (subacute), septic (any site except spine) – *see* Arthritis, pyogenic or pyemic (any site except spine), bacterial NEC, knee. Review the Tabular for correct code assignment.

Rationale: Most of the codes in this chapter have site and laterality designations. A note is available at subcategory M00.8 stating to "Use additional code (B96) to identify bacteria." In this case, it was not specified.

1.97. M08.071 Arthritis, arthritic (acute) (chronic) (nonpyogenic) (subacute), rheumatoid, juvenile (with or without rheumatoid factor), ankle. Review the Tabular for assignment of laterality.
M08.072 Arthritis, arthritic (acute) (chronic) (nonpyogenic) (subacute), rheumatoid, juvenile (with or without rheumatoid factor), ankle. Review the Tabular for assignment of laterality.

Rationale: For juvenile rheumatoid arthritis, there is not a code to identify bilateral; therefore, both codes, to identify right and left, must be assigned.

1.98. M84.551A Fracture, pathological (pathologic), due to neoplastic disease, femur
C79.51 Carcinoma (malignant), metastatic, *see* Neoplasm, secondary. Refer to Neoplasm Table, by site, bone, femur, secondary.
Z85.118 History, personal (of), malignant neoplasm (of), lung
Z92.3 History, personal (of), radiation therapy

Rationale: M84.551A correctly identifies the fracture in the shaft of the right femur. The seventh character A is used as long as the patient is receiving active treatment for the fracture. Examples of active treatment are: surgical treatment, ER encounter, and evaluation and treatment by a new physician. The code Z92.3 can be added to show history of radiation therapy if coding is performed to that degree.

1.99. M80.08XA   Fracture, pathological (pathologic), due to osteoporosis, specified cause NEC – *see* Osteoporosis, specified type NEC, with pathological fracture. Osteoporosis (female) (male), senile – *see* Osteoporosis, age-related, with current pathologic fracture, vertebra(e)

Rationale: In ICD-10-CM, a combination code is utilized to report osteoporosis with an associated pathological fracture. When identifying senile osteoporosis, the code book directs the coder to age-related osteoporosis.

Chapter 14 Coding Cases

1.100. N03.2   Syndrome, nephritic – *see also* Nephritis. Nephritis, nephritic, chronic, with diffuse membranous glomerulonephritis.

Rationale: The indexing of this code is somewhat confusing. If you go to Syndrome, nephritic, there is a note to *see* Nephritis. There are also terms for Nephrotic Syndrome, which causes a different path. The proteinuria and hematuria are symptoms and would not be coded. There are many different choices in the Glomerular Diseases (N00-N08) block. A careful review of the category choices in this block is helpful. Nephritic syndrome is not a specific diagnosis, but a clinical syndrome characterized by several signs. Its prognosis depends on the underlying etiology. Nephritic syndrome and nephrotic syndrome are similar but different.

1.101. N30.01   Cystitis (exudative) (hemorrhagic) (septic) (suppurative), acute, with hematuria
        B96.20   Escherichia (E.) coli, as cause of disease classified elsewhere

Rationale: Suppurative is a nonessential modifier for cystitis, so it is included in the code. There is a combination code for acute cystitis with hematuria (N30.01). The frequent urination and pain are integral to the cystitis and not assigned codes. A note at category N30 states to "Use additional code to identify infectious agent" (B95-B97). This code is never in the first position.

1.102. N92.4   Menorrhagia (primary), preclimacteric or premenopausal

Rationale: Subcategory N92.4, Excessive bleeding in the premenopausal period includes climacteric, menopausal, preclimacteric, or premenopausal menorrhagia or metrorrhagia.

1.103. N17.0   Failure, failed, kidney, acute (*see also* Failure, renal, acute). Failure, renal, acute, with, tubular necrosis
        N40.1   Hypertrophy, prostate – *see* Enlargement, enlarged, prostate, with lower urinary tract symptoms (LUTS)
        N13.8   Obstruction, urinary (moderate)

Rationale: The prostate hypertrophy and urinary obstruction are coded separately in ICD-10-CM. This note is available under subcategory N40.1: Use additional code for associated symptoms, when specified: urinary obstruction (N13.8). There is also a cross reference at code N13.8 stating to code, if applicable, any causal condition first, such as: enlarged prostate (N40.1). Currently, in ICD-9-CM, sequencing guidelines are provided in *Coding Clinic*, 3rd Quarter, 2002 that were used to determine sequencing in this case, but any future ICD-10-CM guidance would determine code assignment. Remember that ICD-9-CM and ICD-10-CM are different.

1.104. N18.3   Disease, diseased, kidney (functional) (pelvis), chronic, stage 3 (moderate)

Z94.0   Status (post), transplant – *see* Transplant, kidney

E89.0   Hypothyroidism (acquired), postsurgical

Z85.850   History, personal (of), malignant neoplasm (of), thyroid

Rationale: The coding guidelines state that "the presence of CKD alone does not constitute a transplant complication. Assign the appropriate N18 code for the patient's stage of CKD and code Z94.0, Kidney transplant status." The note at category N18 states "Use additional code to identify kidney transplant status, if applicable."

1.105. N39.0   Infection, infected, infective, (opportunistic), urinary (tract)

B96.4   Infection, infected, infective (opportunistic), bacterial NOS, as cause of disease classified elsewhere, proteus (mirabilis) (morganii)

Z87.440   History, personal (of), infection, urinary (recurrent) (tract)

Rationale: As in ICD-9-CM, the bacteria causing the urinary tract infection is coded as a secondary diagnosis. The following note at code N39.0 states "Use additional code (B95-B97) to identify infectious agent." The history of UTI does have a separate history code that should be added as an additional diagnosis.

Chapter 15 Coding Cases

1.106. O13.2   Pregnancy (single) (uterine) , complicated by (care of) (management affected by), hypertension, – *see* Hypertension, complicating, pregnancy, gestational (pregnancy induced) (transient) (without proteinuria). Review the Tabular for complete code assignment.

O09.522   Pregnancy (single) (uterine) , complicated by (care of) (management affected by), elderly, multigravida. Review the Tabular for complete code assignment.

Z3A.26   Pregnancy (single) (uterine), weeks of gestation, 26 weeks

Rationale: For these codes, the range of codes is further subdivided by the trimester for the current encounter. The note at the beginning of Chapter 15 defines the second trimester as 14 weeks 0 days to less than 28 weeks 0 days. The Index does not provide complete codes; therefore, it is necessary to review the Tabular for complete code assignment. The Z code identifying the weeks of gestation should also be assigned per the "use additional code" note at the beginning of Chapter 15.

1.107. O21.0   Pregnancy (single) (uterine) , complicated by (care of) (management affected by), hyperemesis (gravidarum) (mild) – *see also* Hyperemesis, gravidarum (mild)

O23.42   Pregnancy (single) (uterine) , complicated by (care of) (management affected by), infection(s), urinary (tract). Review the Tabular for complete code assignment.

B96.20   Infection, infected, infective (opportunistic), bacterial NOS, as cause of disease classified elsewhere, Escherichia coli [E. coli]

Z3A.16   Pregnancy (single) (uterine), weeks of gestation, 16 weeks

Rationale: The hyperemesis gravidarum code for this case is specific to weeks of gestation – "... starting before the end of the 20th week of gestation." Note that there are different options for finding this code in the Index. The UTI code does not require a secondary code for the UTI (as previously seen in ICD-9-CM) because specificity is found in the code, but there is a "use additional code" note to identify the organism.

1.108. O91.22   Mastitis (acute) (diffuse) (nonpuerperal) (subacute), obstetric (interstitial) (nonpurulent), associated with, puerperium

Rationale: In this case, the mastitis is not classified in a pregnancy or delivery complication; however, further indentation in the Index provides the specificity of a postpartum complication.

1.109. O30.003   Pregnancy (single) (uterine) , complicated by (care of) (management affected by), multiple gestations, twin *see* Pregnancy, twin. Review the Tabular for complete code assignment.

O69.81X2   Delivery (childbirth) (labor), complicated, by, cord (umbilical), around neck, without compression. Review the Tabular for seventh character.

Z3A.39   Pregnancy (single) (uterine), weeks of gestation, 39 weeks

Z37.2   Outcome of delivery, twins NEC, both liveborn

Rationale: Complete code assignment for the twin pregnancy is found in the Tabular of ICD-10-CM. The umbilical cord complication is a complication of the delivery rather than the pregnancy and is further subdivided by with or without compression. If both fetus 1 and fetus 2 were found to have nuchal cords, code O69.81X_ would be coded twice with different seventh characters.

1.110. O24.419   Pregnancy (single) (uterine) , complicated by (care of) (management affected by), diabetes (mellitus), gestational (pregnancy induced) *see* Diabetes, gestational (in pregnancy)

Z3A.28   Pregnancy (single) (uterine), weeks of gestation, 28 weeks

Rationale: This sixth character indicates the type of control (namely, diet or insulin) for the gestational diabetes. ICD-10-CM does not provide a specific sixth character for control with oral medication; therefore, the unspecified control code is used.

1.111. O26.12   Pregnancy (single) (uterine) , complicated by (care of) (management affected by), insufficient, weight gain. Review the Tabular for complete code assignment.

O10.012   Pregnancy (single) (uterine) , complicated by (care of) (management affected by), hypertension, *see* Hypertension, complicating, pregnancy, pre-existing, essential. Review the Tabular for complete code assignment.

Z3A.20   Pregnancy (single) (uterine), weeks of gestation, 20 weeks

Rationale: Both of these conditions are indexed under Pregnancy although with the pre-existing hypertension the coder is directed to Hypertension. A review of the Tabular is necessary for complete, correct code assignment.

1.112. O80   Delivery (childbirth) (labor), normal
Z3A.39   Pregnancy (single) (uterine), weeks of gestation, 39 weeks
Z37.0   Outcome of delivery, single, liveborn

Rationale: ICD-10-CM Guidelines define a normal delivery (O80) as a full-term normal delivery with a single, healthy infant without any complications antepartum, during the delivery, or postpartum during the delivery episode. Code O80 is always the principal diagnosis and is not to be used if any other code from Chapter 15 is needed to describe a current complication of the antenatal, delivery, or perinatal period. See the note with code O80 for a full definition of this code. Z37.0 is the only outcome of delivery code appropriate for use with O80.

1.113. O70.1   Delivery (childbirth) (labor), complicated, by, laceration (perineal), perineum, perineal, second degree
O24.12   Pregnancy (single) (uterine), complicated by, diabetes (mellitus), pre-existing, type 2
E11.9   Diabetes, diabetic (mellitus) (sugar), type 2
Z3A.38   Pregnancy (single) (uterine), weeks of gestation, 38 weeks
Z37.0   Outcome of delivery, single, liveborn

Rationale: The patient experienced a second degree perineal laceration (O70.1) during delivery. The patient's type 2 diabetes is identified with O24.12. The 'in childbirth' option is used due to coding guideline I.C.15.a.3. The outcome of delivery was a single liveborn (Z37.0). The Pitocin augmentation is not coded, only failed medical induction of labor.

1.114. O98.712   Pregnancy (single) (uterine) , complicated by (care of) (management affected by), human immunodeficiency [HIV] disease. Review the Tabular for complete code assignment.
B20   AIDS (related complex)
B59   Pneumocystis carinii pneumonia
Z3A.21   Pregnancy (single) (uterine), weeks of gestation, 21 weeks

Rationale: There is a specific ICD-10-CM Coding Guideline for HIV Infections in Pregnancy, Childbirth and the Puerperium (I.C.15.f) which states "During pregnancy, childbirth, or the puerperium, a patient admitted because of an HIV-related illness should receive a principal diagnosis from subcategory O98.7-, Human immunodeficiency [HIV] disease complicating pregnancy, childbirth, and the puerperium, followed by the code(s) for the HIV-related illness(es)." A sixth character of 2 indicates that the patient is in the second trimester. A note appears at the beginning of Chapter 15 of ICD-10-CM that states that "Trimesters are counted from the first day of the last menstrual period. They are defined as follows: 1st trimester: less than 14 weeks, 0 days; 2nd trimester: 14 weeks, 0 days to less than 28 weeks, 0 days; and 3rd trimester: 28 weeks, 0 days until delivery." An instructional note appears under code B20 indicating that code O98.7- is listed first. An instructional note appears under O98.7 which states to "Use an additional code to identify the type of HIV disease."

1.115. O60.14X2   Pregnancy (single) (uterine) , complicated by (care of) (management affected by), preterm labor, third trimester, with third trimester preterm delivery

O36.4XX2   Pregnancy (single) (uterine) , complicated by (care of) (management affected by), fetal (maternal care for), death (near term) or Pregnancy, complicated by, intrauterine fetal death (near term). Review the Tabular for complete code assignment.

O30.103   Pregnancy (single) (uterine) , complicated by (care of) (management affected by), multiple gestations, triplet, *see* Pregnancy, triplet – *see* Tabular for complete code, triplet

O41.1030   Pregnancy (single) (uterine), complicated by (care of) (management affected by), infection(s), amniotic fluid or sac

Z3A.34   Pregnancy (single) (uterine), weeks of gestation, 34 weeks

Z37.61   Outcome of delivery, multiple births, some liveborn, triplets

Rationale: The patient was admitted in early labor with a 34-week gestation (O60.14X2). Review of the Tabular for category O60 (preterm labor) reveals that all codes in category O60 require a seventh character. Seventh characters 1–9 are for cases of multiple gestations to identify the fetus for which the code applies. Code O60.14X2 was sequenced as the principal diagnosis because the preterm labor was the original reason that the patient was admitted. The seventh character, 2, was used to indicate that fetus 2 was responsible for the continued contractions and ultimately the preterm delivery as documented within the case. One of the triplets was an intrauterine fetal death (O36.4XX2) and review of the Tabular indicates that codes from this category also require a seventh character to indicate which fetus was dead. The pregnancy is a triplet pregnancy (O30.103). The patient developed infection of amniotic sac (O41.103). Review of the Tabular for category O41 indicates that all codes from this category also require a seventh character. In this instance, the documentation does not indicate the fetus for which the infection applies; therefore, a seventh character of 0 is used to signify a multiple gestation where the fetus is unspecified. The fever during labor (O75.2) is not coded because the cause is known (infection). The outcome of delivery was triplets, two liveborn and one fetal death (Z37.61).

1.116. O86.0   Complication(s) (from) (of), obstetric, surgical wound NEC, infection; Infection, obstetrical surgical wound (puerperal)

B95.1   Infection, infected, infective (opportunistic) bacterial, as cause of disease classified elsewhere, Streptococcus, group B

Rationale: ICD-10-CM Guidelines state that any complication occurring within the first six weeks (42 days) following delivery is considered to be a postpartum complication. In the Tabular, under subcategory O86, a note instructs the coder to use an additional code (B95-B97) to identify the infectious agent.

1.117. O34.21   Delivery (childbirth) (labor), cesarean (for), previous, cesarean delivery

O64.3XX0   Delivery (childbirth) (labor), complicated, by, obstructed labor, due to, brow presentation

O66.41   Delivery (childbirth) (labor), complicated, by, failed, attempted vaginal birth after previous cesarean delivery

Z3A.39   Pregnancy (single) (uterine), weeks of gestation, 39 weeks

Z37.0   Outcome of delivery, single, liveborn

Rationale: O34.21 is sequenced as the principal diagnosis since it was the reason for the patient's admission. ICD-10-CM Coding Guidelines state "In cases of cesarean delivery, the selection of the principal diagnosis should be the condition established after study that was responsible for the patient's admission. If the patient was admitted with a condition that resulted in the performance of a cesarean procedure, that condition should be selected as the principal diagnosis. If the reason for the admission/encounter was unrelated to the condition resulting in the cesarean delivery, the condition related to the reason for the admission/encounter should be selected as the principal diagnosis, even if a cesarean was performed." The "code first" note under O34 doesn't apply to this scenario because her obstructed labor had nothing to do with conditions classifiable to O34 (which is why only O65.5, and not O66.41, is listed in the note). Notice the note says "code first any associated obstructed labor." There was no obstructed labor associated with the scar from her previous C-section (which is the condition classified to O34). The obstructed labor was due to malpresentation of the fetus, not the O34 condition. In this case, the reason for the C-section was unrelated to the reason for admission, so the reason for admission, and not the reason for the C-section, should be sequenced first. The problem with the baby's malpresentation didn't occur until after admission.

Codes from category O64 require a seventh character to indicate the fetus for which the code applies in the case of multiple gestations. Review of the note under O64, which indicates the seventh character of 0, is for single gestations. The patient has a scar from previous cesarean delivery (O34.21). O66.41 indicates the failed attempt of a vaginal birth after a previous cesarean delivery. The outcome of delivery was a single liveborn (Z37.0).

1.118. O03.4   Abortion (complete) (spontaneous), incomplete (spontaneous)
O13.1   Hypertension, complicating, pregnancy, gestational (pregnancy induced) (transient) (without proteinuria)
Z3A.12   Pregnancy (single) (uterine), weeks of gestation, 12 weeks

Rationale: The abortion was incomplete (O03.4) with no complications. The gestational hypertension (O13.1) was treated during the encounter. The fourth character O13.1 indicates that patient is in the first trimester of pregnancy. The first trimester of pregnancy is defined as less than 14 weeks and 0 days. Code Z3A.12 is added to indicate weeks of gestation.

Chapter 16 Coding Cases

1.119. P36.2   Newborn, (infant) (liveborn) (singleton), sepsis (congenital), due to Staphylococcus, aureus

Rationale: The Z38 category is not assigned, because the birth episode did not occur at this encounter. Code A41.0- is incorrect because this encounter was within the 28 days after birth (perinatal period) and the newborn codes are to be used. See the *Excludes1* note at category A41 – *Excludes1* neonatal (P36.-). This is the only code required because there is no mention of severe sepsis or organ dysfunction. And, the P36.2 code identifies the organism, so no additional code from category B95 is indicated.

1.120. P59.9   Newborn (infant) (liveborn) (singleton), hyperbilirubinemia

Rationale: The birth did not occur at this encounter, so the Z38 category is not assigned. Hyperbilirubinemia without mention of prematurity or specified cause is coded to P59.9. If prematurity was documented, there is a specific code to identify that condition (P59.0).

1.121. Z38.00   Newborn (infant) (liveborn) (singleton), born in hospital
       Q86.0   Syndrome, fetal, alcohol (dysmorphic)

Rationale: According to ICD-10-CM Coding Guidelines, a code from Z38 is assigned as the principal/first listed diagnosis. When the coder reviews code Q86.0, there is an *Excludes2* statement that refers to a possible use of code P04.-. However, when code P04.3 (that with use of alcohol) is referenced, it specifically excludes that with fetal alcohol syndrome.

1.122. Z38.01   Newborn (infant) (liveborn) (singleton), born in hospital, by cesarean
       P04.41   Newborn (infant) (liveborn) (singleton), affected by cocaine (crack)
       P07.14   Weight, 1000–2499 grams at birth (low) – *see* Low, birth weight. Low, birth weight (2499 grams or less) with weight of 1000–1249 grams
       P07.34   Premature, newborn, less than 37 completed weeks – *see* Preterm newborn. Preterm, newborn (infant), gestational age 31 completed weeks (31 weeks, 0 days through 31 weeks, 6 days)
       P74.1   Newborn (infant) (liveborn) (singleton), dehydration

Rationale: There is no documentation of withdrawal, which would be coded P96.1. Following sequencing according to the guidelines, the code for birth weight is sequenced before the code for gestational age. In indexing the premature newborn, note that "preterm infant" is not an option under the term Newborn. It is indexed under Preterm infant, newborn.

Chapter 17 Coding Cases

1.123. Q01.0   Encephalocele, frontal

Rationale: Encephalocele has been expanded in ICD-10-CM from one code to five codes. An encephalocele is defined as a congenital malformation in which brain tissue protrudes through a skull defect. Hydroencephalocele is included in code Q01.0.

1.124. Q37.4   Cleft, (congenital) lip (unilateral), bilateral, with cleft palate, hard with soft

Rationale: Careful review of the documentation is indicated to select the one code that combines these conditions. Cleft lip and palate are congenital defects caused when the bones and tissues don't fuse together in utero. The palate is the roof of the mouth, and consists of the soft (back part near the throat) and the hard (front part behind the teeth) palates. Frequently cleft lip and palate are both present. A cleft lip can be either unilateral or bilateral. The unilateral cleft lip has a gap on one side of the lip under either the left or right nostril, but in a bilateral cleft lip, the gap is on both sides of the lip.

1.125. Q54.2   Hypospadias, penoscrotal

Rationale: In ICD-9-CM, there was one code to identify this condition, whereas in ICD-10-CM codes are available for hypospadias balanic, penile, penoscrotal, perineal, congenital chordee, other hypospadias, and unspecified. Hypospadias refers to a congenital condition in which the urethral meatus lies on the ventral position of the penile shaft and may be located as far down as in the scrotum or perineum.

1.126. Z38.01   Newborn (infant) (liveborn) (singleton), born in hospital, by cesarean
Q20.3   Transposition (congenital) vessels, great (complete) (partial)

Rationale: In this case, the newborn code is listed first. Transposition of the great vessels (TGV) is a congenital heart defect in which the aorta and the pulmonary artery are transposed. Because this is a cyanotic heart defect (too little oxygen), the cyanosis is inherent and not separately coded.

Chapter 18 Coding Cases

1.127. R10.821   Tenderness, abdominal, rebound, right upper quadrant

Rationale: ICD-10-CM provides subcategory R10.81 for abdominal tenderness and subcategory R10.82 for rebound abdominal tenderness. In ICD-9-CM, both conditions were included in subcategory 789.6. Rebound tenderness refers to pain upon removal of pressure rather than application of pressure to the abdomen.

1.128. R40.2111   Coma, with opening of eyes (never)
R40.2211   Coma, with verbal response (none)
R40.2311   Coma, with motor response (none)
R40.2134   Coma, with opening of eyes, in response to sound
R40.2234   Coma, with verbal response, inappropriate words
R40.2344   Coma, with motor response, flexion withdrawal

Rationale: In order to report the scale, all three categories must be identified. The first set of codes identifies the condition as reported by the EMT. The second set of codes corresponds to the neurologist's assessment on day 2. It is appropriate to report more than one set of codes if desired. The seventh character for the first set of codes (1) identifies that this was done by the EMT in the field, and the second set (4) 24 hours or more after hospital admission. This case is used to illustrate the coma scale codes, but they would not be used alone.

1.129. R92.0   Microcalcifications, breast

Rationale: ICD-10-CM has individual codes for mammographic microcalcification found on diagnostic imaging of the breast and mammographic calcification found on diagnostic imaging of breast.

1.130. R00.1   Bradycardia (sinoatrial) (sinus) (vagal)

Rationale: Code R00.1 includes sinoatrial bradycardia. In ICD-9-CM, this condition is classified in the Circulatory chapter, while in ICD-10-CM it is in Chapter 18. There is an *Excludes1* note at category I49, Other cardiac arrhythmias, excluding bradycardia.

1.131. R07.89   Pain(s) (*see also* Painful), chest (central), atypical
I20.9   Angina (attack) (cardiac) (chest) (heart) (pectoris) (syndrome) (vasomotor)
K21.9   Disease, diseased, gastroesophageal reflux (GERD)

Rationale: In the instance where a symptom(s) is followed by contrasting/comparative diagnoses, the symptom code is sequenced first. All the contrasting/comparative diagnoses should be coded as additional codes.

1.132. R50.9   Fever (inanition) (of unknown origin) (persistent) (with chills) (with rigor)

Rationale: ICD-10-CM Diagnostic Coding and Reporting Guidelines for Outpatient Services (IV. H.) states the following for uncertain diagnoses: "Do not code diagnoses documented as 'probable,' 'suspected,' 'questionable,' 'rule out,' or 'working diagnosis,' or other similar terms indicating uncertainty. Rather, code the condition(s) to the highest degree of certainty for that encounter/visit, such as symptoms, signs, abnormal test results, or other reasons for the visit." It would be incorrect to code the viral syndrome in this case. Fever, unspecified includes fever with chills.

1.133. R10.11   Pain(s) (*see* also Painful), abdominal, upper, right quadrant
R11.2   Nausea, with vomiting
R03.0   Elevated, elevation, blood pressure, reading (incidental) (isolated) (nonspecific), no diagnosis of hypertension

Rationale: No conclusive diagnosis was documented; therefore, the symptoms are coded.

Chapter 19 Coding Cases

1.134. T74.4XXA   Syndrome, shaken infant

Rationale: Shaken baby syndrome is a serious form of abuse inflicted upon a child. It usually occurs when a parent or other caregiver shakes a baby out of anger or frustration. There is often no external evidence of injury or physical sign of violence resulting in under diagnosis of this syndrome. Notes at this category state to assign any additional code, if applicable to identify any associated current injury, and the perpetrator, if known (Y07.-).

1.135. S82.852K   Nonunion, fracture – *see* Fracture, by site. Fracture, traumatic (abduction) (adduction) (separation), ankle, trimalleolar (displaced). Review the Tabular for complete code assignment as well as correct seventh character.

Rationale: Aftercare Z codes should not be used for aftercare of fractures. For aftercare of a fracture, assign the acute fracture code with the correct seventh character indicating the type of aftercare. Coding guidelines specify that if displaced versus nondisplaced is not indicated, the default is displaced.

1.136. S52.351B   Fracture, traumatic (abduction) (adduction) (separation), radius, shaft, comminuted (displaced). Review the Tabular for complete code assignment, including the seventh character.

Rationale: A compound fracture is an open fracture and this is stated as a type II open fracture in the documentation. The seventh character B indicates the initial treatment for a type II open fracture.

1.137. G82.21   Paraplegia (lower), complete
S32.029S   Fracture, traumatic (abduction) (adduction) (separation), vertebra, vertebral (arch) (body) (column) (neural arch) (pedicle) (spinous process) (transverse process), lumbar, second. Review the Tabular for correct seventh character.

Rationale: Seventh character S, sequela, is used for complications or conditions that arise as a direct result of an injury. When using seventh character S it is necessary to use both the injury code that precipitated the sequela and the code for the sequela itself. The S is added only to the injury code, not the sequela code. The specific type of sequela (paraplegia) is sequenced first, followed by the injury code.

1.138. S02.65XG   Fracture, traumatic, (abduction) (adduction) (separation), mandible (lower jaw (bone)), angle (of jaw). Review the Tabular for complete code assignment and correct seventh character.

Rationale: As with other fracture aftercare, the code for the acute fracture should be assigned with the seventh character G to indicate the delayed healing.

1.139. S02.0XXA   Fracture, traumatic (abduction) (adduction) (separation), skull, frontal bone. Review the Tabular for complete code assignment.

         S06.5X2A   Hemorrhage, hemorrhagic (concealed), intracranial (nontraumatic), subdural, traumatic – *see* Injury, intracranial (traumatic), subdural hemorrhage, traumatic. Review the Tabular for complete code assignment and correct seventh character.

Rationale: In ICD-10-CM, there is not a combination code for intracranial hemorrhage associated with skull fracture. Both conditions must be identified with separate codes. There is a "code also" note directing the coding professional to code also any associated intracranial injury (S06.-).

1.140. S91.322A   Laceration, heel – *see* Laceration, foot (except toe(s) alone), left, with foreign body. Review the Tabular for correct seventh character.

Rationale: In ICD-10-CM, the Index identifies both the laterality and the presence of the foreign body with the laceration code. The seventh character A is used to indicate the initial encounter.

1.141. S42.431D   Fracture, traumatic (abduction) (adduction) (separation), humerus, lower end, epicondyle, lateral (displaced). Review the Tabular for complete code assignment and the correct seventh character.

Rationale: The documentation indicates that this is the elbow but the epicondyle is coded to the humerus. Indexing Elbow will lead to an incorrect code. The elbow is the lower end of the humerus, and the lateral epicondyle extends medially to form the main part of the lower end of the humerus. This type of fracture is common in children. Even with normal healing, aftercare for fractures is coded to the acute fracture code with the seventh character that indicates routine healing.

1.142. T39.1X1A   Poisoning (acute) - *see* also Table of Drugs and Chemicals, Acetaminophen, Poisoning, Accidental (unintentional). Review the Tabular for the correct seventh character.

         R11.2   Nausea (without vomiting), with vomiting

Rationale: The seventh character is used with the poisoning codes in ICD-10-CM. All manifestations of poisonings should be assigned as an additional code.

1.143. R11.2   Nausea, with vomiting

         R53.83   Fatigue

         T46.0X5A   Table of Drugs and Chemicals, Digoxin, adverse effect

Rationale: The Index directs the coder to T46.0X5 in the Tabular. The seventh character must be assigned to indicate the initial encounter. The Official Coding Guidelines state "Assign the appropriate code for the nature of the adverse effect followed by the appropriate code for the adverse effect of the drug (T36-T50)."

1.144. I13.2   Disease, diseased, heart (organic), hypertensive – *see* Hypertension, heart. Hypertension, hypertensive (accelerated) (benign) (essential) (idiopathic) (malignant) (systemic), heart (disease) with kidney disease (chronic) – *see* Hypertension, cardiorenal (disease), with heart failure, with stage 5 or end stage renal disease

I50.9   Failure, heart (acute) (sudden), congestive (compensated) (decompensated). The "use additional code" statement under code I13.2 indicates the use of this code to identify the type of heart failure.

N18.5   Disease, diseased, kidney (functional) (pelvis), chronic, stage 5. (The "use additional code" statement under code I13.2 indicates the use of this code to identify the stage of the chronic kidney disease.)

T50.1X6A   Refer to Table of Drugs and Chemicals, Lasix, underdosing

Z91.130   Noncompliance, with, medication regimen, underdosing, unintentional, due to patient's age-related debility

Rationale: In ICD-10-CM, underdosing of medication can now be identified. The Coding Guidelines state, "Underdosing refers to taking less of a medication than is prescribed by a provider or a manufacturer's instruction. For underdosing, assign the code from categories T36-T50 (fifth or sixth character 6). Noncompliance (Z91.12-, Z91.13-) or complication of care (Y63.8-Y3.9) codes are to be used with an underdosing code to indicate intent, if known. Codes for underdosing should never be assigned as principal or first-listed codes." There is also a "code first underdosing of medication..." note under code Z91.13. The combination code for heart and kidney disease is used in this situation because both heart and renal disease exist along with the hypertension. According to the Official Coding Guidelines for hypertensive heart disease, the causal relationship is implied with the word "hypertensive." An additional code from category I50 is used to identify the type of heart failure. The "use additional code" note under code I13.2 indicates the use of the N18.5 code to identify the stage of the chronic kidney disease.

1.145. I49.5   Syndrome, sick, sinus

T82.110A   Complication(s) (from) (of), cardiovascular device, graft, or implant, electronic, electrode, mechanical, breakdown. Review the Tabular for assignment of seventh character.

Z53.8   Canceled procedure (surgical), because of, specified reason NEC

Rationale: The complication code, for the broken pacemaker electrode, is assigned as a secondary diagnosis because the sick sinus syndrome was the reason for admission. The Z code for the canceled procedure should also be added.

1.146. T84.51XA   Complication(s) (from) (of), joint prosthesis, internal, infection or inflammation, hip. Review the Tabular for complete code assignment and seventh character.

Rationale: The complication code assigned for this case includes the type of complication, the specific type of prosthesis, and laterality.

1.147. S22.41XA   Fracture, traumatic (abduction) (adduction) (separation), rib, multiple. Review the Tabular for complete code assignment and correct seventh character.

         S62.101A   Fracture, traumatic (abduction) (adduction) (separation), wrist. Review the Tabular for complete code assignment and correct seventh character.

Rationale: In ICD-10-CM, rib fractures are coded as just one or multiple. The chest contusion would not be coded because it is a superficial injury associated with the rib fractures. Both of the codes in this case require a seventh character to identify the initial encounter.

1.148. T40.7X2A   Table of Drugs and Chemicals, Marijuana, Poisoning, Intentional, Self-harm. Review the Tabular for seventh character.

         T40.5X2A   Table of Drugs and Chemicals, Cocaine, Poisoning, Intentional, Self-harm. Review the Tabular for seventh character.

         S01.412A   Laceration, cheek (external). Review the Tabular for complete code assignment and seventh character.

         S01.01XA   Laceration, scalp. Review the Tabular for complete code assignment and seventh character.

Rationale: If an overdose of a drug was intentionally taken or administered and resulted in drug toxicity, it would be coded as a poisoning. The seventh character is required for all of the codes in this case.

Chapter 20 Coding Cases

1.149. V43.53XA   Index to External Causes, Accident, car – *see* Accident, transport, car occupant. Accident, transport, car occupant, driver, collision (with) pickup truck (traffic)

         Y92.411   Index to External Causes, Place of occurrence, highway (interstate)

         Y93.C2   Index to External Causes, Activity (involving) (of victim at time of event), cellular, telephone

Rationale: The transport accident codes have been greatly expanded in ICD-10-CM with much more detail. It takes experience to get used to the External Causes Index and Tabular sections. Just getting familiar with both is a help to coding these conditions correctly. An appropriate seventh character is to be added to each code from category V43. If the code does not contain six characters, the X is used before placing the seventh character. No Status code was selected because this information was not documented.

1.150. Y37.230A   Index to External Causes, Military operations (injuries to military and civilians occurring during peacetime on military property and during routine military exercises and operations) (by) (from) (involving) explosion (of) improvised explosive device [IED] (person-borne) (roadside) (vehicle-borne)

         Y92.139   Index to External Causes, Place of occurrence, military base – *see* Place of occurrence, residence, institutional, military base

         Y99.1   Index to External Causes, External cause status, military activity

Rationale: There is no activity code assigned here because none of the categories is specific to this case. Even though Y93.89 (other activity) is available, it is not assigned in this case because of this note: "They are also appropriate for use with external cause codes for cause and intent if identifying the activity provides additional information on the event." In this case, there is no kind of activity involved. The fact that the person was military personnel injured by an IED is not an activity—it is captured by the Y37 code.

1.151. W54.0XXA   Index to External Causes, Bite, bitten by, dog

         Y92.71   Index to External Causes, Place of occurrence, barn

         Y93.K9   Index to External Causes, Activity (involving) (of victim at time of event), animal care NEC

         Y99.0   Index to External Causes, External cause status, civilian activity done for income or pay

Rationale: In this case, it is possible to report the place of occurrence, activity, and status in addition to the external cause code for bite. When adding the seventh character, if the code does not contain six characters, the X is used before placing the seventh character.

1.152. X10.2XXA   Index to External Causes, Burn, burned, burning (accidental) (by) (from) (on), hot, oil (cooking)

         Y92.511   Index to External Causes, Place of occurrence, restaurant

         Y93.G3   Index to External Causes, Activity (involving) (of victim at time of event), cooking and baking

         Y99.0   Index to External Causes, External cause status, civilian activity done for income or pay

Rationale: The burn was caused by the cooking oil, not the cooker, so code X10.2 is used rather than X15.8. When adding the seventh character, if the code does not contain six characters, the X is used before placing the seventh character.

1.153. S72.002A   Fracture, traumatic (abduction) (adduction) (separation) femur, femoral, neck – *see* fracture, femur, upper end, neck

         W11.XXXA   Index to External Causes, Fall, falling (accidental), from, off, out of, ladder

         Y92.018   Index to External Causes, Place of occurrence, residence (non-institutional) (private), house, single family, specified NEC

         Y93.H9   Index to External Causes, Activity (involving) (of victim at time of event), maintenance, property

         Y99.8   Index to External Causes, External cause status, specified NEC

Rationale: The seventh character of A is used to indicate the initial encounter for the fracture. The X placeholder is used in the external cause code because the seventh character is required. A code from categories Y92, Y93, and Y99 should be used to indicate information about the event. Code Y93.H9 was selected over Y93.E9 (household maintenance) because of the "excludes" note under Y93.E for "activities involving property and land maintenance, building and construction (Y93.H-)." Because the person was on a ladder outside his home, working on a home improvement project, it seems like "property maintenance" might be the best fit.

1.154. S32.019D   Fracture, traumatic (abduction) (adduction) (separation) vertebra, vertebral (arch) (body) (column) (neural arch) (pedicle) (spinous process) (transverse process), lumbar, first

         S32.029D   Fracture, vertebra, vertebral (arch) (body) (column) (neural arch) (pedicle) (spinous process) (transverse process), lumbar, second

         W11.XXXD   Index to External Causes, Fall, falling (accidental), from ladder

Rationale: In ICD-10-CM, fractures of each level of the vertebrae are coded separately. The seventh character D is used to indicate the subsequent encounter for the fracture that is documented as routinely healing. The external cause code, with the appropriate seventh character is assigned for each encounter for which the injury is being treated. Codes from categories Y92 and Y93 are only assigned on the initial encounter, and so are appropriate only with the seventh character A. No external cause status code is assigned because the coding guidelines state that Y99.9 is not assigned if the status is not stated, and this is a subsequent encounter. It is presumed to be inappropriate for use on subsequent encounters because the complete information would not be available in the record, and the details have already been provided at the initial encounter.

1.155. T24.332A   Burn (electricity) (flame) (hot gas, liquid or hot object) (radiation) (steam) (thermal), calf, left, third degree

T21.34XA   Burn (electricity) (flame) (hot gas, liquid or hot object) (radiation) (steam) (thermal), back, third degree

X02.0XXA   Index to External Causes, Fall, falling (accidental), into, fire – *see* Exposure, fire, by type. Exposure (to), fire, flames (accidental) fireplace, furnace or stove – *see* Exposure, fire, controlled, building. Exposure, fire, flames (accidental), controlled (in), building or structure

Y92.003   Index to External Causes, Place of occurrence, residence (non-institutional) (private), bedroom

Y93.02   Index to External Causes, Activity (involving) (of victim at time of event), running

Y99.8   Index to External Causes, External cause status, specified NEC

Rationale: The seventh character A refers to the initial encounter. Only the highest degree of burn (third) on the calf and back are reported. If a code is not a full six characters, a placeholder X must be used to fill the empty characters when the seventh character is required. Notes under category T21.3 and T24.3 state to use additional external cause code to identify the source, place, and intent of the burn. If the percent of body burned was documented, category T31 may be assigned as a secondary code. The rule of nines is not used to calculate this without documentation by the provider. For example, in this case it was documented that the calf was burned, but certainly *not* what percentage of the leg was burned. As with any ICD code, physician documentation is required.

1.156. T22.212D   Burn, (electricity) (flame) (hot gas, liquid or hot object) (radiation) (steam) (thermal) forearm, left, second degree

X10.2XXD   Index to External Causes, Burn, burned, burning (accidental) (by) (from) (on), hot, fat

Z48.00   Change(s) (in) (of) dressing (nonsurgical)

Rationale: The seventh character D is used for both codes to indicate a subsequent encounter for care (the original treatment was rendered "several days ago"). The ICD-10-CM guidelines indicate that these characters must always occupy the seventh character position. If a code is not a full six characters, a dummy placeholder X must be used to fill in the empty characters when the seventh character is required. A place of occurrence and activity code would not be used, as the guidelines state that both a place of occurrence code and activity code is used only once, at the initial encounter for treatment. Coding Guideline I.C.21.c.7 states that aftercare Z codes should not be used for aftercare for injuries. For aftercare of an injury, assign the acute injury code with the seventh character D. In this case, the injury (burn) was sequenced first and not the aftercare code. However, the Z48.00 code might be added to provide additional information. No external cause status code is assigned because the coding guidelines state that Y99.9 is not assigned if the status is not stated, and this is a subsequent encounter. It is presumed to be inappropriate for use on subsequent encounters because the complete information would not be available in the record, and the details have already been provided at the initial encounter.

1.157.

S52.301B	Fracture, traumatic (abduction) (adduction) (separation), radius, shaft. Review tabular for complete code assignment
S52.201B	Fracture, traumatic (abduction) (adduction) (separation), ulna, shaft. Review the Tabular for complete code assignment.
S16.1XXA	Strain, cervical
V43.52XA	Index to External Causes, Accident (to), car – *see* Accident, transport, car occupant, driver, collision (with), car (traffic)
Y92.411	Index to External Causes, Place of occurrence, street and highway, interstate highway

Rationale: In ICD-10-CM, there is not a combination code for fractures of the radius and ulna. These should be coded separately. For codes S52.301B and S52.201B, the sixth character of 1 indicates the laterality—right arm. The seventh character B is used for the fractures as this was the initial encounter for an open fracture and is the correct choice when the extent (Gustilo classification) of the open fracture is not documented. The fifth and sixth digits of code S16.1XXA are placeholders for the use of the seventh character A to indicate the initial encounter. A code from the Y93 category (activity code) is not assigned in this case because none of the codes add any additional detail. The note at the beginning of the activity codes states: "They are also appropriate for use with external cause codes for cause and intent if identifying the activity provides additional information on the event." And in this case, there was no particular "activity" stated. The mere act of "driving" doesn't constitute the intent of the activity codes, as that would just duplicate what is already captured in the base external cause (driver involved in auto collision). No code from category Y99 is assigned because the documentation is not present to indicate if the person was working or not; it would only be assumed that she was not working.

1.158.

S42.401K	Nonunion, fracture – *see* fracture, by site. Fracture, traumatic, humerus, distal end – *see* Fracture, humerus, lower end, lower end
V00.121D	Index to External Causes, Fall, falling (accidental), involving, skates (ice) (in line) (roller) – *see* Accident, transport, pedestrian, conveyance, roller skates (non in-line), fall

Rationale: Although the patient is being treated for a nonunion of a fracture, the external cause code(s) should also be added but the seventh character D should be used to indicate the subsequent encounter.

1.159. L08.9   Infection, infected, infective, skin (Local) (staphylococcal) (streptococcal)

S61.411A   Wound, open, hand, laceration – *see* laceration, hand, right

W25.XXXA   Index to External Causes, Cut, cutting (any part of body) (accidental) – *see also* Contact, with, glass (sharp) (broken)

Y92.511   Index to External Causes, Place of occurrence, restaurant

F10.10   Abuse, alcohol

F15.10   Abuse, amphetamine (or related substance) – *see* Abuse, drug, stimulant NEC

Y99.8   Index to External Causes, External cause status, leisure activity

Rationale: ICD-10-CM does not have a combination code that identifies an infection of an open wound. The skin infection should be listed first as it was the reason for the encounter and the condition that was treated. Since the note under category S61 says "code also any associated wound infection" there is no mandatory sequencing requirement for S61 to be sequenced first. A code from the Y93 category is not assigned because there is no further specification available. There is not enough information available about what she was "doing" at the time of the incident. If this information was available, it would be appropriate to add the Y93 code.

1.160. S06.9X2A   Injury, head, with loss of consciousness. Review Tabular for complete code assignment.

R40.2121   Coma, with, opening of eyes, in response to, pain

R40.2211   Coma, with verbal response (none)

R40.2311   Coma, with motor response (none)

Y04.0XXA   Index to External Causes, Assault (homicidal) (by) (in), fight (hand) (fists) (foot) (unarmed)

Y92.830   Index to External Causes, Place of occurrence, recreation area, park (public)

Y93.01   Index to External Causes, Activity (involving) (of victim at time of event), walking (on level or elevated terrain)

Y99.8   Index to External Causes, External cause status, student activity

Rationale: The seventh character of A is used for the head injury to indicate the initial episode of care. Because the patient was comatose and the three elements of the Glasgow coma scale were documented (eyes open, verbal response, and motor response) each of these can be identified and the seventh character of 1 is used to indicate that the coma scale was completed "in the field" by paramedics. To review information about assigning the Glasgow coma scale, review Chapter 18: Symptoms, signs and abnormal clinical and laboratory findings. The assault was presumed to be an unarmed fight because the documentation indicates a fight, but no weapons were discussed.

1.161. S02.10XA   Fracture, traumatic (abduction) (adduction) (separation), skull, base

S06.5X0A   Hematoma (traumatic) (skin surface intact), subdural (traumatic) – *see* Injury, intracranial (traumatic), subdural hemorrhage, traumatic. Review Tabular for complete code assignment.

S82.855A   Fracture, traumatic, trimalleolar – *see* fracture, ankle, trimalleolar, nondisplaced. Review Tabular for complete code assignment.

W00.1XXA   Index to External Causes, Fall, falling (accidental) due to, ice or snow, from one level to another, on stairs or steps

Y92.018   Index to External Causes, Place of occurrence, residence (non-institutional) (private) house, single family, specified NEC

Y99.8   Index to External Causes, External cause status, specified NEC

Rationale: In ICD-10-CM, there is not a combination code for a skull fracture with a subsequent subdural hematoma; therefore, the two conditions need to be coded separately. In order to select the correct code for the skull fracture, one would need to know or research that basilar is the base of the skull. The seventh character A is used to indicate the initial episode of care for the fractures, hematoma, and fall. A code from the Y93 category would not be assigned here because there is no applicable activity, and according to the ICD-10-CM Coding Guidelines, Y93.9 should not be used if the activity of the patient is not stated or is not applicable. Code Y99.8 was used because the patient was at her own home. If there was documentation that this was a work-related accident, however, that would be coded instead.

1.162. S12.100A   Fracture, traumatic, vertebra, vertebral (arch) (body) (column) (neural arch) (pedicle) (spinous process) (transverse process), cervical, second (axis) – *see* Fracture, neck, cervical vertebra, second (displaced)

S14.112A   Injury, spinal (cord), cervical (neck), complete lesion, C2 level

S06.9X1A   Injury, head, with loss of consciousness. Review Tabular for complete code assignment.

V20.4XXA   Index to External Causes, Accident, transport, motorcyclist, driver, collision (with), animal (traffic)

Y92.410   Index to External Causes, Place of occurrence, street and highway

Y99.8   Index to External Causes, External cause status, leisure activity

Rationale: In a fracture with a spinal cord injury, ICD-10-CM does not have a combination so these conditions need to be coded separately. The note at category S14 states to code also any associated fracture of cervical vertebra. The quadriplegia is not coded separately as this is the current episode of the injury. When you reference quadriplegia, traumatic in the Index, the coder is referred back to the S14 code. The sixth digit of 1 for code S06.9X1A indicates a loss of consciousness of 30 minutes or less. The place of occurrence code is Y92.410 as there is no specific code for a mountain highway. In the Index, under highway (interstate) appears that it may be the correct code since interstate is in parentheses. But on further review, Y92.410 appears to be the best choice. Assigning a place of occurrence code in some cases is not clear in the classification system.

A code from the Y93 category (activity code) is not assigned because none is particularly applicable. Riding a bicycle is similar, but not the same as a motorcycle. There are few choices when it pertains to transport accidents. There is no particular "activity" described in the scenario. Driving his motorcycle does not fall within the intent of the activity codes, as that information is already captured by the V20 code. If he was sending a text message while driving his motorcycle, that would be an activity.

Chapter 21 Coding Cases

1.163. Z38.00   Newborn (infant) (liveborn) (singleton) born in hospital

P55.0   Incompatibility, Rh (blood group) (factor), newborn

Z67.10   Blood, type, A (Rh positive)

Rationale: The newborn code would be listed first, followed by the Rh incompatibility. The blood type of the baby is A+. The mother's blood type is not coded on the newborn's record

1.164. Z02.0   Examination (for) (following) (general) (of) (routine), medical (adult) (for) (of) preschool children, for admission to school

Rationale: ICD-10-CM provides much more specificity for administrative examinations.

1.165. Z44.121   Encounter (with health service) (for) fitting (of) – *see* Fitting (and adjustment) (of). Fitting (and adjustment) (of) artificial, leg – *see* Admission, adjustment, artificial, leg. Admission (for), adjustment (of), artificial, leg, partial

Z89.511   Absence (of) (organ or part) (complete or partial) leg (acquired) (above knee), below knee (acquired)

Rationale: Category Z44 is used for fitting and adjustment of external prosthetic devices, including the removal or replacement of external prosthetic devices. This category is not used for malfunction or other complications of the device. In this case, the acquired absence of the limb was added as an additional code. See Coding Guideline I.C.21.7, which references that a status code should not be used when the aftercare code indicates the type of status, such as using Z43.0, Encounter for attention to tracheostomy, with Z93.0, Tracheostomy status. This is the same type of situation, but the aftercare code indicates that the artificial leg is partial, but not specifically where the amputation occurred. The status code can provide greater specificity about the site; for example, foot, ankle, below knee, above knee. In this case, it was felt that the additional code provided additional information.

1.166. M81.0   Osteoporosis (female) (male), postmenopausal
Z87.310   History, personal (of), fracture (healed) osteoporosis

Rationale: The personal history codes include expanded codes to identify past conditions. The note at category M81 states: Use additional code to identify personal history of (healed) osteoporosis fracture, if applicable (Z87.310). The documentation for the fracture states that it is healed and not causing any complications.

1.167. I21.29   Infarct, infarction, myocardium, myocardial (acute) (with stated duration of 4 weeks or less), ST elevation (STEMI), lateral (apical-lateral) (basal-lateral) (high)

Z92.82   Status (post), administration of tPA (rtPA) in a different facility within the last 24 hours prior to admission to current facility

Rationale: Category I21 has a note: Use additional code, if applicable, to identify: status post administration of tPA (rtPA) in a different facility within the last 24 hours prior to admission to current facility (Z92.82). The coding guidelines specify that this status code is assigned at the receiving facility, not at the transferring facility. The code may be assigned if the tPA was administered within the last 24 hours, even if the patient is still receiving the tPA at the time they are received into the current facility. A note accompanies code Z92.82: Code first condition requiring tPA administration, such as acute cerebral infarction (I63.-); acute myocardial infarction (I21.-, I22.-).

1.168. Z43.6   Attention (to), artificial opening (of), urinary tract NEC
Z90.6   Absence (of) (organ or part) (complete or partial), bladder (acquired)
Z85.51   History, personal (of), malignant neoplasm (of), bladder

Rationale: The reason for the encounter was to check on the patency of the ileal conduit. An ileal conduit is an artificial opening for the urinary tract, not the digestive tract, although the urine is diverted into an isolated segment of the ileum following cystectomy. To create the ileal conduit, the ureters are resected from the bladder, and the ureteroenteric anastomosis is made to drain the urine into a detached section of ileum. The end of the ileum is brought out through a stoma in the abdominal wall.

1.169. S32.411D   Fracture, traumatic (abduction) (adduction) (separation), acetabulum, wall, anterior

V03.90XD   Index to External Causes, Accident (to), pedestrian (on foot), with, transport vehicle – *see* Accident, transport, pedestrian, on foot, collision (with), car

Rationale: Aftercare encounters in ICD-10-CM are coded to the appropriate fracture code with a seventh character D. In the Alphabetic Index, main term Aftercare, subterm Fractures directs the coder to "code to fracture with seventh character D." The sixth character of the fracture code (S32.411D) specifies the laterality of the fracture, right side and the seventh character indicates that this is a subsequent encounter for fracture with routine healing. The accident external cause code can be assigned, once again with seventh character D. No place of occurrence or activity code should be assigned because they are used only on the initial encounter. Code S32.41 (displaced) is the default when not specified, not nondisplaced.

Part II: Site-Specific Cases

Long-Term Care Cases

1.170. N39.0   Infection, infected, infective (opportunistic) urinary (tract)

       B96.20   Infection, infected, infective (opportunistic) bacterial, as cause of disease classified elsewhere, Escherichia coli [E. coli]

       Z79.2   Long-term, (current) (prophylactic), drug therapy (use of), antibiotics

       G35   Sclerosis, sclerotic, multiple (brain stem) (cerebral) (generalized) (spinal cord)

Rationale: The long-term use code is assigned for use of the antibiotics. Instructional notes under N39.0 indicate to use an additional code (B95-B97) to identify infectious agent.

1.171. S52.92XE   Fracture, traumatic (abduction) (adduction) (separation), radius

       S52.202E   Fracture, traumatic (abduction) (adduction) (separation), ulna (shaft)

       X58.XXXD   Index to External Causes, Accident (to)

Rationale: According to the Coding Guidelines, "the aftercare Z codes should not be used for aftercare for injuries." For aftercare of an injury, assign the acute injury code with the appropriate seventh character (in this example, the seventh character E is correct). The seventh character E is used to indicate the subsequent treatment of an open fracture. For an unspecified location, the radius default is unspecified fracture of forearm, while the ulna defaults to fracture of shaft of ulna. It is important to obtain specific fracture sites from the documentation, if possible to assign the most specific codes.

1.172. Z48.812   Aftercare, following surgery (for) (on), circulatory system

       Z95.1   Status (post), aortocoronary bypass

       G89.12   Pain(s) (*see also* Painful), acute, post-thoracotomy

Rationale: In ICD-10-CM, there is not a separate code to identify occupational therapy. The use of the Z48 aftercare code is sufficient in this situation. The aftercare codes are generally first listed to explain the specific reason for the encounter. Pain control or management is not the reason for the encounter, so it is listed as a secondary code.

1.173. G35   Sclerosis, sclerotic, multiple (brain stem) (cerebral) (generalized) (spinal cord)

       S32.9XXD   Fracture, traumatic, (abduction) (adduction) (separation), pelvis, pelvic (bone)

       V00.811D   Index to External Causes, Fall, falling (accidental) from, wheelchair, powered – *see* Accident, transport, pedestrian, conveyance occupant, specified type NEC, wheelchair (powered), fall

Rationale: The seventh character D is assigned for subsequent encounter for fracture with routine healing. An external cause code is assigned to this case. No activity or place of occurrence codes are assigned because this is a subsequent encounter for this injury. Activity and place of occurrence codes are only used on the initial encounter. The reason that the patient continues to reside in the LTC facility is listed in the first position.

1.174. Z45.02   Admission (for), adjustment, device NEC, implanted, cardiac, defibrillator,
                     or Encounter, (with health service) (for) adjustment and management (of),
                     implanted device
         I49.01   Fibrillation, ventricular
         I25.10   Disease, diseased, coronary (artery) – *see* Disease, heart (organic),
                   ischemic, atherosclerotic (of)

Rationale: If indexing Admission (for), adjustment, the Index assists in locating the
specific code; however, when indexing Encounter, the Tabular List must be used to
provide the specific code of Z45.02 for the automatic implantable cardiac defibrillator,
rather than the NEC code provided in the Index.

1.175. S63.004A   Dislocation (articular), wrist (carpal bone)
         W18.30XA   Index to External Causes, Fall, falling (accidental) same level
         Y92.128   Index to External Causes, Place of occurrence, residence, institutional,
                    nursing home, specified NEC
         Y93.01   Index to External Causes, Activity (involving) (of victim at time of event),
                    walking (on level or elevated terrain)
         Y99.8   Index to External Causes, External cause status, leisure activity

Rationale: The Tabular List provides the correct sixth character of 4 for right wrist and
the correct seventh character as A for initial encounter. The seventh character A is also
used for the external cause to indicate the initial encounter.

1.176. G20   Disease, Parkinson's
         E10.9   Diabetes, type 1
         J44.9   Disease, pulmonary, chronic obstructive
         Z60.2   Living alone (problems with)

Rationale: The reason for the admission or encounter is the Parkinson's disease. In
addition, the patient has type 1 diabetes and COPD, coded as secondary diagnoses.
Code Z60.2 is added to show that this patient is not able to live alone.

1.177. R19.7   Diarrhea, diarrheal (disease) (infantile) (inflammatory)
         R11.0   Nausea (without vomiting)
         T45.1X5D Table of Drugs and Chemicals, Fluorouracil, adverse effect column
         C18.4   Carcinoma – *see also* Neoplasm, by site, malignant
                   Neoplasm Table, intestine, large, colon, transverse, in Malignant Primary
                   column

Rationale: The patient first receives treatment for the adverse effect at the hospital
outpatient center. Treatment at the long-term care facility is a subsequent encounter
for the reaction. The adverse reaction to the chemotherapy is coded as a secondary
diagnosis. In this case, an additional secondary diagnosis is the reason why the patient
was receiving chemotherapy, the carcinoma of the transverse colon. The reason why
the patient is a resident in the LTC facility is not provided in this brief case. But following
policy, it would also be coded.

1.178. Z48.01   Aftercare, following surgery, attention to dressings, surgical
         Z89.512   Absence (of) (organ or part) (complete or partial), extremity (acquired),
                   lower, below knee

Rationale: The infection of the stump is not coded because the treatment is complete. The patient was admitted for aftercare dressing changes. Code Z47.81 was not assigned because no documentation was present; however, this code might be appropriate if other services were performed. The fourth character for the left leg is obtained from the Tabular.

1.179. R40.20   Coma

T42.4X2S   Late effect(s) – *see* Sequelae, poisoning – code to poisoning with seventh character S. Table of Drugs and Chemicals, valium, poisoning-intentional self-harm

T51.0X2S   Late effect(s) – *see* Sequelae, poisoning – code to poisoning with seventh character S. Table of Drugs and Chemicals, alcohol, beverage, poisoning-intentional self-harm

Rationale: The sequela (late effect) of the overdose is coded with the acute poisoning codes utilizing the seventh character S. This is in accordance with the Official Coding Guidelines. Consider a physician query for persistent vegetative state.

1.180. M80.021D   Osteoporosis (female) (male), senile – *see* Osteoporosis, age-related, with current pathologic fracture, humerus

Rationale: The seventh character D is used in this case because this is a subsequent encounter for the pathological fracture and there is no documentation of delayed healing, nonunion, or malunion.

1.181. K51.90   Colitis (acute) (catarrhal) (chronic) (noninfective) (hemorrhagic), ulcerative (chronic)

M81.8   Osteoporosis (female) (male), drug-induced – *see* Osteoporosis, specified type NEC

T38.0X5S   Table of Drugs and Chemicals, corticosteroids, adverse effect

Z79.52   Long-term (current) (prophylactic) drug therapy (use of), steroids, systemic

Rationale: Due to the patient's long-term use of corticosteroids and the resulting osteoporosis, the adverse effect code from the Table of Drugs and Chemicals is used. The seventh character S identifies the sequela (or long-term consequences) of the original injury (or in this case, the adverse effect of the drug). The sequela (i.e., colitis) is sequenced first, followed by the code for the adverse effect.

1.182. M86.171   Osteomyelitis (general) (infective) (localized) (neonatal) (purulent) (septic) (staphylococcal) (streptococcal) (suppurative) (with periostitis), acute, tarsus

I96   Gangrene, gangrenous (connective tissue) (dropsical) (dry) (moist) (skin) (ulcer), extremity (lower) (upper)

L89.513   Ulcer, ulcerated, ulcerating, ulceration, ulcerative, decubitus – *see* Ulcer, pressure, by site, pressure (pressure area), ankle

E10.51   Diabetes, diabetic (mellitus) (sugar), type 1, with, peripheral angiopathy

I12.9   Disease, diseased, kidney (functional) (pelvis), chronic, hypertensive – *see* Hypertension, kidney. Hypertension, hypertensive (accelerated) (benign) (essential) (idiopathic) (malignant) (systemic), kidney, with, stage 1 through stage 4 chronic kidney disease

N18.4   Disease, diseased, kidney (functional) (pelvis), chronic, stage 4 (severe)

Z89.512   Absence (of) (organ or part) (complete or partial), limb (acquired) – *see* Absence, extremity (acquired), lower, below knee

E78.0   Hypercholesterolemia (essential) (familial) (hereditary) (primary) (pure)

F10.21   Alcoholism (chronic), with remission

Rationale: The reason for the admission to the nursing home is the osteomyelitis and gangrene which resulted from a decubitus ulcer. When referring to the Alphabetic Index for the Osteomyelitis there is not a subterm for ankle. Instead, the subterms under Osteomyelitis are various bones with the tarsus bone being the correct selection. Because the osteomyelitis and gangrene are documented as due to the decubitus ulcer, these conditions would not be coded as a diabetic complication. Not all ulcers in diabetic patients are diabetic ulcers, and in the absence of documentation of such, the decubitus ulcer is not coded as a diabetic complication

1.183. I50.9   Failure, failed, heart (acute) (senile) (sudden) congestive (compensated) (decompensated)

I48.91   Fibrillation, atrial or auricular (established)

S72.012D   Fracture, traumatic (abduction) (adduction) (separation), femur, femoral, neck, *see* Fracture, femur, upper end, subcapital (displaced)

W06.XXXD   Index to External Causes, Fall, falling (accidental) from, off, out of, bed

Rationale: The sixth character 2 for the left hip is obtained from the Tabular. The seventh character D is used for the subsequent encounter with routine healing. The external cause code is assigned, but no place of occurrence or activity codes are because this is subsequent care. The reason for the readmission is the CHF and atrial fibrillation.

1.184. I69.354   Hemiplegia, following, cerebrovascular disease, cerebral infarction, <u>or</u> Sequelae (of), infarction, cerebral, hemiplegia

I69.321   Dysphasia, following, cerebrovascular disease, cerebral infarction <u>or</u> Sequelae (of), infarction, cerebral, dysphasia

I69.392   Sequelae (of), infarction, cerebral, facial droop

K21.9   Disease, diseased, gastroesophageal reflux (GERD)

M06.9   Arthritis, arthritic (acute) (chronic) (nonpyogenic) (subacute), rheumatoid

G30.0   Disease, diseased, Alzheimer's, early onset, with behavioral disturbance

F02.81

Rationale: The hemiplegia, dysphasia, and facial droop are considered residual conditions of the acute cerebral infarction, and are the reason that the patient is admitted to the nursing home. Coding guidelines state that the residual condition is sequenced first, followed by the cause of the sequela. In this case of cerebrovascular disease, the sequela code has been expanded to include the manifestation and is an exception to the coding guideline

1.185. I69.352   Hemiplegia, following, cerebrovascular disease, cerebral infarction, <u>or</u> Sequelae (of), infarction, cerebral, hemiplegia

I69.398   Alteration (of), altered, sensation, following, cerebrovascular disease, cerebral infarction, <u>or</u> Sequelae, infarction, cerebral, specified effect

R43.9   Sense loss, taste – *see* Disturbance(s), sensation, taste

Rationale: Left dominant hemiplegia is the reason for the admission to the nursing home. Altered sense of taste is coded as a secondary diagnosis. The note at code I69.398 states to use an additional code to identify the sequelae.

1.186. G30.0   Disease, diseased, Alzheimer's, early onset, with behavioral disturbance

F02.81

I63.40   Infarct, infarction, cerebral, due to embolism, cerebral arteries

G81.91   Hemiplegia. Review Tabular for complete code assignment.

R47.01   Aphasia (amnestic) (global) (nominal) (semantic) (syntactic)

Z91.83   Wandering, in diseases classified elsewhere

Rationale: The patient was not hospitalized; therefore, the Alzheimer's disease continues to be the reason for the admission. The infarct is coded as acute, not as sequelae. Secondary diagnoses of right dominant hemiplegia and aphasia are coded. At code F02.81, the note states to use additional code, if applicable, to identify wandering in dementia in conditions classified elsewhere (Z91.83). This code further specifies the behavioral disturbance as wandering off.

1.187. J15.1   Pneumonia, in (due to) Pseudomonas
G20   Dementia (degenerative) (primary) (old age) (persisting), in (due to) Parkinson's disease (Parkinsonism)
F02.80
I34.0   Regurgitation, mitral (valve) – *see* Insufficiency, mitral. Insufficiency, insufficient, mitral (valve)
M40.209   Kyphosis, kyphotic (acquired)
J45.909   Asthma, asthmatic (bronchial) (catarrh) (spasmodic)
E11.9   Diabetes, diabetic (mellitus) (sugar) type 2

Rationale: ICD-10-CM does not classify therapies. Acute conditions are coded, or if resolved, limited aftercare codes are available for other conditions excluding injuries. In reviewing the Index for Dementia due to Parkinson's, note that the nonessential modifier, (Parkinsonism), listed with Parkinson's disease is *incorrect*. Parkinsonism is *not* synonymous with Parkinson's disease. Parkinsonism dementia (G31.83) and dementia due to Parkinson's disease (G20) describe different conditions. The documentation does not state whether the mild asthma is intermittent or persistent, and therefore it must be coded to J45.909.

1.188. T84.50XD   Complication(s) (from) (of), joint prosthesis, internal, infection or inflammation, hip. Review Tabular for complete code assignment.
B95.2   Infection, infected, infective (opportunistic), bacterial, as cause of disease classified elsewhere, enterococcus
Z16.21   Resistance, resistant, organism (s), to, drug, vancomycin
Z95.828   Presence (of), vascular implant or device, access port device
             Hypertrophy, prostate – *see* Enlargement, enlarged, prostate
N40.1   Enlargement, enlarged, prostate, with lower urinary tract symptoms (LUTS
N13.8   Obstruction, obstructed, obstructive, urinary, specified NEC
F43.24   Depression (acute) (mental), situational
I10   Hypertension, hypertensive (accelerated) (benign) (essential) (idiopathic) (malignant) (systemic)
I48.91   Fibrillation, atrial or auricular (established)
Z79.01   Long-term (current) (prophylactic) drug therapy (use of) anticoagulants
Z51.81   Monitoring (encounter for), therapeutic drug level

Rationale: For code T84.50xD, the seventh character D is used to identify the subsequent encounter. The Tabular notes state that the coder should "use additional code to identify infection." ICD-10-CM provides many combination codes, but a drug-resistant organism is not one of those. The coder must select the infection with the organism and then a code from category Z16 to specify that the organism is drug resistant. Enlargement of the prostate, N40.1, directs the coder to "Use additional code for associated symptoms, when specified." Therefore, the coder should code N13.8, Urinary obstruction. It is difficult to find the correct code in the Index. Under Obstruction, urinary, due to hyperplasia (hypertrophy) of prostate, the instruction is to *see* Hyperplasia, prostate, specified type, with obstruction. When searching that term, there is no entry. The code is available with N40.1. Depression, situational in the Index directs the coder to F43.21 but the Tabular List allows the coder to refine the code to F43.24, Situational depression with agitation (disturbance of conduct). The reason that code Z79.2, Long-term (current) drug therapy (use of), antibiotics was not assigned is because of the wording "will require," which indicates that the patient has not yet begun the antibiotic therapy. If there is a question about the appropriateness of the documentation, the physician may be queried. Regarding code Z95.828, there is also a code Z45.2 Admission (for) device, vascular access. It was elected in this scenario to assign the Z95.828 because of the note at Encounters for other specific healthcare (Z40-Z53): Categories Z40-Z53 are intended for use to indicate a reason for care. In this case, there was no documentation that the encounter was for adjustment and/or management of the PICC line.

1.189.

Z47.81	Aftercare, following surgery (for) (on), amputation
E11.51	Diabetes, diabetic (mellitus) (sugar), type 2, with peripheral angiopathy
E11.43	Diabetes, diabetic (mellitus) (sugar), type 2, with gastroparesis
I08.0	Regurgitation, mitral (valve) – *see* Insufficiency, mitral. Insufficiency, insufficient, mitral (valve), with aortic valve disease
K40.90	Hernia, hernial (acquired) (recurrent), inguinal (direct) (external) (funicular) (indirect) (internal) (oblique) (scrotal) (sliding)
M15.9	Disease, diseased, joint, degenerative – *see* Osteoarthritis. Osteoarthritis, generalized
J44.9	Disease, diseased, pulmonary, chronic obstructive
Z79.4	Long-term (current) (prophylactic) drug therapy (use of) insulin
Z89.439	Absence (of) (organ or part) (complete or partial), foot (acquired)

Rationale: The documentation does not specify which foot was amputated; therefore the sixth character 9 is assigned from the Tabular. Both peripheral vascular disease and gastroparesis are due to type 2 diabetes. Codes are assigned for both conditions. The patient uses insulin and code Z79.4 is assigned. Code Z89.439, Acquired absence of the foot, is assigned to identify the level of the amputation. Also, there is a "use additional code" note under code Z47.81 to identify the limb amputated (Z89.-).

Home Healthcare Cases

1.190.

S01.81XD	Laceration, face – *see* Laceration, head, specified site
X58.XXXD	Index to External Causes, Accident (to)

Rationale: As stated in the Official Coding Guidelines: "Superficial injuries such as abrasions or contusions are not coded when associated with more severe injuries of the same site."

1.191. Z48.812   Aftercare, following surgery (for) (on), circulatory system
       Z48.01   Aftercare, following surgery (for) (on), attention to, dressings, surgical
       I25.10   Atherosclerosis, coronary artery
       Z95.0   Status (post), pacemaker, cardiac

Rationale: The aftercare following surgery on the circulatory system as well as aftercare for the dressing change are assigned. The code for coronary artery disease without angina is assigned, as no angina is documented.

1.192. T78.40XA   Allergy, allergic (reaction) (to). Review Tabular for complete code assignment.
       T45.1X5A   Allergy, allergic (reaction) (to), drug, medicament & biological (any) (external) (internal), correct substance properly administered – *see* Table of Drugs and Chemicals, by drug, adverse effect, fluorouracil
       C80.1   Cancer, unspecified site (primary) (secondary)

Rationale: Without documentation of the specific adverse effect, the code for the allergic reaction (T78.40XA) is assigned. The seventh character A is used as the documentation does not indicate that the patient has received prior treatment for this allergic reaction. The unspecified cancer code is used as the documentation does not indicate the type of cancer being treated. The Coding Guidelines state that this code should be used "when no determination can be made as to the primary site of a malignancy."

1.193. S72.21XD   Aftercare, fracture – code to fracture with seventh character D. Fracture, traumatic, hip – *see* Fracture, femur, neck. Fracture, femur, neck – *see* Fracture, femur, upper end, neck. Fracture, femur, upper end, subtrochanteric (displaced)
       Z48.01   Admission (for), change of, surgical dressing
       W10.0XXD   Index to External Causes, Fall, falling, from, off, out of, escalator

Rationale: Unlike ICD-9-CM, ICD-10-CM does not have an aftercare code for healing traumatic fractures. Instead, the fracture code continues to be utilized for subsequent encounters with a seventh character, which designates that this encounter is for subsequent care of the fracture. The fracture code is five characters in length with an X placeholder added for the sixth character prior to adding the seventh character. ICD-10-CM Coding Guideline A.5 states "Certain ICD-10-CM categories have applicable seventh characters. The applicable seventh character is required for all codes within the category, or as the notes in the Tabular List instruct. The seventh character must always be the seventh character in the data field. If a code that requires a seventh character is not six characters, a placeholder X must be used to fill in the empty character(s)." An external cause code is used with injury codes. Activity and place of occurrence codes are only assigned at the initial encounter.

1.194. Z47.1   Aftercare, following surgery (for) (on), joint replacement
       Z96.642   Status (post), organ replacement, by artificial or mechanical device or prosthesis of, joint, hip – *see* Presence, hip joint implant. Presence (of), hip-joint implant (artificial) (functional) (prosthesis)
       R26.2   Gait, abnormality, walking difficulty NEC
       Z51.81   Monitoring (encounter for), therapeutic drug level
       Z79.01   Therapy, drug, long-term (current) (prophylactic), anticoagulants
       Z48.01   Change(s) (in) (of), dressing, surgical

Rationale: The main reason for this home health encounter was for aftercare following a joint replacement (Z47.1). In the Tabular under Z47.1, there is an instructional note to "Use additional code to identify the joint (Z96.6-)." Note under Z51.81 instructs to code also any long-term (current) drug therapy.

1.195. J44.9   Disease, diseased, pulmonary, chronic obstructive
Z99.81   Dependence (on) (syndrome), oxygen (long term) (supplemental)

Rationale: The reason for this home health encounter was the COPD (J44.9). Z99.81 is coded as an additional diagnosis for the home oxygen.

1.196. L03.113   Cellulitis (diffuse) (phlegmonous) (septic) (suppurative), upper limb. Review Tabular for complete code assignment
Z79.2   Long-term (current) (prophylactic) drug therapy (use of), antibiotics
Z45.2   Admission (for), adjustment (of), device, vascular access

Rationale: The reason for this encounter was to continue the treatment of the cellulitis (L03.113). Code Z79.2 is added as a secondary diagnosis for the continued use of the antibiotics and Z45.2 is added for the maintenance of the PICC line (vascular access device). In this scenario, Z45.2 was assigned rather than Z95.828, Presence of other vascular implants and grafts. Even though there is an *Excludes2* note under Z45 that states: *Excludes2*: presence of prosthetic and other devices (Z95-Z97), it was felt that the addition of code Z95.828 does not provide any additional specificity to this scenario.

1.197. Z48.3   Aftercare, following surgery (for) (on), neoplasm
C50.511   Refer to Neoplasm Table, by site (breast), malignant, primary site, lower-outer quadrant. Review Tabular for complete code assignment.
Z48.01   Admission (for), change of, surgical dressing
Z90.11   Absence (of) (organ or part) (complete or partial), breast(s) (and nipple(s)) (acquired)

Rationale: The reason for this encounter was to provide aftercare following surgery for the malignant neoplasm. In the Tabular there is a note under Z48.3 that instructs the coding professional to use an additional code to identify the specific neoplasm. Z48.01 is also coded as a secondary diagnosis for the dressing changes. Absence of the breast is coded as Z90.1 with the fifth character 1 determined from the Tabular List.

1.198. Z47.1   Aftercare, following surgery (for) (on), joint replacement
Z96.651   Status (post), organ replacement, by artificial or mechanical device or prosthesis of, joint, knee – *see* Presence (of), knee joint implant (functional) (prosthesis)
R26.9   Abnormality, gait – *see* Gait. Gait abnormality

Rationale: The reason for this encounter was to provide aftercare following surgery for the malignant neoplasm. In the Tabular, there is a note under Z48.3 that instructs the coding professional to use an additional code to identify the specific neoplasm. Z48.01 is also coded as a secondary diagnosis for the dressing changes. Absence of the breast is coded as Z90.1 with the fifth character 1 determined from the Tabular List.

1.199. Z47.1   Aftercare, following surgery (for) (on), joint replacement

       T81.4XXA   Infection, infected, infective (opportunistic), postoperative wound. Review Tabular for complete code assignment.

       R26.9   Abnormality, gait – *see* Gait. Gait abnormality

       Z48.01   Aftercare, following surgery, attention to dressings, surgical

       Z96.642   Status (post), organ replacement, by artificial or mechanical device or prosthesis of, joint, hip – *see* Presence (of), hip joint implant (functional) (prosthesis)

Rationale: Home care is providing service for the gait abnormality and the infected surgical wound. The seventh character A is used with code T81.4 to identify the initial treatment for the wound infection. The patient has a hip-joint prosthesis and the aftercare code for that condition should be used. The original hip fracture is not coded in this case because the fracture is gone and the joint replacement is being treated with aftercare.

1.200. Z46.6   Admission (for), adjustment (of), device, urinary <u>or</u> Change(s) (in) (of), indwelling catheter

       N31.9   Neurogenic, bladder

Rationale: The patient is seen specifically for changes of the indwelling urinary catheter. Both the "admission for" and "change" entries in the Index direct the coder to Z46.6.

1.201. Z48.815   Aftercare, following surgery (for) (on), digestive system

       Z48.01   Aftercare, following surgery (for) (on), attention to dressings, surgical

       Z48.03   Aftercare, following surgery (for) (on), attention to drains

Rationale: The cholecystitis is not coded because it has been resolved. Several aftercare codes fully describe this encounter.

1.202. I50.9   Failure, failed, heart (acute) (senile) (sudden), congestive (compensated) (decompensated)

       I73.9   Insufficiency, insufficient, vascular, peripheral

       E03.9   Hypothyroidism (acquired)

Rationale: The patient is seen for all three diagnoses. Code sequencing cannot be determined from the documentation.

1.203. E10.65   Diabetes, diabetic (mellitus) (sugar), poorly controlled – code to Diabetes, by type, with hyperglycemia, type 1

       Z71.3   Counseling (for), dietary

       Z46.81   Counseling (for), insulin pump use, <u>or</u>
                      Encounter (with health service) (for), training, insulin pump

Rationale: The patient's ketoacidosis is a life-threatening condition which was resolved prior to discharge and is not coded by the HHA. The note in the Index states that diabetes inadequately controlled, out of control, or poorly controlled is coded to diabetes by type with hyperglycemia. Code Z96.41, Presence of insulin pump, is not coded because the information that the pump is present is contained in code Z46.81, Counseling, insulin pump use.

1.204. Z48.812   Aftercare, following surgery (for) (on), circulatory system

       I25.10   Disease, diseased, coronary (artery) – *see* Disease, heart (organic), ischemic, atherosclerotic (of)

       Z95.1   Status (post), aortocoronary bypass

Rationale: The patient is being seen by the HHA for aftercare following cardiac surgery, Z48.812 and has an aortocoronary bypass graft in place, Z95.1. The coronary artery disease is still present and coded.

1.205. Z48.3   Aftercare, following surgery (for) (on), neoplasm
C18.7   Neoplasm Table, by site, intestine, large, colon, sigmoid (flexure) in Malignant Primary column
Z43.3   Colostomy, attention to

Rationale: The Index contains entries for Aftercare following surgery on a neoplasm. For this case, the code for aftercare following surgery on the neoplasm is assigned as the first-listed code and codes for the neoplasm of the sigmoid colon and the colostomy status are assigned as secondary diagnoses. The Z43.3 is assigned rather than Z93.3 (Status colostomy) because they are doing teaching and cleansing and toilet care.

1.206. S72.002D   Fracture, traumatic (abduction) (adduction) (separation), hip – *see* Fracture, traumatic, femur, upper end, neck
R26.9   Abnormality, gait – *see* Gait. Gait abnormality
W19.XXXD   Fall, falling (accidental)

Rationale: The fracture is not stated as open or closed. The coder should not confuse the open treatment with an open fracture. Coding Guideline 1.C.19.c directs the coder to code a closed fracture when open or closed is not specified. An external cause of injury code is used with the fracture code. Activity and place of occurrence codes are not used for subsequent encounters.

1.207. T81.4XXD   Infection, infected, infective, postoperative wound
Z47.1   Aftercare, following surgery (for) (on), joint replacement
T81.31XD   Dehiscence (of), operation wound, external operation wound (superficial)
B95.62   Infection, infected, infective, staphylococcal, as cause of disease classified elsewhere, aureus, methicillin resistant (MRSA) <u>or</u> MRSA, infection, as the cause of diseases classified elsewhere
Z96.642   Presence (of), implanted device, joint, hip
M15.9   Osteoarthritis, generalized
R26.9   Abnormality, gait – *see* Gait. Gait abnormality

Rationale: This patient is receiving aftercare following a joint replacement, but the surgical wound infection represents the most acute condition and requires the most intensive skilled service. The osteoarthritis is coded for this case because other joints are still affected.

1.208. Z48.3   Aftercare, following surgery (for) (on), neoplasm
C50.911   Neoplasm Table, by site (breast), malignant primary column
I69.398   Sequelae (of), stroke, specified effect NEC
M62.81   Weak, weakening, weakness (generalized), muscle
Z90.11   Absence (of) (organ or part) (complete or partial), breast(s) (nipple(s)) (acquired)

Rationale: The neoplasm is determined from the Neoplasm Table under Breast. The fifth and sixth characters are determined from the Tabular List, which directs the coder to use an additional code to identify the sequelae of weakness, muscle.

1.209. I69.341   Monoplegia, following, cerebrovascular disease, cerebral infarction, lower limb <u>or</u> Sequelae, infarction, cerebral, monoplegia, lower limb

         R26.9   Abnormality, gait – *see* Gait. Gait abnormality

         Z99.3   Status (post), wheelchair confinement

Rationale: The patient is described as wheelchair dependent or chairfast. The Index entry for Status (post) directs the coder to Z99.3, Wheelchair confinement.

Hospital Inpatient Cases

1.210. A41.51   Sepsis (generalized), Escherichia coli (E. coli)

         N39.0   Infection, infected, infective (opportunistic), urinary (tract)

         B95.1   Infection, infected, infective (opportunistic), bacterial NOS, as cause of disease classified elsewhere, streptococcus, group B

         B96.20   Infection, infected, infective (opportunistic), bacterial NOS, as cause of disease classified elsewhere, Escherichia coli [E. coli]

         J44.9   Disease, diseased, pulmonary, chronic obstructive

         I69.920   Aphasia (amnestic) (global) (nominal) (semantic) (syntactic) following, cerebrovascular disease

         I69.951   Sequelae (of), disease, cerebrovascular, hemiplegia

         N28.9   Insufficiency, insufficient, renal (acute)

Rationale: Urine culture results were documented as group B streptococcus and E. coli. The EKG showed tachycardia, but unless the physician indicates this was a significant finding, the tachycardia would not be coded. During the course of hospitalization, the patient underwent "fluid rehydration." The coding professional may want to query the physician to determine if dehydration is an additional diagnosis and should be reported. The patient is on tube feedings. The coder should review the remainder of the health record to determine if the patient has a gastrostomy (Z93.1). Additional physician query might be generated to gather more specificity about the renal insufficiency, because if this condition was actually acute kidney failure from the sepsis, the code would change, and severe sepsis would be additionally assigned.

1.211. D64.81   Anemia (essential) (general) (hemoglobin deficiency) (infantile) (primary) (profound), due to (in) (with), antineoplastic chemotherapy

         C25.0   Carcinoma (malignant) – *see also* Neoplasm Table, by site, malignant Neoplasm Table, Pancreas, head, malignant primary column

         T45.1X5A   Table of Drugs and Chemicals, Antineoplastic NEC

Rationale: The anemia is sequenced first because the treatment is directed at the anemia. The neoplasm and adverse effect codes are coded as secondary diagnoses. The seventh character A is assigned to T45.1X5- because this is the patient's initial encounter for treatment of the adverse effect.

1.212. C79.31   Neoplasm Table, by site, (brain NEC), secondary
         C80.1   Neoplasm Table, by site (unknown site or unspecified), malignant primary
         G30.1   Disease, diseased, Alzheimer's, late onset
         F02.80
         S00.83XA   Contusion (skin surface intact), head, specified part NEC
         F32.9   Depression (acute) (mental)
         J43.9   Emphysema (atrophic) (bullous) (chronic) (interlobular) (lung) (obstructive) (pulmonary) (senile) (vesicular)
         W05.0XXA   Index to External Causes, Fall, falling (accidental) from, off, out of, wheelchair, non-moving
         Y92.129   Index to External Causes, Place of Occurrence, residence, institutional, nursing home
         Y99.8   Index to External Causes, External cause status, specified NEC

Rationale: The symptom of ataxia is a manifestation of the brain metastasis. Coding Guidelines direct that codes for symptoms that are inherent to a disease process should not be reported. The principal diagnosis is the brain metastasis. Code C80.1, Malignant neoplasm, unspecified is used when no determination can be made as to the primary site of the malignancy. In the Alphabetic Index, Dementia, senile, Alzheimer's type refers the coder to Disease, Alzheimer's, late onset, resulting in G30.1 and F02.80.

1.213. E11.649   Diabetes, diabetic (mellitus) (sugar), type 2, with hypoglycemia
         C34.11   Neoplasm Table, by site, (lung), upper lobe malignant, primary
         E11.21   Diabetes, diabetic (mellitus) (sugar), type 2, with nephropathy
         E11.40   Diabetes, diabetic (mellitus) (sugar), type 2, with neuropathy
         R16.0   Hepatomegaly, *see also* Hypertrophy, liver
                     Hypertrophy, hypertrophic, liver
         E78.5   Hyperlipemia, hyperlipidemia
         Z79.4   Long-term (current) (prophylactic), drug therapy (use of), insulin

Rationale: The inpatient admission was due to the hypoglycemia which was complicating the type 2 diabetes; therefore, E11.649 is the correct principal diagnosis (with hypoglycemia and without coma) and code Z51.11 would be inappropriate since the chemotherapy was never administered. Additionally, it would be inappropriate to code Z53.09 (Procedure and treatment not carried out because of other contraindication) because the chemotherapy was not planned during the inpatient admission. The patient was initially scheduled for outpatient chemotherapy, which did not occur due to the hypoglycemia.

1.214. I50.9   Failure, failed, heart (acute) (senile) (sudden), congestive (compensated) (decompensated)
         E86.0   Dehydration
         D69.49   Thrombocytopenia, thrombocytopenic, primary NEC
         N39.0   Infection, infected, infective (opportunistic), urinary (tract)
         E11.9   Diabetes, diabetic (mellitus) (sugar), type 2

Rationale: The principal diagnosis should be the CHF because it was present on admission and was the main focus of treatment during the inpatient stay. The petechial hemorrhage and hematomas are not coded because they are part of the thrombocytopenia.

1.215. I11.0   Hypertension, hypertensive, heart, with, heart failure (congestive)
I50.1   Failure, failed, heart (acute) (senile) (sudden), with, acute pulmonary
edema – *see* Failure, ventricular, left
J15.1   Pneumonia, in (due to) Pseudomonas NEC
J44.9   Disease, diseased, pulmonary, chronic obstructive
Z87.891   History, personal (of), nicotine dependence
Z66   Status (post), do not resuscitate (DNR)

Rationale: ICD-10-CM provides a combination code for hypertension and heart failure when a causal relationship is stated (due to hypertension) or implied (hypertensive). The pulmonary edema is not coded separately, as it is a manifestation of the heart failure. See Index:

    Edema, pulmonary, see lung
    Edema, lung
        With heart condition or failure – *see* failure, ventricular, left

1.216. J18.1   Pneumonia, lobar (disseminated) (double) (interstitial)
I50.33   Failure, failed, heart (acute) (senile) (sudden), diastolic (congestive),
acute (congestive), and (on) chronic (congestive)
I10   Hypertension, hypertensive
I20.9   Angina
F41.9   Anxiety
I25.2   Infarct, Infarction, myocardium, myocardial, healed or old

Rationale: The documented symptoms on admission support pneumonia as the principal diagnosis. Additionally, the documentation supports the pneumonia to be lobar. Acute on chronic diastolic CHF, hypertension, angina, anxiety, and history of MI all meet the definition of other (secondary) diagnoses and should be coded.

1.217. O24.410   Pregnancy (single) (uterine), complicated by (care of) (management affected by), diabetes (mellitus), gestational (pregnancy induced) – *see* Diabetes, gestational
Diabetes, diabetic (mellitus) (sugar), gestational (in pregnancy), diet controlled
O99.89   Pregnancy (single) (uterine), complicated by (care of) (management affected by), disorders of, specified NEC
M62.08   Diastasis, muscle, specified site NEC
Z3A.40   Pregnancy (single) (uterine), weeks of gestation, 40 weeks

Rationale: Gestational diabetes codes to subcategory O24.4 and is further subclassified whether it is in pregnancy, in childbirth, or in the puerperium. For this encounter, the patient is still in pregnancy, resulting in assignment of O24.410, Gestational diabetes mellitus in pregnancy, diet controlled. The sixth character of gestational diabetes codes classifies whether it is diet controlled, insulin controlled, or unspecified controlled. The patient's pregnancy has been complicated by diastasis recti, or a rupture of the abdominal wall muscle. This is a specified disorder of the pregnancy. A note at subcategory O99.8 states to use an additional code to identify the condition. Code O71.89 (diastasis recti complicating delivery) is not assigned because there was no delivery at this encounter. The Z3A.40 code is added to indicate weeks of gestation.

1.218. P38.9   Omphalitis (congenital) (newborn)

B95.62   Infection, infected, infective (opportunistic), staphylococcal NEC, as cause of disease classified elsewhere, aureus, methicillin resistant (MRSA)

B95.4   Infection, infected, infective (opportunistic), bacterial NOS, as cause of disease classified elsewhere, Streptococcus, specified NEC

Rationale: Both infectious causes of the omphalitis, Staphylococcus aureus (MRSA) and Group H Streptococcus, should be coded in this case.

1.219. T43.622A   Overdose, overdosage (drug) – *see* Table of Drugs and Chemicals, by drug, poisoning. Table of Drugs and Chemicals, Amphetamines, NEC

T51.0X2A   Overdose, overdosage (drug), – *see* Table of Drugs and Chemicals, by drug, poisoning. Table of Drugs and Chemicals, Alcohol, beverage

F10.229   Dependence (on) (syndrome) alcohol (ethyl) (methyl) (without remission), with, intoxication

F15.229   Dependence (on) (syndrome), amphetamine(s) (type) *see* Dependence, drug, stimulant, NEC, with, intoxication

R00.0   Tachycardia

F90.9   Disorder (of), attention-deficit hyperactivity (adolescent) (adult) (child)

F91.1   Disorder (of), aggressive, unsocialized

E86.0   Dehydration

Y90.2   Index to External Causes, Blood alcohol level, 40–59 mg/100 ml

Rationale: The seventh character A is required to identify the initial encounter for the amphetamine and alcohol overdose. A note under F10 reminds the coder to assign a code for the alcohol level, which is found in the Index to External Causes. The column, Poisoning, intentional, self-harm was selected because a suicide attempt was documented.

1.220. T84.032A   Complication(s) (from) (of), joint prosthesis, internal, mechanical, loosening, knee. Review the Tabular for complete code assignment.

G20   Parkinsonism (idiopathic) (primary)

I11.0   Hypertension, hypertensive, heart (disease), with heart failure (congestive)

I50.9   Failure, failed, heart, congestive

H40.1430   Glaucoma, capsular – *see* Glaucoma, open angle, primary, capsular. See Tabular for complete code assignment.

I25.2   Infarct, Infarction, myocardium, myocardial, healed or old

R94.39   Findings, abnormal, inconclusive, without diagnosis, stress test

Rationale: The mechanical complication (aseptic loosening) of the knee prosthesis is sequenced first because it is the reason for the encounter. I50.9 is coded in addition to I11.0 as a result of an instructional note appearing under I11.0 to use an additional code to identify the type of heart failure. The sixth character of the glaucoma code 3 specifies the laterality of the condition, which in this case is bilateral. The seventh character 0 indicates that the stage of the glaucoma is unspecified. An external cause code is not assigned because the external cause is included in the T-code. See Coding Guideline I.C.19.g.4.

1.221. D25.0   Leiomyoma, uterus (cervix) (corpus), submucous
N80.0   Endometriosis, uterus (internal)
N80.1   Endometriosis, ovary
N80.3   Endometriosis, pelvic peritoneum
N73.6   Adhesions, adhesive, peritoneum, peritoneal, pelvic, female
K91.72   Complication(s) (from) (of), intraoperative (intraprocedural), puncture or laceration (accidental) (unintentional) (of), digestive system, during procedure on other organ
D62   Anemia, blood loss, acute
Y92.234   Index to External Causes, Place of occurrence, hospital, operating room

Rationale: The leiomyoma (D25.0) is documented as the reason for the procedure and is sequenced as the principal diagnosis. The patient experienced an intraoperative complication (K91.72). ICD-10-CM differentiates between intraoperative and postprocedural complications. In this instance, the complication of care code is located within the Diseases of the Digestive System chapter rather than within the External Cause of Morbidity chapter of ICD-10-CM. A place of occurrence code provides information and is coded. Coding Guideline I.C.20.c states that activity codes are not applicable to poisonings, adverse effects, misadventures, or late effects. Additionally, I.C.20.k states that the external cause status codes are not applicable to poisonings, adverse effects, misadventures, or late effects. An additional external cause code (misadventure) is not assigned because of Coding Guideline I.C.19.g.4. The complication code includes the necessary information and there is no additional misadventure code that applies to accidental puncture. The complication code assigned includes enough specificity.

1.222. Z38.00   Newborn
Q25.1   Coarctation of aorta (preductal) (postductal)
Q21.0   Defect, defective, ventricular septal
Q69.1   Polydactylism
Q66.89   Deformity, foot, congenital, specified type NEC
Q68.1   Deformity, hand, congenital

Rationale: The newborn was born at this hospital and delivered vaginally; therefore, Z38.00 is assigned. The Index entry for polydactylism is not specific to finger or thumb. The fourth digit for thumb is determined from the Tabular List. There is no Index entry for cleft hand or foot. The Index entry Deformity provides codes for both feet and hands. There is another Index option for the Cleft Deformities that produces different codes than the ones obtained by following Deformity. Cleft – *see* Imperfect closure, Organ or site not listed – *see* anomaly by site. Under Anomaly, anomalous, there are choices for hand (Q74.0) and foot (Q74.2). After review of the Tabular, the Q66.89 and Q68.1 seem to provide better specificity.

Physician-Related Cases

1.223. D27.1   Sertoli-Leydig cell tumor – *see* Neoplasm, benign. Neoplasm, neoplastic – *see* also Neoplasm Table. Neoplasm Table, ovary, benign column. Review the Tabular for complete code assignment.

Rationale: The Index entry for Sertoli-Leydig cell tumor of a specified site directs the coder to code Neoplasm, benign. The site of left ovary is coded as D27.1.

1.224. R76.11   Findings, abnormal, inconclusive, without diagnosis, tuberculin skin test (without active tuberculosis)

         G70.00   Myasthenia gravis

         M41.124   Scoliosis (acquired) (postural), adolescent (idiopathic) *see* Scoliosis, idiopathic, thoracic

Rationale: The positive TB skin test is the reason for today's encounter and is coded first. The patient has myasthenia gravis and scoliosis as secondary diagnoses.

1.225. Z01.419   Examination (for) (following) (general) (of) (routine), annual (adult) (periodic) (physical), gynecological

         M1A.9XX1   Gout, chronic

         Z23   Vaccination (prophylactic), encounter for

Rationale: The Pap smear is not coded separately. The Index directs the coder to Z01.419 when the Pap smear is part of a routine gynecological exam. Chronic gout is coded as M1A.9 with a seventh character of 1 for with tophus (tophi); add two X placeholders to add the seventh character. Code Z23 is used to code the fact that an immunization was given. A coding note directs the coder that procedure codes are required to identify the types of immunizations given.

1.226. C71.7   Ependymoma (epithelial) (malignant), specified site – *see* Neoplasm, malignant. Neoplasm Table, Brain, midbrain, primary

         G97.48   Complications (from) (of), intraoperative (intraprocedural), puncture or laceration (accidental) (unintentional) (of), brain, during a nervous system procedure

         M62.81   Weak, weakening, weakness (generalized), muscle

         Y92.234   Index to External Causes, Place of occurrence, hospital, operating room

Rationale: The Neoplasm Table contains an entry for midbrain under the heading of brain. The Tabular confirms that category C71 represents malignant neoplasm of the brain stem. The patient had a laceration of brain during the procedure. Intraoperative laceration of the brain during a nervous system procedure is coded as G97.48. The physician does not state that there was hemorrhage and G97.3- for intraoperative hemorrhage has an *Excludes1* note that directs the coder to use G97.4- for intraoperative hemorrhage caused by puncture or laceration. A misadventure external cause code is not assigned to this case because of Coding Guideline I.c.19.g.4, which states "As with certain other T codes, some of the complications of care codes have the external cause included in the code. The code includes the nature of the complication as well as the type of procedure that caused the complication. No external cause code indicating the type of procedure is necessary for these codes." It is correct to assign a place of occurrence code. Guideline I.C.20.k states that the external cause status codes are not applicable to poisonings, adverse effects, misadventures, or late effects.

1.227. A69.23   Arthritis, arthritic, (acute) (chronic) (nonpyogenic) (subacute) due to or associated with Lyme disease

         S40.861S   Bite(s), (animal) (human), arm (upper), superficial NEC, insect. Review the Tabular for complete code assignment.

         E66.01   Obesity, morbid

         Z68.41   Body, bodies, mass index (BMI), adult, 40–44.9

         W57.XXXS   Index to External Causes, Bite, bitten by, insect, (nonvenomous)

Rationale: ICD-10-CM provides a combination code for arthritis due to Lyme disease, A69.23, rather than assigning individual codes for Lyme disease and arthritis. The Lyme disease and subsequent arthritis are a sequela of the tick bite and the bite code with the appropriate seventh character S is assigned. An external cause of injury code is assigned to accompany the tick bite code. Obesity and BMI are coded as secondary diagnoses due to the physician discussion.

1.228. D21.22   Fibroma - *see also* Neoplasm, connective tissue, benign. Neoplasm
            Table, Connective tissue, foot, benign
   D21.21   Neoplasm Table, Connective tissue, foot, benign column
   E11.40   Diabetes, diabetic, (mellitus) (sugar), type 2 with neuropathy

Rationale: The fifth character for the plantar fibroma codes are found in the Tabular. In this case, ICD-10-CM does not provide an option for bilateral and the code needs to be assigned twice. Diabetes mellitus, type 2 with neuropathy, unspecified is a combination code in ICD-10-CM. The physician did not document that the diabetes is inadequately controlled, out of control, or poorly controlled at this visit. Hyperglycemia was not coded at this encounter, although a query could be implemented if desired.

1.229. Z30.2   Multiparity (grand), requiring contraceptive management – *see*
            Contraception. Contraception, contraceptive, sterilization
   N90.89   Tag (hypertrophied skin) (infected), vulva

Rationale: Multiparity is not coded separately as the Index directs the coder to Contraceptive management when the desire is sterilization. Rather, Z30.2, Encounter for sterilization is coded.

1.230. K12.2   Cellulitis (diffuse) (phlegmonous) (septic) (suppurative), mouth (floor)
   K12.0   Ulcer, ulcerated, ulcerating, ulceration, ulcerative, aphthous (oral)
            (recurrent)
   B08.5   Herpangina

Rationale: The physician documents three separate diagnostic statements that all must be coded. There are no *Excludes1* notes between any of the conditions documented. The choice of first-listed diagnosis is left to the coder, as all are equally evaluated and treated.

1.231. B37.3   Candidiasis, candidal, vagina
   B35.4   Tinea (intersecta) (tarsi) corporis
   E28.2   Syndrome, ovary, polycystic

Rationale: Either vaginal candidiasis or the tinea corporis could be the first-listed diagnosis. The physician does not state which condition was the primary focus of care received that day. Polycystic ovarian syndrome is coded as a secondary diagnosis because treatment was continued.

1.232. S83.231A   Tear, torn (traumatic) meniscus (knee) (current injury), medial, complex
   M71.21   Baker's cyst – *see* Cyst, Baker's
   M22.41   Chondromalacia (systemic), patella
   W19.XXXA   Index to External Causes, Fall, falling (accidental)
   Y92.830   Index to External Causes, Place of occurrence, park (public)
   Y93.02   Index to External Causes, Activity (involving) running
   Y99.8   Index to External Causes, External cause status, leisure activity

Rationale: The meniscal tear is a current injury, based on the statement that the physician is diagnosing a new problem. Therefore, the Index entry of Articular cartilage, old is not correct. Tear, meniscus, medial, complex leads the coder to the correct code of S83.23- with a sixth digit of 1 for the right knee and a seventh digit of A for the initial encounter. Chondromalacia of the patella is coded as M22.4- with a fifth digit of 1 for the right knee.

1.233. C78.7   Carcinoma – *see also* Neoplasm by site, malignant. Neoplasm Table – liver, malignant secondary column

Z85.068   History, personal (of), malignant neoplasm (of), small intestine

Z66   Status (post), do not resuscitate (DNR)

Z90.49   Absence (of) (organ or part) (complete or partial), duodenum (acquired)

Z92.21   History, personal (of), chemotherapy for neoplastic condition

Rationale: Z51.5, Encounter for palliative care is not assigned because the patient was seen for evaluation of secondary malignant neoplasm of the liver. The patient is sent to the hospice program where palliative care would be coded.

1.234. F90.2   Disorder (of), attention-deficit hyperactivity (adolescent) (adult) (child), combined type

F82   Disorder (of), developmental, coordination (motor)

Rationale: ICD-10-CM does not contain a code for coordination disorder. A coordination disorder is a developmental disorder of coordination or F82.

1.235. Q77.4   Achondroplasia (osteosclerosis congenita) <u>or</u> Osteosclerosis congenita

G47.33   Apnea, apneic (spells) sleep, obstructive (adult) (pediatric)

Q76.426   Lordosis, congenital, lumbar region

Z82.79   History, family (of), chromosomal anomaly <u>or</u>
              History, family (of), congenital malformations and deformations

Rationale: Achondroplasia is an inherited chromosomal abnormality with potential malformations of long bones. The spine can also be affected. Lordosis was noted on the patient's initial newborn bone survey, and is therefore coded as congenital. The sleep apnea is coded as G47.33 because this is new since this last visit, rather than sleep apnea of newborn, which is coded as P28.3. All family histories of congenital malformations, deformations, and chromosomal abnormalities are coded as Z82.79.

1.236. H81.02   Vertigo, labyrinthine – *see* subcategory H81.0

R51   Headache

Rationale: Labyrinthine vertigo is coded with a fifth digit of 2 because the physician indicates that the patient's symptoms involve the left ear. "Rule out temporal arteritis" is not coded. This statement indicates uncertainty and is, therefore, not coded.

1.237. R51   Pain(s) (*see also* Painful), face, facial

R68.84   Pain(s) (*see also* Painful), jaw

G51.0   Bell's palsy, paralysis, <u>or</u> Palsy, Bell's – *see also* Palsy, facial

H65.92   Otitis (acute), media (hemorrhagic) (staphylococcal) (streptococcal), nonsuppurative

Rationale: The coder does not code the uncertain diagnosis of "Rule out superimposed trigeminal neuralgia" but rather codes the facial pain and jaw pain. The Index directs the code to H65.9- for nonsuppurative otitis media. The coder selects the fifth digit of 2 for the left ear from the Tabular.

1.238. L03.012   Paronychia – *see also* Cellulitis, digit
                  Cellulitis (diffuse) (phlegmonous) (septic) (suppurative), digit, finger – *see*
                  Cellulitis, finger (intrathecal) (periosteal) (subcutaneous) (subcuticular)
        J41.0   Cough (affected) (chronic) (epidemic) (nervous), smokers'
        Z72.0   Tobacco (nicotine), use

Rationale: Cellulitis of the left thumb is L03.01- with a sixth digit of 2 for the left finger. The Index does not provide an entry for tobacco or nicotine under the heading of Abuse, but category J41.0 does direct the coder to use an additional code to identify tobacco use, Z72.0.

1.239. O99.283   Pregnancy (single) (uterine), complicated by (care of) (management affected by), endocrine diseases
        O24.410   Diabetes, diabetic (mellitus) (sugar), gestational (in pregnancy), diet controlled
        E06.3   Thyroiditis, Hashimoto's (struma lymphomatosa)
        Z3A.34   Pregnancy (single) (uterine), weeks of gestation, 34 weeks

Rationale: The physician documents that the Hashimoto thyroiditis is complicating pregnancy. No entry exists for thyroid disorders or Hasimoto thyroiditis. The entry for Endocrine disorders is chosen and verified in the Tabular. The coding note under subcategory O99.2 states that it includes conditions in E00-E90. Coding Guideline I.C.15.a.1 states that additional codes may be used with Chapter 15 codes to further specify conditions and, therefore, code E06.3 is added. The guideline also tells us that Chapter 15 codes are sequenced first. Code Z3A.4 is added to indicate weeks of gestation.

1.240. M79.641   Pain(s) (*see also* Painful), hand, *see* Pain, limb, upper, hand
        R20.2   Paresthesia, *see also* Disturbance(s), sensation (cold) (heat) (localization) (tactile discrimination) (texture) (vibratory), skin, paresthesia
        Z33.1   Pregnancy (childbirth) (labor) (puerperium), incidental finding

Rationale: The physician establishes the onset of her hand pain prior to the pregnancy and, therefore, the pregnancy is coded as an incidental finding. Coding Guideline I.C.15.a.1 states that it is the provider's responsibility to state that the condition being treated is not affecting the pregnancy, which the provider does by stating, "incidental pregnancy."

1.241. A04.7   Colitis (acute) (catarrhal) (chronic (noninfective) (hemorrhagic), Clostridium difficile
        E86.0   Dehydration
        I73.9   Disease, diseased, peripheral vascular NOS

Rationale: Colitis caused by C. diff is a combination code in ICD-10-CM. The colitis and the infection should not need to be coded separately. Dehydration is not integral to colitis and should be coded separately as E86.0. Peripheral vascular disease is coded as a secondary diagnosis because the physician is ordering evaluation and prophylaxis.

1.242. F32.9   Depression (acute) (mental), major
        Z63.4   Bereavement (uncomplicated)

Rationale: The physician documented the patient's diagnosis as major depression, a specific form of depression and also documented a secondary diagnosis of bereavement. The physician did not document psychotic symptoms; therefore, F32.9 is the correct code.

1.243. E66.01   Obesity, due to, excessive calories, morbid

I10   Hypertension, hypertensive (accelerated) (benign) (essential) (idiopathic) (malignant) (systemic)

E78.0   Hypercholesterolemia (essential) (familial) (hereditary) (primary) (pure)

Rationale: The obesity is the reason for this encounter and is the first listed diagnosis. The hypertension and hypercholesterolemia are coded as additional diagnoses.

1.244. H66.003   Otitis (acute), media (hemorrhagic) (staphylococcal) (streptococcal), suppurative, acute

J06.9   Infection, infected, infective (opportunistic) respiratory (tract), upper (acute)

Rationale: The otitis is described as acute and suppurative but with no mention of eardrum rupture; therefore, H66.003, not H66.013, is the correct code. A diagnosis code for conjunctivitis is not added due to the statement in the plan which attributes the eye problems to backup from her nose rather than conjunctivitis.

1.245. E11.43   Diabetes, diabetic (mellitus) (sugar) type 2, with, gastroparesis

K31.84   Gastroparesis

Z79.4   Therapy, drug, long-term (current) (prophylactic), insulin or
Long-term (current) (prophylactic) drug therapy (use of), insulin

Rationale: The patient is type 2 diabetic which codes to category E11. ICD-10-CM provides combination codes for diabetes and its manifestations/complications. There is a note at the beginning of category E11 that instructs the coding professional to "use an additional code to identify any insulin use (Z79.4)." The addition of code K31.84, Gastroparesis, while not mandatory, does specify the type of neuropathy.

1.246. N18.6   Disease, diseased, renal (chronic) (functional) (pelvis), end-stage (failure)

Z99.2   Dependence (on) (syndrome), on, renal dialysis (hemodialysis) (peritoneal) or Presence (of), arterial-venous shunt (dialysis)

Rationale: The patient did not receive renal dialysis on this outpatient visit. The encounter was for the ESRD.

1.247. C67.3   Neoplasm Table, by site, bladder (urinary), malignant, primary site, wall, anterior

N40.0   Hypertrophy, hypertrophic, prostate – *see* Enlargement, enlarged, prostate

Z92.21   History, personal (of), chemotherapy for neoplastic condition

Rationale: According to ICD-10-CM Coding Guideline I.C.21.c.8, Follow-up, "A follow-up code may be used to explain repeated visits. Should a condition be found to have recurred on the follow-up visit, then the diagnosis code for the condition should be assigned in place of the follow-up code." Additionally, since there is a recurrence of the cancer, the history should not be used.

1.248. M15.0   Arthritis, arthritic (acute) (chronic) (nonpyogenic) (subacute) degenerative – *see* Osteoarthritis
Osteoarthritis, generalized, primary

M47.817   Osteoarthritis, spine – *see* Spondylosis
Spondylosis, without myelopathy or radiculopathy, lumbosacral region

I25.10   Arteriosclerosis, arteriosclerotic (diffuse) (obliterans) (of) (senile) (with calcification), coronary (artery)

I10   Hypertension, hypertensive (accelerated) (benign) (essential) (idiopathic) (malignant) (systemic)

Rationale: Either M15.0 or M47.817 may be sequenced as the first listed diagnosis as both are the reason for this office visit. Note that in the Tabular, under the section for Osteoarthritis (M15-19), there is an *Excludes2* note for osteoarthritis of the spine (M47.-). Coding Guideline I.A.12.b indicates that when an *Excludes2* note is pertinent for a code, it is acceptable to use both the code and the excluded code together when the patient has both conditions at the same time. Note: If the physician is queried about how long the patient has been on Celebrex, code Z79.1 could also be coded, if it is determined to be long-term use.

1.249. Answer, First visit:

E30.0	Delay, delayed, puberty (constitutional)
Z60.4	Problem (with) (related to), social, exclusion and rejection

First visit: In the Tabular, under category R62, there is an *Excludes1* note – *Excludes1*: delayed puberty (E30.0), so R62.52 is not assigned. ICD-10-CM code E34.3 would not be used, as an endocrine disorder is not documented and the lab results have not been received.

Answer, Second visit:

E23.0	Deficiency, deficient, growth hormone (idiopathic) (isolated)

Second Visit: Code E34.3 cannot be used with E23.0. In the Tabular, under code E34.3, there is an *Excludes1* note with "pituitary short stature (E23.0)." Coding Guideline A.12.a, *Excludes1*, states that an *Excludes1* note indicates that the code excluded should never be used at the same time as the code above the *Excludes1* note. An *Excludes1* is used when two conditions cannot occur together, such as a congenital form versus an acquired form of the same condition.

1.250.

T83.51XA	Complication(s) (from) (of), catheter (device), urethral, indwelling, infection and inflammation
N39.0	Infection, infected, infective (opportunistic), urinary (tract)
B96.20	Infection, infected, infective (opportunistic), Escherichia (E) coli, as cause of disease classified elsewhere

Rationale: A complication code is assigned when the infection is documented as resulting from the indwelling catheter. In the Tabular, an instructional note appears under subcategory T83.5 to use an additional code to identify the infection, which in this case is N39.0, Urinary tract infection. Additionally, in the Tabular under N39.0 there is a note to use an additional code to identify infectious agent which in this case is B96.20, E. coli. An external cause code is not assigned to this case because of Coding Guideline I.c.19.g.4 which states "As with certain other T codes, some of the complications of care codes have the external cause included in the code. The code includes the nature of the complication as well as the type of procedure that caused the complication." There is no documentation available to justify place of occurrence/activity codes.

1.251.

I13.2	Failure, failed, heart (acute) (senile) (sudden), hypertensive – *see* Hypertension, heart. Hypertension, hypertensive (accelerated) (benign) (essential) (idiopathic) (malignant) (systemic), heart (disease) (conditions in I51.4-I51.9 due to hypertension), with kidney disease (chronic) – *see* Hypertension, cardiorenal (chronic). Hypertension, cardiorenal, with heart failure, with stage 5 or end stage renal disease
I50.9	Failure, heart (acute) (senile) (sudden), congestive (compensated) (decompensated)
N18.5	Disease, diseased, kidney (functional) (pelvis, chronic, stage 5)

Rationale: The combination code for hypertensive heart and renal disease (cardiorenal) is assigned because the hypertension was documented as the cause of the heart disease. An additional code for the CHF (I50.9) is assigned due to an instructional note appearing under I13.2 which states "Use additional code to identify type of heart failure (I50.-)." Additionally, a secondary code for the stage 5 CKD is assigned due to a second instructional note stating "use additional code to identify the stage of CKD (N18.5, N18.6)."

Hospital Outpatient Cases

1.252. A60.01   Herpes, herpesvirus, herpetic, penis
A60.02   Herpes, herpesvirus, herpetic, scrotum
R94.5   Findings, abnormal, inconclusive, without diagnosis, function study, liver
Z21   HIV, positive, seropositive
F11.229   Dependence (on) (syndrome), heroin – *see* Dependence, drug, opioid, with, intoxication
Z72.51   Problem (with) (related to), life style, high risk sexual behavior (heterosexual)

Rationale: HSV-2 or herpes simplex virus 2 is coded to two sites. Documentation of lesions of both the penis and the scrotum should be reported. The "suspected hepatitis" is not coded on this emergency room record as the coding guidelines state: "Do not code diagnoses documented as 'probable,' 'suspected,' 'questionable,' 'rule out,' 'working diagnosis' or other similar terms indicating uncertainty." Codes for the drug addiction and lifestyle risks would be added as they are clearly delineated by the attending physician and affect the management of the patient. In following the coding guidelines for HIV, Z21, Asymptomatic human immunodeficiency virus [HIV] infection status, is to be applied when the patient without any documentation of symptoms is listed as being "HIV positive," "known HIV," "HIV test positive," or similar terminology.

1.253. Z51.11   Chemotherapy (session) (for), cancer
C25.7   Neoplasm Table, by site, pancreas, neck, malignant, primary site
E86.0   Dehydration
R11.2   Nausea, with vomiting
T45.1X5A   Table of Drugs and Chemicals, Anticancer agents NEC, adverse effect

Rationale: The reason for the encounter (chemotherapy) is the first-listed diagnosis. Even though the nausea and vomiting led up to the dehydration, it is not always an integral component of the dehydration; therefore, it is also coded. The neoplasm is coded as the reason for chemotherapy.

1.254. D57.219   Disease, diseased, sickle cell, Hb-C with crisis (vasoocclusive pain)
E11.9   Diabetes, diabetic (mellitus) (sugar), type 2
Z63.8   Inadequate, inadequacy, family support

Rationale: It would not be necessary to code the inguinal pain or fever as these are symptoms of the sickle-cell crisis. The hemochromatosis is not coded because it was not treated. The avascular necrosis was not confirmed and should not be coded.

1.255. D50.0   Anemia (essential) (general) (hemoglobin deficiency) (infantile) (primary) (profound), blood loss (chronic)

       E11.9   Diabetes, diabetic (mellitus) (sugar), type 2

       I25.10   Disease, diseased, coronary (artery) *see* – disease, heart, ischemic, atherosclerotic; Disease, heart, ischemic, atherosclerotic (of)

       Z95.1   Status (post), aortocoronary bypass

       Z57.5   Exposure (to) (*see also* contact, with), occupational toxic agents (gases) (liquids) (solids) (vapors) in industry NEC

Rationale: The physician documents "chronic blood loss anemia"; therefore, it is appropriate to code this. The weakness is a symptom of the anemia and should not be coded. The additional diagnoses of ASHD, diabetes, and status bypass may be coded because they were treated and/or applicable to the case.

1.256. P28.81   Arrest, arrested, respiratory, newborn

       P29.81   Arrest, arrested, cardiac, newborn

       P07.18   Low, birth weight, with weight of, 2000–2499 grams

Rationale: The code for the birth weight reflects the weight at birth, not the current weight. ICD-10-CM code P28.5, Respiratory failure of newborn, is not coded due to the *Excludes1* note under code P28.5 – "*Excludes1*: respiratory arrest of newborn (P28.81)." The P07.18 code is assigned since this is within the 28 days after birth. Status codes (subcategory Z91.7) are available to classify status of low birth weight and immaturity once the patient is no longer a neonate.

1.257. R07.9   Pain(s) (*see also* Painful), chest (central)

       R06.02   Short, shortening, shortness, breath

       I10   Hypertension, hypertensive (accelerated) (benign) (essential) (idiopathic) (malignant) (systemic)

       E10.65   Diabetes, diabetic (mellitus) (sugar), out of control – code to Diabetes, by type, with hyperglycemia. Diabetes, diabetic, type 1, with hyperglycemia

       E10.51   Diabetes, diabetic (mellitus) (sugar), type 1, with peripheral angiopathy

Rationale: This is an outpatient encounter; therefore, the symptoms are coded rather than the "rule out" diagnoses. ICD-10-CM Diagnostic Coding and Reporting Guidelines for outpatient services state "Do not code diagnoses documented as 'probable,' 'suspected,' 'questionable,' 'rule out,' 'working diagnosis' or other similar terms indicating uncertainty. Rather, code the condition(s) to the highest degree of certainty for that encounter/visit, such as symptoms, signs, abnormal test results, or other reason for the visit."

1.258. T25.211A   Burn (electricity) (flame) (hot gas, liquid or hot object) (radiation) (steam) (thermal), ankle, right, second degree

       X12.XXXA   Index to External Causes, Burn, burned, burning (accidental) (by) (from) (on), hot liquid

       Y92.010   Index to External Causes, Place of occurrence, residence (non-institutional) (private), house, single family, kitchen

       Y93.G3   Index to External Causes, Activity (involving) (of victim at time of event), cooking and baking

       Y99.8   Index to External Causes, External cause status, leisure activity

Rationale: The documentation states that the patient was cooking dinner at home. The external cause status for this is leisure. The burn code and the external cause code are coded with the seventh character A for initial encounter because she was seen in the ED today.

1.259. K57.92   Diverticulitis (acute)

Z80.0   History, family (of), malignant neoplasm (of), gastrointestinal tract <u>or</u> History, family (of), malignant neoplasm (of), digestive organ

I10   Hypertension, hypertensive (accelerated) (benign) (essential) (idiopathic) (malignant) (systemic)

Rationale: The physician does not establish the exact location of the diverticulitis; therefore, the main entry of Diverticulitis (acute) is chosen. Family history does not have an entry for the colon; therefore, the entry for gastrointestinal tract or digestive organ is chosen. Family history of colon cancer and hypertension are coded as additional diagnoses.

1.260. H05.012   Cellulitis (diffuse) (phlegmonous) (septic) (suppurative), orbit, orbital

H00.024   Hordeolum (eyelid) (externum) (recurrent), internum, left, upper

Rationale: The reason for the encounter is the orbital cellulitis and the hordeolum is coded as a secondary diagnosis.

1.261. R09.1   Pleurisy (acute) (adhesive) (chronic) (costal) (diaphragmatic) (double) (dry) (fibrinous) (fibrous) (interlobar) (latent) (plastic) (primary) (residual) (sicca) (sterile) (subacute) (unresolved)

B97.89   Infection, infected, infective (opportunistic) virus, viral, as a cause of disease classified elsewhere

G35   Sclerosis, sclerotic, multiple (brain stem) (cerebral) (generalized) (spinal cord)

Rationale: The patient presented with pleuritic pain as the reason for the encounter. The Index does not contain an entry for viral pleurisy; therefore, Infection, viral, as a cause of disease classified elsewhere is added as a secondary diagnosis. Multiple sclerosis is also added as a secondary diagnosis.

1.262. M12.39   Rheumatism (articular) (neuralgic) (nonarticular), palindromic, multiple site

N39.46   Incontinence, urge, and stress (female) (male)

Rationale: Coding Guideline 1.C.13.a instructs the coder to code the multiple sites code for diseases when multiple bones, joints, or muscles are involved. In this case, two joints are involved and therefore, code M12.39 is assigned. The physician documents both urge and stress incontinence, which together are known as mixed incontinence. Urge incontinence is coded to N39.41 which has an *Excludes1* note for mixed incontinence. Under code N39.46 for mixed incontinence, it lists urge and stress incontinence.

1.263. G44.001   Headache, cluster, intractable

Rationale: The physician does not state whether this is chronic or episodic; therefore, code G44.001 for intractable cluster headache is assigned.

1.264. Z52.3   Donor (organ or tissue), bone, marrow
        R50.82   Fever (inanition) (of unknown origin) (persistent) (with chills) (with rigor), postoperative
        R11.2   Nausea, with vomiting

Rationale: Guideline IV.A.2, Observation Stay, instructs the coder to assign the reason for the encounter (bone marrow donor status) as the first-listed diagnosis and complications as secondary diagnoses (postop fever and nausea with vomiting). Code Z52.3 describes the patient's status as a live bone marrow donor. The symptoms of fever and the combination code of nausea with vomiting are found in Chapter 18: Symptoms, signs and abnormal clinical and laboratory findings, not elsewhere classified (R00-R99), because no definitive diagnosis was established.

1.265. K80.51   Jaundice (yellow), obstructive – *see also* Obstruction, bile duct
                    Obstruction, obstructed, obstructive, bile duct or passage (common) (hepatic) (noncalculous), with calculus
        R00.0   Tachycardia

Rationale: Jaundice is not coded separately because the Index directs obstructive jaundice to be coded as obstruction of the bile duct by calculus. The tachycardia was a pre-existing condition and is not a postoperative complication.

1.266. N76.4   Abscess (connective tissue) (embolic) (fistulous) (infective) (metastatic) (multiple) (pernicious) (pyogenic) (septic), labium (majus) (minus) <u>or</u> Abscess, vulva
        Z88.2   History, personal (of), allergy (to) sulfonamides

Rationale: The Index entry for Abscess, skin refers the coder to Abscess, by site. Therefore, the correct code is N76.4 for labium or vulva. The allergy to Bactrim is not a current reaction and, therefore, the correct Index entry is History, personal, allergy to sulfonamides. Bactrim is a sulfonamide, which codes to a more specific code than the entry for drugs or antibiotic agent. The physician states that the abscess is "from what appears to be staph." This statement indicates uncertainty and is therefore not coded.

1.267. J20.9   Bronchitis (diffuse) (fibrinous) (hypostatic) (infective) (membranous) (with tracheitis), acute or subacute (with bronchospasm or obstruction)
        D86.0   Sarcoidosis, lung
        M25.50   Arthralgia, *see also* Pain, joint
        R03.0   Elevated, elevation, blood pressure reading (incidental) (isolated) (nonspecific), no diagnosis of hypertension

Rationale: The sarcoidosis is documented as pulmonary in the history. Even though the patient has cervical lymphadenopathy, the physician does not specify that the lymphadenopathy is related to the sarcoidosis. Therefore, the Index entry for Sarcoidosis, lung provides the correct code of D86.0. The physician and the patient do not specify which joints are painful. Therefore, the Index entry Pain, joint provides the correct code of M25.50. The patient does not have a current diagnosis of hypertension, but only has an elevated blood pressure reading today.

1.268. J06.9   Infection, infected, infective (opportunistic) respiratory (tract), upper (acute), viral NOS

      D70.9   Neutropenia, neutropenic (chronic) (genetic) (idiopathic) (immune) (infantile) (malignant) (pernicious) (splenic)

      M31.30   Granulomatosis, Wegener's

Rationale: The reason for the encounter is the viral URI and neutropenia. The Wegener's granulomatosis is a secondary diagnosis. Viral URI is a combination code in ICD-10-CM.

1.269. H04.553   Stenosis, stenotic, nasolacrimal duct, *see also* Stenosis, lacrimal duct

      Q93.5   Syndrome, Angelman

Rationale: Stenosis of the nasolacrimal duct directs the coder to Stenosis, lacrimal duct. This is a 22-year-old patient and the diagnosis is not stated as congenital; therefore, code H04.55- is chosen, with a sixth character of 3 for bilateral acquired stenosis. Microcephaly is not coded separately because it is a component of Angelman syndrome, coded as Q93.5. Angelman syndrome is a rare neurological disorder primarily affecting the nervous system. Most affected children also have epilepsy and microcephaly. (Source: Genetics Home Reference. http://ghr.nlm.nih.gov/)

1.270. I49.3   Contractions(s), contracture, contracted, premature, ventricular

Rationale: The only code assigned for this case is I49.3 to identify the premature ventricular contractions. There is an *Excludes1* note under category R00, Specified arrhythmias (I47-I49), which excludes the use of code R00.8 for this case.

1.271. K56.1   Intussusception (bowel) (colon) (enteric) (ileocecal) (ileocolic) (intestine) (rectum)

      K52.9   Gastroenteritis (acute) (chronic) (noninfectious)

      R68.11   Excess, excessive, excessively crying of infant

Rationale: The abdominal pain is integral to both gastroenteritis and intussusception and is not coded separately. Although an acutely ill infant will cry, the physician documented excessive crying, potentially trying to explain severity and intensity of service. Excessive crying of infant is coded as R68.11 due to the age of the patient. Although ICD-10-CM does not give a specific definition of infant versus child, many pediatricians use 24 months as an arbitrary cut-off age for infant.

1.272. K02.9   Caries, dental

      F88   Delay, delayed, development, global

      Z94.4   Transplant(ed) (status), liver

Rationale: The physician does not provide documentation of the location of the dental caries; therefore, the unspecified code is assigned. Status post liver transplant is located in the Index under Transplant(ed), with code Z94.4 being assigned for liver transplant.

AHIMA ICD-10 Products

Available at www.ahimastore.org

Books from AHIMA Press
- *Implementing ICD-10-CM/PCS for Hospitals* (AC201009)
- *Pocket Guide of ICD-10-CM and ICD-10-PCS* (AC203010)
- *ICD-10-CM and ICD-10-PCS Preview,* Second Edition (AC206009)
- *ICD-10-CM and ICD-10-PCS Preview Exercises,* Second Edition (AC216011)
- *ICD-10-CM Coder Training Manual 2014* (AC206814)
- *ICD-10-PCS Coder Training Manual 2014* (AC206814)
- *Transitioning to ICD-10-CM/PCS: The Essential Guide to General Equivalence Mappings (GEMs)* (AC202810)
- *Root Operations: Key to Procedure Coding in ICD-10-PCS (*AC211010)
- *ICD-10-PCS: An Applied Approach,* Second Edition (AC201113)
- *Basic ICD-10-CM/PCS Coding Exercises,* Fourth Edition (AC210512)
- *Diagnostic Coding for Physician Services: ICD-10-CM*, 2014 Edition (AC201213)
- *Basic ICD-10-CM/PCS Coding,* 2013 (AC200512)
- *Clinical Coding Workout with Answers,* 2013 Update (AC201514)

AHIMA Online Education
AHIMA offers a complete program of online ICD-10 training for organizational and non-coding staff, acute-care coders, and specialty coding settings
- ICD-10-CM Overview: Deciphering the Code
- ICD-10-PCS Overview: Deciphering the Code
- ICD-10-CM Coding Course Collection (28 hours)
- ICD-10-PCS Coding Course Collection (23 hours)
- Coding Proficiency Assessments
- ICD-10-CM Coder Readiness Assessment
- ICD-10-PCS Coder Readiness Assessment
- ICD-10 A&P System Coding Assessments and Courses

AHIMA Meetings, Audio Seminars, and Webinars
- Annual ICD-10/Computer-Assisted Summit
- Academy for ICD-10-CM/PCS Trainers (multiple dates and locations throughout the year)
- Coder Workforce Training for ICD-10 (multiple dates and locations throughout the year)
- Private Academies (Contact AHIMA's Business Innovation Group.)
- Annual Clinical Coding Meeting
- AHIMA Annual Convention and Exhibits

AHIMA is constantly developing products and resources to meet the needs of HIM professionals. Check ahima.org for updates and announcements of new products.